Medicine and Maladies

Faux Titre

ÉTUDES DE LANGUE ET LITTÉRATURE FRANÇAISES

VOLUME 422

The titles published in this series are listed at *brill.com/faux*

Medicine and Maladies

Representing Affliction in Nineteenth-Century France

Edited by

Sophie Leroy

BRILL
RODOPI

LEIDEN | BOSTON

Cover illustration: Honoré Daumier, 'Une heureuse trouvaille. – Parbleu je suis ravi … vous avez la fièvre jaune … c'est la première fois de ma vie que j'ai le bonheur d'en soigner une!', published in *Le Charivari*, 11 September 1844. Courtesy of the Benjamin A. and Julia M. Trustman collection of Honoré Daumier lithographs, Robert D. Farber University Archives and Special Collections Department, Brandeis University © Brandeis University.

Library of Congress Cataloging-in-Publication Data

Names: Medicine and maladies (Conference) (2014 : University of Bristol) | Leroy, Sophie, 1988– editor.
Title: Medicine and maladies : representing affliction in nineteenth-century France / edited by Sophie Leroy.
Description: Leiden ; Boston : Brill Rodopi, 2018. | Series: Faux titre ; volume 422 | In English and French. | Based on the conference, Medicine and Maladies, held at the University of Bristol in September, 2014. | Includes bibliographical references and index.
Identifiers: LCCN 2018014172 (print) | LCCN 2018024403 (ebook) | ISBN 9789004368019 (E-books) | ISBN 9789004367999 (hardback : alk. paper)
Subjects: LCSH: French literature—19th century—History and criticism—Congresses. | Medical literature—France—History—19th century—Congresses. | Literature and medicine—Congresses. | Medicine in literature—-Congresses. | Diseases in literature—Congresses.
Classification: LCC PQ283 (ebook) | LCC PQ283 .M38 2018 (print) | DDC 840.9/3561—dc23
LC record available at https://lccn.loc.gov/2018014172

Typeface for the Latin, Greek, and Cyrillic scripts: "Brill". See and download: brill.com/brill-typeface.

ISSN 0167-9392
ISBN 978-90-04-36799-9 (hardback)
ISBN 978-90-04-36801-9 (e-book)

This book is printed on acid-free paper and produced in a sustainable manner.

Contents

Acknowledgements

The original idea for this edited volume was conceieved following the conference *Medicine and Maladies*, held at the University of Bristol in September 2014. I would like to thank the School of Modern Languages at the University of Bristol, the Bristol Institute for Research in the Humanities and Arts, and the *Society of Dix-Neuviémistes* for their generous financial support of that initiating conference. Special thanks are due to all anonymous peer-reviewers for their deep engagement with individual chapters and for their encouragement and support during the production of this book. Many thanks to Christa Stevens at Brill for her patience and advice in seeing the manuscript through to publication.

Finally, I am very grateful to the invited contributors to this volume for their participation and co-operation as the manuscript was being prepared.

List of Illustrations

Notes on Contributors

Cyril Barde

ancien élève de l'École Normale Supérieure LSH, est professeur agrégé de lettres modernes en classes préparatoires. Il prépare une thèse sur les rapports entre littérature et Art Nouveau autour de 1900, sous la direction de Jean-Nicolas Illouz (Université Paris VIII).

Mélanie Bhend

est chargée de cours à l'Université de Nottingham depuis 2013. Elle y enseigne la langue française aux étudiants de Bachelor et de Master, ainsi que la littérature française aux étudiants de première année. En 2017, elle a achevé sa thèse de doctorat portant sur la représentation conceptuelle et esthétique de la folie et du discours du fou dans des textes littéraires mettant en scène un narrateur fou en France durant l'âge d'or de la psychiatrie (1830-1870). Ses domaines de recherche sont la littérature (plus particulièrement le XIXe siècle), la narratologie et l'histoire de la psychiatrie. Elle privilégie la recherche interdisciplinaire et fait partie du groupe 'Nottingham Health Humanities'.

Géraldine Crahay

est Assistant Teaching Fellow à l'Université de Durham. Elle a fait une licence et une maîtrise en langues et littératures françaises et romanes à l'Université de Liège et a achevé en 2015 une thèse de doctorat à l'Université de Bangor sur le malaise masculin et les ambiguïtés sexuelles dans les textes scientifiques et les romans de la monarchie de Juillet. De manière générale, sa recherche porte sur les études de genre, et en particulier la masculinité, les ambiguïtés sexuelles, l'hermaphrodisme et l'homosexualité au XIXe siècle. Elle a publié un article sur l'homosexualité dans *Mademoiselle de Maupin* dans la revue *Nineteenth-Century French Studies*.

Larry Duffy

is Senior Lecturer in French at the University of Kent. He is the author of *Le Grand Transit Moderne: Mobility, Modernity and French Naturalist Fiction* (Rodopi, 2005), *Flaubert, Zola and the Incorporation of Disciplinary Knowledge* (Palgrave, 2015), and numerous articles on Flaubert, Zola, Maupassant, Mérimée, and Houellebecq.

Elizabeth Emery
is Professor of French at Montclair State University where she teaches medieval and nineteenth-century French literature and culture. She is the author of books, articles, and essay anthologies related to the reception of medieval art and architecture in nineteenth-century France and America, and has recently published books exploring the late nineteenth-century phenomenon of writers' private homes turned into public museums: *Photojournalism and the Origins of the French Writer House Museum (1881–1914)* (Ashgate Press, 2012) and *En toute intimité ... Quand la presse* people *de la Belle Epoque s'invitait chez les célébrités* (Parigramme, 2015). She serves as Book Review coeditor for *Nineteenth-Century French Studies*.

Philippa Lewis
is a Leverhulme Early Career Fellow at the University of Bristol where she is working on a cultural history of shyness in modern France. She completed her PhD at the University of Cambridge, and has published articles on nineteenth-century French literature and culture in *Modern Language Review* and *Nineteenth-Century French Studies*. She was Teaching Associate in French at St. John's College, Cambridge, from 2013 to 2014, and has previously worked as a translator for Classiques Garnier.

Julie Müller
est maître de conférence à l'université de Hambourg. Ses recherches portent principalement sur l'histoire de la médecine et interrogent les interactions entre littérature, science et religion au XIXe siècle. Elle termine actuellement sa thèse de doctorat intitulée : 'Alcoolisme et acédie : le monstre alcoolique dans la pensée clinique du XIXe siècle (1850–1900)'. Elle est l'auteure de plusieurs articles portant sur l'histoire de l'alcoolisme, mélancolie et neurasthénie, notamment dans l'oeuvre de Zola et Proust.

Joanna Rajkumar
agrégée de lettres modernes, docteur ès lettres et sciences humaines en littératures comparées (Université Paris Ouest), auteur d'une thèse sur 'Les limites du langage d'un siècle à l'autre chez Baudelaire, Hofmannsthal, Michaux', à paraître aux Classiques Garnier sous le titre *Lignes sans réponses*. Elle enseigne actuellement en Classes Préparatoires aux Grandes Ecoles (CPGE) en littérature et en cinéma en région parisienne. Ses recherches portent sur la poésie et sur les relations entre littérature, arts et cinéma. Elle a notamment publié

différents articles sur l'indicible en poésie et au cinéma, les mythes (Ganymède, Salomé, Frankenstein), le geste, le rêve, les marionnettes et la danse.

Natasha Ruiz-Gómez
is Senior Lecturer in the History of Art at the University of Essex. She specializes in French art and visual culture of the long nineteenth century and is especially interested in the relationship between art and science. Her work has appeared in *Art History, Medical Humanities, Modern & Contemporary France* and *Thresholds*, as well as in the several anthologies. Her current projects include a book manuscript in which she examines the artistic but purportedly objective practices of Doctor Jean-Martin Charcot and his protégés at the Hôpital de la Salpêtrière.

Steven Wilson
is Lecturer in French Studies at Queen's University Belfast. His research interests lie in nineteenth-century French literature and the medical humanities, and include the illness narrative (especially autopathography), literary representations of contagion, disease and the figure of the clinician, and discourses of public health in French medico-literary cultures. He has published journal articles on representations of prostitution in Balzac, Sand, Baudelaire, Zola and Rachilde, is guest editor of a special issue of *L'Esprit Créateur* (Summer 2016) on the theme of 'French Autopathography', and is currently working on a monograph-length study on contagion narratives in nineteenth-century France.

Susannah Wilson
is Professor in French Studies at the University of Warwick. Her research interests focus on nineteenth- and early twentieth-century French culture and literature, with specialist interest in representations of mental health and illness; gender and criminality; psychoanalytical theory; the history of the French psychological sciences; and all forms of 'self-writing', including autobiography, memoir, and correspondence. She has a particular interest in the period and idea of the *fin-de-siècle*. Her latest book, *Voices from the Asylum: Four French Women Writers, 1850–1920* (Oxford University Press, 2010), investigates the lives and first-hand written accounts of nineteenth-century women writers incarcerated in French psychiatric hospitals. Susannah held a British Academy Postdoctoral Fellowship from 2011–2014 and is currently the recipient of a British Academy Rising Star Engagement Award. She is now working on a book project exploring morphine use in the French cultural imagination.

Introduction

Sophie Leroy

Medicine and Maladies: Representing Affliction in Nineteenth-Century France probes the transgressive capacities of nineteenth-century literary and medical discourses. Established and emerging scholars from the United Kingdom, the United States, France, and Germany offer fresh readings of nineteenth-century fictional narratives, clinical case studies, medical reports, memoirs, poetry, philosophical writings, and debates around visual art. Central to the analysis which runs through this edited volume is the porous relationship between medical science and the arts, with the eleven contributors demonstrating how representations of affliction shaped wider French cultural imaginations of the healthy and the pathological.

The nineteenth century represents a crucial turning point in the history of modern medicine, with shifts in the philosophical understandings of health and illness; the invention of new technologies and medical equipment; and improved capacities to visualize or represent disease. French science played a fundamental role in these changes, both through individual innovations and the establishing of new scholarly collectives. Significant developments in this period include the invention of the stethoscope in 1816 by René Laennec, the creation of the Académie Royale de Médecine by Louis XVIII in 1820, the publication of the journal *Annales d'hygiène publique et de médecine légale* (1829–), the revolutionizing work of Louis Pasteur on bacteria during the 1860s and the 1870s, and growing social concerns with sanitization and public health. These and other advances in clinical medicine announced major shifts in scientific understandings of physiological processes which found expression in transformed attitudes towards the physician, medical diagnoses, and broader perceptions of sickness and health.

The contributors to *Medicine and Maladies* address how specific nineteenth-century transformations in the sciences of behaviour, temperament, and pathology were shaped by, and interrelated with, a range of aesthetic and socio-political contexts. More specifically, chapters reveal the instability of traditional disciplinary distinctions by exposing the relations that cross and weave between the fields of psychology, pharmacy, philosophy, literary criticism, and art history. Chapters examining the interactions between nineteenth-century French medical thought and practice, on the one hand, and aesthetic domains of literature and art, on the other, offer new perspectives on the interdisciplinary and intermedial dimensions of French encounters with the pathological.

 | DOI:10.1163/9789004368019_002

Critics and researchers in French studies have long explored the status and role of medicine in nineteenth-century France. An important edited volume to engage with this question is *French Medical Culture in the Nineteenth Century* (1994).[1] Adopting an historical approach to medical developments, the scholarship included in this edited volume demonstrates the extension and wider 'medicalization' of nineteenth-century France, drawing attention to the dominant role of Paris and its institutions as centres for the production and diffusion of medical culture and to the establishment of new kinds of regulations around medical industry and practice. One of the only chapters in this volume to focus on the relationship between medical and literary discourse is Jan Goldstein's work on male hysteria and Flaubert. However, whilst Goldstein's intervention usefully opens up the notion of hysteria beyond gendered confines through a close reading of Flaubert's writing, it also mobilizes some rigid distinctions between literary and medical fields. As Goldstein claims: 'Literary discourse and medical discourse intersected repeatedly in France during the nineteenth century, but it is striking that, at the points of intersection, the traffic went one way only'.[2] The argument put forward by Goldstein reveals a common tendency amongst historians of nineteenth-century France to recognize the influence of medical science upon literary narratives, but to suggest that this was a one-way process in which traffic moves from the medical domain to the literary. This perspective is also pervasive within French literary studies, appearing for example in Jean-Louis Cabanès's *Le Corps et la maladie dans les récits réalistes (1856–1898)* (1991).[3] Cabanès analyses novelistic explorations of the diseased body in the second half of the nineteenth century, and argues for the scientific basis of literary realism in which detailed descriptions of physical symptoms echo the findings of clinical discourse. By way of contrast, *Medicine and Maladies* offers a number of readings of specific medical debates and texts that challenge and complicate this image of a unidirectional relationship and trouble the apparent stability of different disciplinary fields.

1 Ann La Berge, and Mordechai Feingold (eds), *French Medical Culture in the Nineteenth Century* (Oxford: Rodopi, 1994).

2 Jan Goldstein, 'The Uses of Male Hysteria: Medical and Literary Discourse in Nineteenth-Century France', in Ann La Berge, and Mordechai Feingold (eds), *French Medical Culture in the Nineteenth Century*, pp. 210–47 (p. 213).

3 Jean-Louis Cabanès's two-volume study of the sick body in relation to realist narrative, *Le Corps et la maladie dans les récits réalistes (1856–1898)* (Paris: Klincksieck, 1991), examines the influence of medical knowledge and scientific descriptions of pathological conditions on the novels of Zola, Huysmans, Maupassant, and the Goncourt brothers.

The connections between literary and medical discourses are reflected in other works of literary and cultural theory. Jann Matlock adopts a fluid reading of the different discourses (novels, hospital archives, memoirs, and scientific writings) that attempt to configure female sexuality in her *Scenes of Seduction: Prostitution, Hysteria, and Reading Difference in Nineteenth-Century France* (1994).[4] Turning to studies of prostitution, the discursive treatment of hysteria, and fictional narratives of desire, Matlock reveals how the pathological body of the hysteric and prostitute should above all be critically understood as textual products that are constituted through discursive circulations and narrative devices, the movements of which trouble interpretative assumptions about the radical separation and difference between literary and scientific discourses. Cultural imaginaries of specific pathological conditions which demonstrate further these interrelationships between literature, culture, and history have been well documented.[5] In *Eccentricity and the Cultural Imagination in Nineteenth-Century Paris* (2009), for example, Miranda Gill undertakes a study of the phenomenon of eccentricity in the nineteenth-century French collective imagination. In this work, Gill analyzes diverse textual sources through which the figure of the eccentric was shaped; a process that Gill demonstrates in terms of the evolution of contested social meanings that travelled between and across different disciplines.[6]

Studies of the history of madness, hysteria, and genius-insanity debates in nineteenth-century France have been particularly productive in cultivating interdisciplinary analyses of cultural texts and fostering study around institutional systems, treatment, and the socio-political framing of mental pathologies.[7] Nicole Edelman, in her *Les Métamorphoses de l'hystérique: Du*

---

4 Jann Matlock, *Scenes of Seduction: Prostitution, Hysteria and Reading Difference in Nineteenth-Century France* (New York: Columbia University Press, 1994).

5 General contributions to the cultural history of disease include the edited volume *Framing and Imagining Disease in Cultural History* (Basingstoke: Palgrave Macmillan, 2003), ed. by G. S. Rousseau, with Miranda Gill, David Haycock, Malte Herwig, which engages with the representation of a range of maladies across a number of historical periods and geographical boundaries.

6 Miranda Gill, *Eccentricity and the Cultural Imagination in Nineteenth-Century Paris* (Oxford: Oxford University Press, 2009).

7 See *Paradigmes de l'âme: littérature et aliénisme au XIXe siècle*, ed. by Jean-Louis Cabanès, Didier Philippot, and Paolo Tortonese (Paris: Presses Sorbonne nouvelle, 2012); Michael Finn, *Hysteria, Hypnosis, the Spirits and Pornography: Fin-de-Siècle Cultural Discourses in the Decadent Rachilde* (Newark: University of Delaware Press, 2009); Jacqueline Carroy, *Hypnose, suggestion et psychologie. L'invention de sujets* (Paris: PUF, 1991). Ann Jefferson tracks the multiple meanings and shifting understandings of genius across the eighteenth, nineteenth,

début du XIXe siècle à la Grande Guerre (2003), offers a historical reading of the shifting descriptions and classifications of hysteria over the course of the long nineteenth century.[8] Working with scientific documents, medical case-studies, and religious and literary texts, Edleman covers key moments in the transformations of perceptions of hysteria: from the corporeal dysfunction and treatment of hysteria as a 'névrose génitale' by Philippe Pinel in the early decades of the century, to the neurological issues underpinning hysteria in medical texts from 1830–1850, to the psychoanalytic writings of Sigmund Freud. In *Les Romans de la Salpêtrière. Réception d'une scénographie clinique: Jean-Martin Charcot dans l'imaginaire fin-de-siècle* (2008), Bertrand Marquer focuses on Charcot's research on hysteria, the status of mental pathologies at the end of the nineteenth century, and the imaginary of the clinic.[9] Combining a socio-historical study of the influence of Charcot's medical theories with careful readings of literary representations of the doctor from the *fin de siècle*, Marquer shows how the nervous disorders were linked by writers to social evolution and political affairs. The political dimensions of mental pathologies are powerfully demonstrated in Janet Beizer's *Ventriloquized Bodies: Narratives of Hysteria in Nineteenth-Century France* (1994). Beizer examines the discursive power of patriarchal knowledges to present hysteria as an object of clinical intervention and control, but also to erase and devocalize the hysterical body. By mobilizing narratological and psychoanalytical perspectives, Beizer is able to stress the fluid and dispersed nature of the textuality of hysteria.[10] In Beizer's terms, hysteria's text 'is not a place but a mobile discursive practice that defies containment in space or time'.[11] Indeed, it is through attention to the writing and metaphors of hysteria that Beizer reveals how this mental pathology could not be contained within disciplinary boundaries, but was subject to multiple practices of discursive control.

What this diverse body of scholarship in French studies uncovers is the fluidity of medical culture and textual practice. Following on from these studies, the contributions of *Medicine and Maladies* are devoted to close analyses of

---

and twentieth centuries in *Genius in France: An Idea and its Uses* (Princeton and Oxford: Princeton University Press, 2015).

8 Nicole Edelman, *Les Métamorphoses de l'hystérique: Du début du XIXe siècle à la Grande Guerre* (Paris: La Découverte, 2003).

9 Bertrand Marquer, *Les Romans de la Salpêtrière. Réception d'une scénographie clinique: Jean-Martin Charcot dans l'imaginaire fin-de siècle* (Geneva: Droz, 2008).

10 Janet Beizer, *Ventriloquized Bodies: Narratives of Hysteria in Nineteenth-Century France* (Ithaca and London: Cornell University Press, 1994).

11 Ibid., p. 10.

how illness is represented in fictional and non-fictional narratives. Given these research foci, this volume's attention to the tangled relationship between medical practice, the history of medicine, literature, and art also contributes to ongoing discussions in the field of the 'medical humanities', which engages with the humanization of healthcare, scientific epistemology in philosophical, psychological and literary writing, phenomenological experiences of illness, and the cultural history of disease. Whilst the term 'medical humanities' can be traced to the 1980s and 90s, it is increasingly an important contemporary research initiative characterized by interdisciplinarity. In recent years, textbook studies — produced in part to accompany the growing number of courses in the medical humanities offered in higher education — outline a range of perspectives and approaches that explore scientific knowledge, the history of medicine, clinical practice, and bioethics.[12] Alongside qualitative studies and engagement with health-care policies, the value of literature and culture in medical education has also received sustained attention.[13] Perhaps unsurprisingly, as the field of the medical humanities originates in North America, much existing research is written for an Anglophone audience and centred on Anglophone contexts and source materials.[14]

The turn to the interdisciplinary themes of the medical humanities has helped to extend the range of possible ways of addressing the history, politics, and aesthetics of the medical beyond the shadow of Michel Foucault in French and Francophone scholarship. In recent years, there has been a shift in French trends from the history of medicine (*histoire de santé*) towards 'les humanités médicales'. The support of international funding bodies indicates

---

12 The 'medical humanities' has been described as witnessing 'a moment of emergence' in *The Edinburgh Companion to the Critical Medical Humanities*, ed. by Sarah Atkinson, Jane Macnaughton, and Jennifer Richards (Edinburgh: Edinburgh University Press, 2016), p. 14. Introductory studies to the medical humanities include: *Medical Humanities: An Introduction*, ed. by Thomas R. Cole, Nathan S. Carlin, and Ronald A. Carson (Cambridge: Cambridge University Press, 2015); *Medical Humanities*, ed. by Martyn Evans and Ilora G. Finlay (London: MMJ, 2001); *Medical Humanities Companion Volume One: Symptom*, ed. by Martyn Evans, Rolf Ahlén, Iona Heath, and Jane McNaughton (Oxford: Radcliffe, 2008); *Medical Humanities Companion Volume Two: Diagnosis*, ed. by Rolf Ahlén, Martyn Evans, Pekka Louhiala, and Raimo Puustinen (Oxford: Radcliffe, 2008).

13 International and interdisciplinary research networks, like 'Cognitive Futures in the Arts and Humanities', and journals dedicated to the field of the medical humanities, such as *Medical Humanities*, *Journal of Medical Humanities*, and *Literature and Medicine*, indicate the growing body of research in this area.

14 See, *Medicine, Health and the Arts: Approaches to the Medical Humanities*, ed. by Victoria Bates, Alan Bleakley, and Sam Goodman (Oxford: Routledge, 2014).

the rigour within French literary and visual studies across the Channel and *outre-mer* for research projects underlining the value of the arts and humanities in this fast-developing field.[15] Within nineteenth-century French studies, these include explorations of the relationship between literature and medicine in first-person illness narratives;[16] gastrointestinal health;[17] and the history of emotions and emotional wellbeing.[18] The growing number of monograph publications in key areas of cultural history, disability studies, and gender studies similarly attest to the overlap between medical concepts and material culture in critical approaches to representations of the clinical gaze, afflicted body, and social pathologies.[19]

Building upon discussions occupying both scholars of nineteenth-century France and researchers in the field of the medical humanities, *Medicine and Maladies* aims to develop critical insight into nineteenth-century French medical practices and perceptions of illness. Each chapter makes an original contribution to growing work on the status of 'new' sciences of the nineteenth century, such as psychiatry and pharmacy; neurological theories of the mind and 'behaviour'; psychiatric practices; first-person accounts of disease; and, representations of affliction in popular media. Alongside fresh readings of canonical works, one of the defining characteristics of this edited volume is the mobilization of non-canonical material, whether scientific treatises by marginal psychologists, fictional works by underexplored novelists, or everyday objects. While contemporary studies have tended to engage primarily with connections between narrative and medical discourse, our approach is intermedial with a number of chapters analyzing visual representations of disease. Encompassing

---

15 See, *inter alia*, Bertrand Marquer's project 'La Littérature de l'estomac' (2015–2020), supported by the Institut Universitaire de France. At the time of going to press, Steven Wilson was awarded an Arts and Humanities Research Council Leadership Fellowship for a new project 'Global Disease: Language(s) and the Literary Imagination'.

16 See Steven Wilson, 'French Autopathography', *L'Esprit Créateur*, Vol. 56, no. 2 (2016).

17 See Manon Mathias, 'Recycling Excrement in Flaubert and Zola', *Forum for Modern Language Studies*, 2017, <doi:10.1093/fmls/cqx040> [accessed 10 December 2017]; Bertrand Marquer, *L'Autre siècle de Messer Gaster? Physiologies de l'estomac dans la littérature du XIXe siècle* (Paris: Éditions Hermann, coll. "Hors collection", 2017).

18 On jealousy, see Masha Belenky *The Anxiety of Dispossession: Jealousy in Nineteenth-Century French Culture* (Cranbury, NJ: Rosemont Publishing Corp., 2008).

19 Hannah Thompson analyses representations of the diseased body and disability in French realist texts in *Taboo: Corporeal Secrets in Nineteenth-Century France* (Oxford: Legenda, 2013). In her most recent monograph, *Reviewing Blindness in French Fiction, 1789–2013* (London: Palgrave Macmillan, Literary Disability Studies, 2017), Thompson investigates depictions of blindness in French literary texts.

art history and practice, the visual evidence considered draws on material cultural production as well as 'high art': from social representations of affliction in the form of caricatural images to Auguste Rodin's celebrated sculpture of Honoré de Balzac, from imagery as propaganda in postcard illustrations of the alcoholic to representations of disease in Art Nouveau. What emerges from the rich and diverse engagement with iconographic sources, cultural history, and textual narrative in the chapters of *Medicine and Maladies* is a broader questioning of the cultural resources and traditions that shape understandings of affliction across the nineteenth century.

Medicine and Maladies is structured in such a way as to present and evoke the possible interrelationships between different disciplinary approaches and forms of representation, and to thereby maintain and develop readings across multifarious sources, rather than bracketing debates into discrete domains. The edited volume has three parts divided according to thematic and historical concerns to facilitate the interdisciplinary and intermedial connections to be found in critical readings of medical discourse: Part One, 'Documenting Medical Affliction'; Part Two, 'Writing Pathological Experiences'; and Part Three, 'Reading Body, Mind, and Environment'. Questions of the sick and suffering body as well as the relationship between the medical sciences and the humanities in nineteenth-century French culture are central to the readings developed here. Can cultural representations of disease enhance understandings of nineteenth-century medical theory? How do scientific terms and concepts inform cultural texts? How might representations of affliction appropriate, critique, or develop medical discourse and how might literary or aesthetic depictions of disease transform, or enhance, the investigations of medical experts? More specifically, authors explore, for example, how cultural assumptions about gender and sexuality shape understandings of the female body and examine the ways in which corporeal experiences of illness enable narrative.

In Part One, 'Documenting Medical Affliction', authors turn their focus to non-fictional texts and the particular historical moments in which they appeared, actively analysing how medical definitions and theories were shaped by specific cultural conditions. In the opening chapter Géraldine Crahay offers an analysis of medical treaties documenting sexual difference by physicians including Pierre-Jean-Georges Cabanis, Jacques Louis Moreau de la Sarthe, Charles François Menville, and the anthropologist Julien-Joseph Virey. Crahay sets out to show how this body of scientific knowledge, published between 1802 and 1845, deploys a binary rhetoric (positive, negative; hot, cold; rational, emotional) to highlight anatomical differences between the sexes and expose differences between masculine and feminine behaviours. After outlining the fundamental dichotomy underpinning both the biological distinctions between males and females and the socially and culturally constructed conceptions of men and women in these male-authored works, Crahay examines medical interest in the ambivalent figure of the 'femme masculine' (*femme hommasse*). Extending the notion of 'masculinité féminine' developed by Judith Halbestram, Crahay explores how the medical establishment depicted women whose atypical behaviours evaded scientific categories and troubled the codes of femininity and female sexuality. Crahay shows that male practitioners — repulsed by women whose conduct went against the norms of sensuality — staged problematic figures such as the *virago, vieille fille, lesbienne*, or *tribade* as sick, unbalanced, sterile, or cancerous. While literary writings contemporary with these medical texts explored sexual ambiguity, the scientific writings of physicians, Crahay argues, upheld rigid dichotomies between the sexes and presented as deviant those who threatened biological distinctions, successful reproduction, and social codes, values, and conventions.

In Chapter 2, Larry Duffy focuses on the similarities and differences that shape texts produced by medical and pharmaceutical professionals, and that span non-literary and literary discourse. With a particular focus on the Napoleonic period, Duffy compares the content of the pharmaceutical *journal de campagne* with medical narratives produced during Napoleon's military campaigns. The writings of author-pharmacists Charles-Louis Cadet de Gassicourt and Pierre-Irénée Jacob are considered alongside texts produced by the army surgeon Dominique de Larrey, as Duffy explores the distinctions between the pharmaceutical memoir and clinical accounts of battlefield surgeries, case histories, and amputation practices. Duffy argues that the 'discursive polyvalency' and broad thematic scope of the texts produced by pharmacists involved in the Napoleonic Campaigns demonstrate the generic mobility of pharmaceutical narratives. The writings of nineteenth-century military pharmacists, long before canonical realist texts such as Flaubert's *Madame Bovary* (1856), troubled the boundaries between disciplines, professions, discursive fields, and genres.

Issues surrounding the definition and treatment of the alcoholic in the course of the nineteenth century are the subject of Julie Müller's historical exploration, in Chapter 3, of transitioning perceptions of excessive alcohol consumption. Tracing shifts in understandings and approaches to drinking from antiquity to the end of the nineteenth century, Müller turns to scientific theories such as Magnus Huss's influential medical study of 1849, which introduced the description of alcoholism as a disease, and Charles Bouchard's theory of autointoxication. Müller reviews the major scientific currents shaping ideas of the drunkard, changes to penal and juridical systems regarding the management of alcoholics, varying attitudes towards the individual's responsibility for bodily urges, and common links between alcoholism and *fin-de-siècle* theories of degeneration. Arguing that scientific writings on alcoholism, and its symptoms of vice, violence, vulgarity, and idleness, reveal connections between the discourse of individual physicians and Christian religious doctrine, Müller demonstrates how the ancient figure of the *ivrogne* informed late-nineteenth-century representations of the intoxicated body. Along with medical texts, Müller discusses the circulation of shared vocabularies and stylistic tropes across fictional and non-fictional genres, and draws on literary and visual materials, including postcard illustrations and novels, to track shifting cultural perspectives of the alcoholic.

In Chapter 4, Philippa Lewis explores the pathologization of timidity at the *fin de siècle*. Working in pliant ways across cultural history, literary criticism, philosophy, and psychological theory, Lewis casts a fresh gaze on the problem of shyness at a specific moment of emerging specialization of the medical field. Through a comparative reading of Ludovic Dugas's *La Timidité: étude psychologique et morale* (1898) and Paul Hartenberg's *Les Timides et la timidité* (1901), Lewis considers the epistemological uncertainty that surrounds timidity and examines the ideological functions of shyness 'norms'. Discussions of the *fin-de-siècle* figure of the *timide*, Lewis shows, brought into play issues of gender, sexuality, race, class, and national decline. Mindful of the social and cultural contexts underpinning Hartenberg and Dugas's scientific descriptions, Lewis can fully probe developments in the understandings and treatments of the *timide* put forward in each of these medical texts. Key to Lewis's reading is an awareness of how both Dugas and Hartenberg enhance their work with examples from novels and literary culture. By highlighting entanglements between medical and literary texts, porous connections between disciplines (science and literature), and overlaps between discourses (medical, psychiatric, literary, and philosophical), Lewis reveals how theories of shyness blur disciplinary and professional boundaries.

Shifting the emphasis from historical context to individual experience, the chapters of Part Two, 'Writing Pathological Experiences', focus on representations of disease in cultural texts and ask how the narrative strategies that writers adopt shape notions of selfhood, depict the doctor-patient relationship, and inform understandings of illness. Each of the four chapters examines the strategies of resistance used by writers in texts that depict the embodied experience of sufferers and probes the links between sickness and expression.

In Chapter 5, Mélanie Bhend explores how the self is at stake in the narratives of individuals writing from within French psychiatric hospitals. Analyzing two accounts published in the 1860s, Bhend turns her attention to an overlooked period in the development of attitudes towards conceptions of madness and the clinically insane following advances in psychiatric medicine. Placing the patient's voice at the centre of her study of Karl-des-Monts's epistolary narrative *Un martyre dans une maison de fous* (1863) and Hector Malot's novel *Un beau-frère* (1869), Bhend addresses depictions of the insane asylum from the perspective of the incarcerated individual and examines how, in both the autobiographical text and fictional first-person written account, thematic imagery shapes the ways in which experiences of madness and confinement are conceptualized and communicated. If the images of monstrosity and bestiality deployed in both texts reinforce cultural ideas of the clinically insane, Bhend argues that one finds in Karl-des-Monts and Malot resistance to institutional power structures. Both writers present the reader with a subjective experience of the asylum system and expose the ineffectiveness of the asylum as a cure for madness. Yet, Bhend claims, the reliability of the accounts voiced by those imprisoned in the system of *aliénistes* varies according to the author's choice of narrative form.

Chapter 6, 'La Maladie comme métaphore chez Baudelaire', attends to the figures of speech and symbolic expressions of affliction that span Baudelaire's correspondence, literary criticism, and prose poetry. At the heart of Joanna Rajukmar's analysis is the question of how metaphors convey sickness and obscure descriptions of malady. Alert to the biographical context that informed Baudelaire's approach to medicine and the medical profession, Rajkumar illustrates how Baudelaire's use of generic linguistic formulations, silences, and empty diagnoses expose the doctor as a charlatan, rather than an individual with access to specialist medical knowledge. Tracing the metaphorical expression 'jet(er) (s)a langue aux chiens', Rajkumar examines, through tropes of animality and linguistic contamination, Baudelaire's struggle to articulate his own experience of illness. Her exploration of the limitations and capacities of language reveals the poet as the victim of the medical doctor's clichéd discourse and as reliant on the same ambivalent dimensions of language. Focusing on 'Madame Bistouri', Rajkumar is concerned with the double meanings and contradictions that make it difficult to distinguish between doctor and prostitute, male and female, patient and practitioner, healthy and pathological, and, crucially, between the character of the physician-narrator and the voice of the poet.

In Chapter 7, Susannah Wilson demonstrates how wasting women refuse to act according to established convention, troubling the family unit and the institutional structures that shape society. Wilson's comparative reading of texts by the Goncourt brothers and by the physician Dr Georges Gasne addresses questions relating to the multiplicity of forms and approaches that can be used to convey the attitudes and the prejudices encountered by the 'jeune fille'. She turns first to the portrayal of the eponymous heroine of the Goncourt's novel *Renée Mauperin* (1864) before considering the circumstance of Béatrice Gill, the subject of a medical case study of 'hysterical anorexia' in 1900. In both the Goncourt's and Gasne's writing, the figure of the wasting woman is presented as ambivalent and subverts the traditional ideas of weakness and vulnerability that accompany traditional depictions of the emaciated female body. In these narratives — the first a fictional text and the second a medical account that incorporates a letter by the patient — adolescent women, in various ways, resist bourgeois norms and male domination. Rather than cede narrative control to the medical practitioner, Wilson argues that these two narratives of wasting women expose the patient's voice. The phenomenological experience of self-starvation and its emotional and physical symptoms are not silenced but discursively articulated. By confronting others with her condition of physical frailty, Wilson contends, the patient can be read as a source of power and knowledge; a figure of rebellion against the constraints imposed by patriarchal structures, expectations of the family, and bourgeois femininity.

Concern with returning the patient's voice to the centre of the medical discourse is also crucial to Steven Wilson's study, in Chapter 8, of the evocation of pain in Alphonse Daudet's *La Doulou: 1887–1895*. Published posthumously in 1930, Daudet's notebook offers a first-person written account of the author's experience of living with a long-term medical condition. Wilson begins by introducing contemporary perspectives on pain by Elaine Scarry and Joanna Bourke before drawing on this theoretical framework to examine Daudet's articulation of symptoms, feelings, and embodied experiences of syphilis. Analyzing Daudet's use of metaphors of invasion and infiltration, conflict, and physical martyrdom, Wilson discusses the capabilities and limitations of figurative language in the communication of pain. For Wilson, the patient articulates pain and charts the degeneration of the body in ways that medicine cannot describe. Thus, Wilson argues, the patient's subjective experience of the three symptomatic stages of syphilis offers valuable insight into the mental and physical deterioration caused by this chronic illness and provides an important contribution to scientific knowledge of the disease.

The relationship between writing the self and writing disease is an area of scholarship with strong connections to on-going research in the medical humanities, with work on 'illness narratives' the subject of recent journal special issues.[20] Returning the patient to the centre of medical enquiry, these chapters

20 Close readings of first-person representations of illness or disability that span from nineteenth-century artist Adèle Lanzier to twentieth-century writings on HIV/AIDS and cancer, and the twenty-first century films of André Techiré and Julian Schnabel are

explore the sick individual as a key source of medical knowledge and make specific contributions to debates on writing about experiences of illness. The works in question — whether novels, autobiographical narratives, poetry, or medical case studies — have a common interest in the patient's perspective: Karl-des-Monts and Hector Malot expose the voice of the incarcerated individual; Baudelaire presents the patient threatened by the loss of voice; literary and clinical accounts of anorexia nervosa reveal tensions between the voices of the male narrator, author, or doctor and the voice of the adolescent female patient; and Daudet's first-person accounts of pain communicate the voice of the suffering subject. What emerges are analyses concerned with how corporeal experience is translated into language and how patient narratives might extend scientific knowledge of hysteria, madness, *anorexie hystérique*, or syphilis.

In Part Three, 'Reading Body, Mind, and Environment', the final three chapters examine links between medical discourse, social problems, and political uncertainty in the final decades of the nineteenth century. Discussing examples drawn from literature and art criticism, authors consider the impact of external influences (heredity and environment) on internal states and the ways internal imbalances are made manifest as corporeal abnormalities or psychological instabilities (nervous disorders, behavioural traits, emotional responses, hysterical afflictions). In addition, each of these chapters suggests that the health of the individual might be symbolic or symptomatic of broader social problems. For example, across literary and journalistic discourses the sustained association of physical symptoms of disease with discussions of national decline strengthened connections between illness, (moral) corruption, and (social) degeneration in the collective imagination.

In a close reading of Octave Mirbeau's novel *L'Abbé Jules* (1888), in Chapter 9, Elizabeth Emery probes the outbursts of rage that characterize the reactions of the eponymous protagonist, Jules Dervelle, in order to demonstrate how Mirbeau's fiction can be read as a critique of social conventions and medical classification. Working from Galen's theories of the humours and Debreyne's hygiene manuals, Emery demonstrates what she terms Mirbeau's 'poetics of physiological difference'. As well as attending to the significant overlaps between the discourses of medical science and Mirbeau's incorporation of medical terminology in his representation of Jules's 'exalted' temperament, Emery investigates how Mirbeau undermines medical treatises related to behaviour and resists the pathologization of behavioural difference. Resisting 'Naturalist' readings of *L'Abbé Jules*, Emery shows that Mirbeau is governed

---

pursued by the contributors to Steven Wilson's special issue to *L'Esprit Créateur*, 56, 2 (2016).

not by the need to identify 'types' but by the drive to represent the complexities and fluctuations of individual temperament. Thus, Emery discerns in Mirbeau's complex literary portrayal of the processes behind human behaviour a precursor to twenty-first century debates on 'neuronormativity'. In terms of narrative style, form, and content Emery's analysis draws attention to the modernity of Mirbeau's writing and argues that it both goes beyond literary models and reaches forward to debates of interest in medical science today.

Theories of regional type, degeneration, and genius are the focus of Chapter 10 in which Natasha Ruiz-Gómez examines the relation between physiological enquiry and aesthetic production in Auguste Rodin's *Monument to Balzac* (1898). Attentive to process, Ruiz-Gómez details how Rodin's preliminary studies were informed by a naturalist approach and scientific outlook, influenced by work on physiognomy and by the idea of hereditary pathology. While physiognomic principles shaped Rodin's initial research, Ruiz-Gómez investigates how by the mid-1890s emerging medical discourses on nervous disorders altered Rodin's creative process and definitive method. By charting the progression of the clay works, plaster models, and casts that Rodin produced in preparation for the final version, Ruiz-Gómez shows how the *Monument* became a study of genius. She considers how, in the context of scientific theories of degeneration and new medical sciences of the nineteenth century, the sculpture of Balzac demonstrates Rodin's transition from naturalistic observation to subjective interpretation, artistic innovation, and creative genius.

Finally, in Chapter 11, Cyril Barde focuses on the aesthetic and sociopolitical discussions of Art Nouveau around 1900. Critical commentary on the graphic portrayals of organic forms and vegetal matter in Art Nouveau, Barde reveals, echo the discourses of degeneration that informed the nineteenth-century medical imaginary. Turning to the reactions of journalists and art critics in caricature illustrations and in written articles, Barde explores audience responses to this style and technique of art and architecture. As Barde demonstrates, critics consistently interpreted the vegetal themes of Art Nouveau as manifestations of disease, rather than celebrations of organic materials and the natural world: discursive tropes of exhaustion and suffocation (asthma, parasitism); neurosis and psychological illness (hysteria, deliria); and, viral or bacterial infection (contagion) shaped the critics' accounts of viewing experiences. The illness metaphors present in audience responses to the decorative arts and visual practices of the *fin de siècle*, Barde argues, did not just signify an aesthetic response mobilized against earlier artistic movements. Rather, these discourses reveal how innovations in the field of the decorative arts were considered symptomatic of the physical and mental health of both the individual body and the domestic interior. Accordingly, Barde contends, the socio-political dimensions of audience responses to Art Nouveau — the body of the spectator as convulsive, contorted, infiltrated, infected — act as metaphors for the ailing social body and illustrate anxieties about the perceived threat that external ideas and influences posed to late nineteenth-century France.

Across the chapters of *Medicine and Maladies*, examples drawn from a rich and diverse corpus show the transgressive capacities of nineteenth-century French literary and medical discourse. Contextualized readings of works of literary and visual culture, including novels by the Goncourt brothers and Mirbeau, Baudelaire's versification, and Daudet's personal experience of syphilis, are combined with close readings of understudied writings by medical practitioners and theorists such as Dominique de Larrey and Paul Hartenberg. Not only do medical definitions and concepts permeate literary narratives and inform artistic practice, but works of literature and art provide doctors and practitioners with 'evidence' that is referenced in scientific texts that document and describe pathological conditions.

Collectively, we contribute to the vibrant dialogues occurring internationally about the relationships between aesthetics and medicine and a complex picture of affliction in nineteenth-century France emerges.

Bibliography

Ahlén, Rolf, Martyn Evans, Pekka Louhiala, and Raimo Puustinen (eds), *Medical Humanities Companion Volume Two: Diagnosis* (Oxford: Radcliffe, 2008)

Atkinson, Sarah, Jane Macnaughton, and Jennifer Richards (eds), *The Edinburgh Companion to the Critical Medical Humanities* (Edinburgh: Edinburgh University Press, 2016)

Bates, Victoria, Alan Bleakley, and Sam Goodman (eds), *Medicine, Health and the Arts: Approaches to the Medical Humanities* (Oxford: Routledge, 2014)

Beizer, Janet, *Ventriloquized Bodies: Narratives of Hysteria in Nineteenth-Century France* (Ithaca and London: Cornell University Press, 1994)

Belenky, Masha, *The Anxiety of Dispossession: Jealousy in Nineteenth-Century French Culture* (Cranbury, NJ: Rosemont Publishing Corp., 2008)

Cabanès, Jean-Louis, *Le Corps et la maladie dans les récits réalistes (1856–1898)*, 2 vols (Paris: Klincksieck, 1991)

——, Didier Philippot, and Paolo Tortonese (eds), *Paradigmes de l'âme: littérature et aliénisme au XIXe siècle* (Paris: Presses Sorbonne nouvelle, 2012)

Carroy, Jacqueline, *Hypnose, suggestion et psychologie. L'invention de sujets* (Paris: PUF, 1991)
Cole, Thomas R., Nathan S. Carlin, and Ronald A. Carson (eds), *Medical Humanities: An Introduction* (Cambridge: Cambridge University Press, 2015)
Edelman, Nicole, *Les Métamorphoses de l'hystérique: Du début du XIXe siècle à la Grande Guerre* (Paris: La Découverte, 2003)
Evans, Martyn, and Ilora G. Finlay (eds), *Medical Humanities* (London: MMJ, 2001)
Evans, Martyn, Rolf Ahlén, Iona Heath, and Jane McNaughton (eds), *Medical Humanities Companion Volume One: Symptom* (Oxford: Radcliffe, 2008)
Finn, Michael, *Hysteria, Hypnosis, the Spirits and Pornography: Fin-de-Siècle Cultural Discourses in the Decadent Rachilde* (Newark: University of Delaware Press, 2009)
Gill, Miranda, *Eccentricity and the Cultural Imagination in Nineteenth-Century Paris* (Oxford: Oxford University Press, 2008)
Goldstein, Jan, 'The Uses of Male Hysteria: Medical and Literary Discourse in Nineteenth-Century France', in *French Medical Culture in the Nineteenth Century*, ed. by Ann La Berge and Mordechai Feingold, pp. 210–47
Jefferson, Ann, *Genius in France: An Idea and its Uses* (Princeton and Oxford: Princeton University Press, 2015)
La Berge, Ann, and Mordechai Feingold (eds), *French Medical Culture in the Nineteenth Century* (Oxford: Rodopi, 1994)
Marquer, Bertrand, *L'Autre siècle de Messer Gaster? Physiologies de l'estomac dans la littérature du XIXe siècle* (Paris: Éditions Hermann, coll. "Hors collection", 2017)
——, *Les Romans de la Salpêtrière. Réception d'une scénographie clinique: Jean-Martin Charcot dans l'imaginaire fin-de-siècle* (Geneva: Droz, 2008)
Mathias, Manon, 'Recycling Excrement in Flaubert and Zola', *Forum for Modern Language Studies*, 2017 <doi: 10.1093/fmls/cqx040> [accessed 10 December 2017]
Matlock, Jann, *Scenes of Seduction: Prostitution, Hysteria and Reading Difference in Nineteenth-Century France* (New York: Columbia University Press, 1994)
Rousseau, G. S., Miranda Gill, David Haycock, and Malte Herwig (eds), *Framing and Imagining Disease in Cultural History* (Basingstoke: Palgrave Macmillan, 2003)
Thompson, Hannah, *Reviewing Blindness in French Fiction, 1789–2013* (London: Palgrave Macmillan, Literary Disability Studies, 2017)
——, *Taboo: Corporeal Secrets in Nineteenth-Century France* (Oxford: Legenda, 2013)
Wilson, Steven, 'French Autopathography', *L'Esprit Créateur*, 56, 2 (2016)

PART 1

Documenting Medical Affliction

CHAPTER 1

'Voyez les femmes les plus hommasses, ces *viragines* audacieuses' : la domestication de la femme masculine dans les traités savants de la première moitié du dix-neuvième siècle

Géraldine Crahay

Le médecin et philosophe Pierre-Jean-Georges Cabanis affirmait, dans ses *Rapports du physique et du moral de l'homme* (1802), que l'homme et la femme sont faits pour la perpétuation de l'espèce et que cette dernière n'est possible que si l'homme séduit la femme en attaquant et si elle se laisse séduire en se défendant, avant de céder au parti le plus avantageux, c'est-à-dire au plus fort.[1] La qualité que la femme doit, elle, posséder pour mener à bien ce jeu de séduction duquel dépend la survie de l'espèce humaine est la faiblesse : 'La principale grâce de l'homme est dans sa vigueur', assure Cabanis : 'l'empire de la femme est caché dans des ressorts plus délicats ; on n'aime point qu'elle soit si forte'.[2] La force de la femme, qu'elle soit physique, morale ou intellectuelle, suscite l'inquiétude, voire le dégoût du médecin, et cet avis devrait selon lui être universellement partagé par la gent masculine, comme l'indique le pronom indéfini et généralisant *on*. Cette femme forte peut être définie comme une femme masculine, c'est-à-dire une femme présentant des caractéristiques physiques et comportementales généralement attribuées aux hommes. À des degrés divers, les femmes masculines suscitent la polémique, car elles enfreignent, d'une manière ou d'une autre, les conventions sociales du dix-neuvième siècle associées aux sexes.

L'idée de masculinité féminine, ou *female masculinity*, est développée par Judith Halberstam dans son livre éponyme, dans lequel elle envisage de conceptualiser la masculinité sans les hommes.[3] Elle déclare en effet que la masculinité est souvent incorrectement associée au sexe masculin (ou *maleness*) alors

1 Pierre-Jean-Georges Cabanis, *Rapports du physique et du moral de l'homme* (Paris : Crapart, Caille et Ravier, 1802), I, pp. 347–48. L'orthographe des textes scientifiques a été modernisée et corrigée si nécessaire.

2 Ibid., p. 351.

3 Judith Halberstam, *Female Masculinity* (Durham, NC : Duke University Press, 1998), p. 2.

 | DOI:10.1163/9789004368019_003

que le sexe masculin n'en est qu'une incarnation parmi plusieurs.[4] Les *gender studies* et notamment l'important essai de Judith Butler *Gender Trouble* (1990) ont en effet mis en évidence le décalage qui existe entre sexe et genre. Le sexe est une réalité biologique tandis que le genre en est sa construction culturelle et sociale :

> Originally intended to dispute the biology-is-destiny formulation, the distinction between sex and gender serves the argument that whatever biological intractability sex appears to have, gender is culturally constructed: hence, gender is neither the causal result of sex nor as seemingly fixed as sex.[5]

Autrement dit, la masculinité, ou genre masculin, n'est pas forcément le propre du sexe masculin, bien que la langue française entretienne la confusion.[6]

La séparation moderne des concepts de genre et de sexe de même que la reconnaissance du fait que le sexe et le genre d'une personne ne correspondent pas toujours (chez les individus dits transgenres, par exemple) sont des positions qui ne sont pas acceptées par les savants français du début du dix-neuvième siècle. Ces derniers sont guidés par un principe de séparation stricte des sexes. Ils conçoivent ce que Thomas Laqueur appelle un modèle à deux sexes (*two-sex model*), ou incommensurabilité, une invention des Lumières qui est fondée sur un principe d'opposition entre le sexe masculin et le sexe féminin.[7] Auparavant, c'est-à-dire depuis l'Antiquité grecque, et notamment depuis Aristote et Galien, c'est le modèle à un sexe (*one-sex model*) qui prévalait. Les organes génitaux féminins étaient considérés comme identiques à ceux des hommes mais étaient internes plutôt qu'externes. Le vagin d'une femme, par exemple, équivalait en quelque sorte au pénis masculin. En raison de leur caractère interne, les organes génitaux féminins étaient perçus comme inférieurs à ceux des hommes, instituant entre les deux sexes un rapport d'hiérarchie plutôt que d'opposition.

---

4 Halberstam, *Female Masculinity*, p. 2.

5 Judith Butler, *Gender Trouble : Feminism and the Subversion of Identity* (New York : Routledge, 1990), p. 6.

6 Comme il n'y a pas de véritable équivalent à l'adjectif anglais *male*, l'adjectif *masculin* fait référence à la fois au sexe et au genre d'un individu.

7 Thomas Laqueur, *Making Sex : Body and Gender from the Greeks to Freud* (Cambridge, MA : Harvard University Press, 1990), pp. 2–3. Voir aussi Thomas Laqueur, 'Orgasm, Generation, and the Politics of Reproductive Biology', *The Making of the Modern Body : Sexuality and Society in the Nineteenth Century*, éd. par Catherine Gallagher et Thomas Laqueur (Berkeley : University of California Press, 1987), pp. 1–41 (pp. 4–6, 23).

D'après le principe de séparation des sexes — que nous appellerons également dichotomie sexuelle — l'homme et la femme ont des organes génitaux radicalement différents, voire opposés. Cette différence n'est pas uniquement génitale. En vérité, elle crée une différence physiologique, morale et comportementale entre l'homme et la femme. Les savants de la première moitié du dix-neuvième siècle se sont tout particulièrement intéressés à la constitution des femmes, à leurs habitudes et à leur mentalité — en un mot à leur féminité — afin de déterminer le rôle décisif que la différence entre hommes et femmes joue au moment de la reproduction. Si une femme est physiquement et psychologiquement masculine, elle constitue une aberration médicale et menace le système de la séparation des sexes.

Nous expliquerons dans un premier temps le concept de séparation des sexes et l'importance que joue l'opposition entre l'homme et la femme dans la procréation en nous basant sur quatre textes scientifiques de la première moitié du dix-neuvième siècle : le cinquième mémoire des *Rapports du physique et du moral de l'homme* (1802) de Pierre-Jean-Georges Cabanis, intitulé 'De l'influence des sexes sur le caractère des idées et des affections morales' ; l'*Histoire naturelle de la femme* (1803) du médecin Jacques Louis Moreau de la Sarthe ; le traité *De la Femme* de l'anthropologue Julien-Joseph Virey (1823) ; et l'*Histoire médicale et philosophique de la femme* (1845) du médecin Charles François Menville de Ponsan.[8] Dans un second temps, nous relèverons les différents types de femmes masculines qui sont mentionnés dans ces textes, à savoir la prostituée, la femme du peuple, la lesbienne, la femme âgée, la vieille fille et la femme intellectuelle. Il faut préciser que la femme masculine constitue pour les savants un sujet presque insignifiant ; elle n'apparaît dès lors que dans les marges de leurs textes, comme anecdote ou contre-exemple.[9] Nous soutiendrons cependant que, sous cette apparente insignifiance, se cache la

8 Jacques Louis Moreau de la Sarthe, *Histoire naturelle de la femme suivie d'un traité d'hygiène appliquée à son régime physique et moral aux différentes époques de la vie*, 2 vols (Paris : Duprat, 1803) ; Julien-Joseph Virey, *De la Femme, sous ses rapports physiologique, moral et littéraire*, 2e éd. (Paris : Crochard Libraire, 1825 [1823]) ; et Charles François Menville de Ponsan, *Histoire médicale et philosophique de la femme considérée dans toutes les époques principales de sa vie avec tous les changements qui surviennent dans son physique et son moral avec l'hygiène applicable à son sexe et toutes les maladies qui peuvent l'atteindre aux différents âges*, 3 vols (Paris : Amyot-Labé, 1845). Toute référence future au traité *De la Femme* figurera dorénavant dans le corps du texte de l'article et sera abréviée *F.*

9 La femme masculine ne jouit donc pas dans les traités savants de la même visibilité que celle dont bénéficient l'homosexuel et le 'pervers', que Michel Foucault a étudiée dans *Histoire de la sexualité, I : la volonté de savoir* (Paris : Gallimard, 1976), et en particulier dans son chapitre 'L'implantation perverse' (pp. 50–67).

crainte de l'émancipation des femmes. Il s'agira donc de déterminer comment la femme masculine est présentée implicitement comme une menace contre le système patriarcal et la séparation des sexes et, dès lors, de mettre en évidence les stratégies discursives — c'est-à-dire les moyens langagiers par lesquels le savoir est employé et détourné pour imposer une certaine vision du monde — qui sont utilisées par les savants pour dénigrer l'intégrité des femmes réputées masculines en limitant leur portée contestataire.[10]

La dichotomie sexuelle dans la première moitié du dix-neuvième siècle

Le principe d'opposition entre les sexes est essentiel dans les textes scientifiques du début du dix-neuvième siècle, mais il existait déjà dans *Émile ou de l'éducation* (1762) de Rousseau, qui a eu une influence considérable sur les savants de son temps.[11] Ce principe est basé uniquement sur l'examen des organes génitaux internes et externes, car ceux-ci constituaient à l'époque les seules preuves tangibles du sexe d'un individu (là où interviennent aujourd'hui d'autres facteurs, tels que les chromosomes et les hormones, alors inconnus). Un homme est pourvu d'un pénis, d'un scrotum, et de testicules ; la femme a un vagin, un utérus, et des ovaires. Ces organes génitaux suffisent en principe à déterminer le sexe d'un individu. Les savants affirment également, d'une part, que ces organes ont une influence 'incontestable' sur les autres organes[12] et, d'autre part, que cette influence est plus grande chez les femmes que chez les hommes. Virey assure même : 'Tout individu femelle est uniquement créé pour la propagation ; ses organes sexuels sont la racine et la base de toute sa structure' (*F*, 2). De même, Moreau de la Sarthe déclare : 'Les irradiations, la réaction puissante des organes de la reproduction ont encore plus d'empire sur la constitution des femmes'.[13]

10 Sur le discours comme stratégie de pouvoir, voir Foucault, *Histoire de la sexualité, I*, pp. 132–33, et en particulier : 'C'est bien dans le discours que pouvoir et savoir viennent s'articuler. Et pour cette raison même, il faut concevoir le discours comme une série de segments discontinus, dont la fonction tactique n'est ni uniforme ni stable' (p. 133).

11 Jean-Jacques Rousseau affirme dans *Émile ou de l'éducation*, éd. par André Charrak (Paris : Garnier-Flammarion, 2009), p. 515 : 'En tout ce qui tient au sexe la femme et l'homme ont partout des rapports et partout des différences'. En ce qui concerne l'influence de Rousseau, Moreau de la Sarthe, *Histoire naturelle de la femme*, II, p. 346, rappelle la révolution instaurée par le philosophe en ce qui concerne l'allaitement maternel.

12 Cabanis, *Rapports du physique et du moral de l'homme*, I, p. 320.

13 Moreau de la Sarthe, *Histoire naturelle de la femme*, I, pp. 203–04.

L'influence des organes génitaux sur les autres organes détermine d'autres signes corporels de masculinité ou de féminité. Ce sont des caractéristiques physiques, qu'on appelle de nos jours caractères sexuels secondaires, qui différencient chaque sexe et participent à l'identité sexuelle d'un individu sans jouer de rôle significatif dans la reproduction. Si les organes sexuels d'un individu sont ambigus — si cet individu est hermaphrodite, ou intersexué, c'est-à-dire qu'il possède des caractéristiques génitales appartenant aux deux sexes — le sexe 'véritable' de cette personne peut être identifié grâce à l'influence qu'il exerce sur son apparence physique. Cabanis, Moreau de la Sarthe, Virey et Menville de Ponsan dressent des portraits de l'homme et de la femme fondés sur l'opposition de ces traits physiques : l'homme est chaud, la femme est froide ; il est sec, elle est humide ; il a le teint hâlé, elle a le teint pâle ; il a une voix grave, elle a une voix aiguë, et ainsi de suite.[14] Virey note ainsi : 'L'un est actif, l'autre passif ; l'un est chaud et sec, ardent par sa constitution, l'autre humide et plus froid ; le premier commande et triomphe, le second succombe et supplie' (*F*, 187).

De plus, l'importance du corps et de la physiologie d'un individu se mesure également à l'influence qu'ils exercent sur sa personnalité et son comportement. La femme, par exemple, est physiquement et psychologiquement plus sensible que l'homme.[15] Cette sensibilité est déterminée par sa constitution réputée plus faible et son système nerveux. Sa sensibilité affecte ses goûts visuels, olfactifs, musicaux, culinaires et tactiles. Moreau de la Sarthe affirme ainsi qu'une femme préfère les couleurs claires, le parfum des fleurs et les musiques douces, et qu'elle repousse les mets très assaisonnés et les objets et tissus rugueux.[16] La sensibilité d'une femme affecte également son émotivité et son instinct, et elle est responsable de sa passivité et de sa versatilité.[17] Le caractère de la femme est donc perçu comme plus 'naturel', plus instinctif, plus émotif et plus passif que celui de l'homme.

Ces différences physiques et psychologiques sont considérées comme étant dues aux fonctions que chaque sexe est amené à exercer dans la société. Ainsi que le résume Cabanis :

---

14 Cabanis, *Rapports du physique et du moral de l'homme*, I, p. 316 ; Moreau de la Sarthe, *Histoire naturelle de la femme*, I, pp. 88–210 ; Virey, *De la Femme*, pp. 69–70, 172, 175, 176, 178, 180–82, 195 ; et Charles François Menville de Ponsan, *Histoire médicale et philosophique de la femme*, I, pp. 17–21.

15 Cabanis, *Rapports du physique et du moral de l'homme*, I, pp. 334–35, 350 ; Moreau de la Sarthe, *Histoire naturelle de la femme*, I, pp. 112–13, 118 ; et Virey, *De la Femme*, vii, pp. 103–04.

16 Moreau de la Sarthe, *Histoire naturelle de la femme*, I, pp. 79–81, 114–18.

17 Ibid., pp. 693–95 ; Virey, *De la Femme*, pp. 220–23.

> la nature n'a pas simplement distingué les sexes par les seuls organes, instruments directs de la génération : entre l'homme et la femme il existe d'autres différences de structure, qui se rapportent plutôt au rôle qui leur est assigné.[18]

Comme l'explique Pierre Bourdieu, il y a une inversion — qui confine à l'absurde — des causes et des effets dans la représentation du rapport entre corps biologiques et fonctions sociales dans les discours scientifiques du dix-neuvième siècle : selon la croyance de l'époque, c'est parce que l'homme et la femme seraient prédestinés à remplir des rôles différents dans la société que leur physiologie serait différente, et non l'inverse.[19] Selon Moreau de la Sarthe et ses confrères, la mission 'naturelle' d'une femme est d'être mère.[20] En effet, la mollesse de son corps et la douceur de son caractère la prédestineraient aux soins prodigués aux enfants. Cabanis n'hésite pas affirmer :

> La faiblesse de la femme [...] est surtout nécessaire, ou du moins très utile, pour la conception, pour la grossesse, pour l'accouchement, pour la lactation de l'enfant nouveau-né, pour les soins qu'exige son éducation pendant les premières années de sa vie.[21]

L'homme, plus fort et plus rationnel, est quant à lui jugé inapte à la garde des enfants en raison de sa maladresse et de sa lourdeur.[22] Il exerce dès lors 'naturellement' une activité physique et intellectuelle, dans la sphère publique.[23] Toutes ces différences 'naturelles' sont donc nécessaires. Cabanis résume ainsi les portraits de l'homme et de la femme : 'Il faut que l'homme soit fort, audacieux, entreprenant ; que la femme soit faible, timide, rusée', avant d'ajouter solennellement : 'Telle est la loi de la nature'.[24]

Il convient de s'interroger sur le bien-fondé d'une telle déclaration. Pourquoi, en effet, cette opposition entre les physiologies et comportements masculins et féminins est-elle à ce point nécessaire ? Pourquoi une femme doit-elle être faible à tout instant, même lorsqu'elle met au monde un enfant, alors que les

18 Cabanis, *Rapports du physique et du moral de l'homme*, I, pp. 315–16.

19 Pierre Bourdieu, *La Domination masculine* (Paris : Seuil, 'Points/Essais', 2002 [1998]), p. 39.

20 Moreau de la Sarthe, *Histoire naturelle de la femme*, II, pp. 156, 186.

21 Cabanis, *Rapports du physique et du moral de l'homme*, I, p. 349.

22 Ibid., I, p. 356.

23 Ibid., I, p. 349 ; Virey, *De la Femme*, p. 174.

24 Cabanis, *Rapports du physique et du moral de l'homme*, I, p. 348.

femmes meurent encore souvent en couches à l'époque de Cabanis ?[25] Et pourquoi l'homme doit-il être fort à n'importe quel moment ? La déclaration de Cabanis est trop catégorique pour ne pas révéler une certaine angoisse liée au rôle de la femme dans la société sur laquelle nous reviendrons. Les savants justifient leur position en invoquant la reproduction. Selon Virey, elle n'est possible que si l'homme et la femme se complètent mutuellement, autrement dit si chacun apporte les qualités dont l'autre est privé lors de l'acte sexuel. Il souligne donc le principe de complémentarité entre l'homme et la femme : 'L'homme sans la femme n'est point un être complet' (*F*, 2). D'après l'anthropologue, un homme et une femme sont complémentaires en raison de leur opposition physiologique et émotionnelle :

> Comment donc s'établit l'amour le plus pénétrant, le plus parfait entre les sexes ? C'est lorsque la femme est le plus femelle, et que l'homme est le plus viril ; c'est quand un mâle brun, velu, sec, chaud et impétueux, trouve l'autre sexe délicat, humide, lisse et blanc, timide et pudique. L'un doit donner, et l'autre est constituée pour recevoir ; le premier, par cette raison, doit avoir un principe de surabondance, de force, de générosité, de libéralité, qui aspire à s'épancher ; la seconde, au contraire, étant constituée *en moins*, doit, par sa timidité tendre à recueillir, à absorber, avec une sorte de besoin et d'économie, le *trop* de l'autre, pour établir l'égalité, le niveau complet. Ainsi le résultat de l'union conjugale, ou le but de la procréation d'un nouvel être, ne peut être rempli que par cette unité physique et morale dont parlent Pythagore et Platon, au moyen de laquelle les deux sexes s'égalent, se saturent pour ainsi dire réciproquement. (*F*, 195 ; souligné dans le texte)

Les hommes sont en quelque sorte représentés par le signe mathématique *plus* ; les femmes, par le signe *moins*. Les différences entre les hommes et les femmes leur permettent dès lors de remplir leurs fonctions reproductives et d'engendrer une progéniture idéalement virile. Ceci implique d'une part de donner naissance majoritairement à des garçons. Le rapport filles/garçons en France est de 96 filles pour 100 garçons selon Virey (*F*, 138). Le surplus de naissances masculines est compensé par un taux de mortalité plus élevé chez les hommes, qui meurent d'exercer leurs activités viriles, telles que la guerre

25 'Un résultat bien important de l'arithmétique politique nous apprend que la plus grande mortalité des femmes est entre 20 et 35 ans ; c'est-à-dire dans la période où l'accouchement et ses suites multiplient davantage pour elles les chances d'une mort accidentelle et prématurée', déclare Moreau de la Sarthe dans *Histoire naturelle de la femme*, II, p. 341.

et des métiers plus dangereux (*F*, 140).[26] D'autre part, il s'agit de donner naissance à des garçons bien virils. Une femme qui ne correspond pas à l'idéal du *moins* et qui domine son mari enfantera ainsi des garçons efféminés. Or, selon Virey, la virilité est le signe d'une nation supérieure tandis que l'efféminement conduit à 'l'abâtardissement de la race' (*F*, 148) tant redouté par les Français du dix-neuvième siècle.[27] Selon ce point de vue, l'Orient est considéré comme étant féminisé et, de là, inférieur à l'Occident.[28] Il ne s'agit donc pas d'y voir un modèle pour les relations de sexe et de genre. Et pourtant, le harem oriental génère à cette époque d'innombrables fantasmes parmi les hommes (et les femmes) de l'Ouest.[29] Virey doit donc combattre les préjugés favorables de ses lecteurs envers le harem et n'a pas de mots assez forts pour dénigrer la polygamie comme modèle de virilité (*F*, 142–48). Pour ce faire, il ne substitue pas un compte-rendu anthropologique exact du harem à ce fantasme, mais crée une nouvelle image de la polygamie, à connotation négative, qui met en évidence ses conséquences dégénératives. La polygamie est en effet jugée peu virile, car l'autorité du mari polygame est divisée entre ses femmes : 'Oui, l'Indien asservi, au milieu de ces êtres fantasques et jaloux de leur empire, qui font payer si cher et leur fraîcheur et leurs charmes, ne vit ni le plus libre ni le plus heureux' (*F*, 144). Pis : sa semence est aussi divisée entre les épouses et va dès lors engendrer une descendance féminisée (*F*, 147–48).

Le modèle des relations entre les sexes chez Virey est nationaliste, puisque qu'il est occidental et plus particulièrement français, mais il est également prescriptif puisqu'il se réfère à un idéal 'naturel' (qui suit l'exemple de la nature ; *F*, 132) qui devrait être atteint par tous les couples. Pourtant, malgré l'imperfection proclamée des cultures polygames (*F*, 142), le texte de Virey révèle l'inquiétude du savant quant à la supériorité de la nation française. Cette dernière pourrait bien être menacée par la dégénérescence due au manque de complémentarité entre les sexes. Toute infraction à la dichotomie sexuelle menace le bon fonctionnement de la reproduction et donc l'intégrité de la 'race' française. Il s'agit non seulement de prescrire le comportement sexuel

---

26 Voir Robert A. Nye, *Masculinity and Male Codes of Honor in Modern France* (Berkeley : University of California Press, 1998), pp. 86–87.

27 Nye, *Masculinity*, pp. 72–95.

28 Sur la représentation de l'Orient dans la culture occidentale, voir Edward W. Said, *Orientalism : Western Conceptions of the Orient* (Londres : Penguin Books, 1995). Sur la féminisation de l'Orient, voir Meyda Yeğenoğlu, *Colonial Fantasies : Towards a Feminist Reading of Orientalism* (Cambridge : Cambridge University Press, 1998), pp. 56, 92.

29 Mary Roberts, *Intimate Outsiders : The Harem in Ottoman and Orientalist Art and Travel Literature* (Durham, NC, et Londres : Duke University Press, 2007), p. 9.

et psychologique approprié, mais aussi de dénoncer les comportements 'déviants' afin de consolider, voire de restaurer, la suprématie nationale.

La masculinisation de la femme

La femme masculine, on s'en doute, ne s'intègre pas dans le schéma de la dichotomie sexuelle. Mais, au fait, d'où vient la femme masculine, ou plutôt : comment une femme devient-elle masculine ? En effet, pour les savants du dix-neuvième siècle, on ne naît pas femme masculine ; on le devient. La réponse se trouve en partie dans le principe de la complémentarité des sexes. Durant l'acte sexuel, ainsi que nous l'avons vu, la femme absorbe le surplus de sperme produit par son partenaire selon Virey (*F*, 195) et acquiert quelques caractéristiques masculines comme l'énergie, la force, la robustesse, l'assurance, voire la hardiesse, qui la différencient de la jeune fille (*F*, 85).[30] La masculinisation est donc le sort de toute femme mariée : '[e]lle est maintenant, par rapport à la jeune vierge, ce que l'homme est à l'égard de la femme'.[31] Néanmoins, ce processus de masculinisation se produit en petite proportion (*F*, 181) et n'a donc pas d'influence profonde sur sa féminité.

Lorsque la quantité de semence masculine est excessive, elle est dangereuse pour la femme, car elle peut conduire à un développement exagéré des caractéristiques masculines. La prostituée, ou du moins la femme aux mœurs légères, est ainsi désignée comme 'hommasse' par Virey (*F*, 86, 104, 181) en raison de ses nombreuses relations avec les hommes et des grandes quantités de sperme qu'elle reçoit. Virey en dresse un portrait peu flatteur :

> Voyez les femmes les plus hommasses, ces *viragines* audacieuses, dont tous les organes sont très développés, tels que les parties sexuelles dilatées, les mamelons du sein ouverts, dont la parole est haute, criarde, arrogante, dont les gestes sont provocants, dont la marche est délibérée, l'air hardi, la trogne masculine, même le ton grenadier. En effet, les courtisanes, les vivandières se présentent avec ce maintien et ces qualités demi-viriles, comme si elles étaient déjà transformées à moitié en l'autre sexe à force de cohabiter avec les hommes, et il en est plusieurs auxquelles pousse un peu de barbe au menton, surtout en avançant en âge. (*F*, 86 ; souligné dans le texte)

30 Voir aussi Menville de Ponsan, *Histoire médicale et philosophique de la femme*, I, p. 242.

31 Menville de Ponsan, *Histoire médicale et philosophique de la femme*, I, p. 242.

L'association entre la courtisane et la vivandière, qui ne va pas de soi *a priori*, s'explique peut-être par le fait que les vivandières et les lavandières officiaient souvent comme prostituées au sein des troupes et devaient donc aussi recevoir une grande quantité de sperme durant leurs rencontres avec les soldats.[32] Le texte de Virey montre paradoxalement que les femmes masculines se caractérisent par des traits physiques incontestablement féminins tels que la poitrine volumineuse, les gros mamelons et la voix criarde, alors que leurs gestes, leur démarche, leur air et leur ton sont résolument masculins. Ceci laisse à penser que la masculinité des femmes hommasses n'est pas seulement due à l'absorption de sperme, comme le soutient Virey (mais aussi Menville de Ponsan), mais également à un principe d'imitation selon lequel les femmes vivant dans la promiscuité avec des hommes en viennent à copier leur attitude. Il y a donc une contradiction au sein du texte de Virey, car il montre — sans toutefois l'affirmer explicitement — que la masculinisation n'est pas uniquement un procédé biologique.

Ailleurs, Virey indique de la même manière que les femmes du peuple sont hommasses. Elles deviennent masculines à force d'exercer des tâches exténuantes, apparemment réservées aux hommes :

> Aguerries par les travaux, habituées aux fortes émotions, les paysannes, par exemple, les femmes laborieuses du peuple, sont peu maladives ; les passions exercent moins de ravages sur elles ; enfin, dans la vieillesse, plusieurs de ces *viragines* deviennent hommasses, acquièrent de la barbe, des traits masculins, une voix rauque, une allure presque martiale. (*F*, 104 ; souligné dans le texte)

Cet extrait révèle le fait que le raisonnement de Virey est basé sur deux présupposés. En premier lieu, la Femme au dix-neuvième siècle, c'est surtout la femme bourgeoise, oisive, confinée dans la sphère domestique. Cette femme fantasmée ne travaille pas, ou très peu, se contentant de quelques travaux d'aiguille et de la supervision des soins du ménage, car c'est son mari qui est le soutien de famille. Les femmes du peuple, elles, doivent travailler pour vivre ; elles sont habituées aux travaux physiques harassants aux champs ou à l'usine. Pour cette raison, elles sont considérées comme étant moins femmes que les femmes des classes supérieures. En second lieu, il semblerait que Virey envisage ici la virilité sous l'angle de l'inné, bien qu'il ait montré ailleurs qu'elle s'acquérait par l'absorption de sperme. Les qualités réputées viriles de force

32 Jean-Paul Bertaud, 'L'armée et le brevet de virilité', dans *Histoire de la virilité, II : le triomphe de la virilité. Le XIXe siècle*, éd. par Alain Corbin (Paris : Seuil, 2011), pp. 63–79 (p. 75).

et robustesse qui caractérisent les femmes du peuple apparaissent 'naturelles' pour le savant et déterminées par leur statut social, plutôt qu'acquises et développées par une existence rude. Le texte de Virey n'assume guère les paradoxes du raisonnement de son auteur, qui oscille entre l'idée d'une virilité inhérente à la condition de l'homme et parcimonieusement transmise à la femme, et celle d'une virilité développée par contact avec ou par imitation de la rigueur du monde masculin.

Masculinité féminine et homosexualité

Dans les deux extraits précédents, les femmes hommasses sont qualifiées de *viragines*. La sixième édition du *Dictionnaire de l'Académie française* (1835) définit une virago comme une 'fille ou femme de grande taille, qui a l'air d'un homme' et ajoute 'ne se dit que par dérision'.[33] La connotation péjorative est évidente. La femme masculine est blâmée pour son allure virile, car elle enfreint les impératifs de faiblesse et de délicatesse imposés à la femme par les hommes et qui, comme on l'a vu chez Cabanis, sont censés constituer l'essence de la condition féminine. Paradoxalement, une femme qui a été virilisée par ses nombreuses interactions avec les hommes devrait être incapable d'attirer les hommes parce qu'elle est jugée 'révolt[ante]' pour les sens (*F*, 176–77) — en dépit du fait que les prostituées, pourtant décrites comme masculines, n'ont aucune difficulté à séduire de nouveaux clients. Virey ajoute plus loin : 'Jamais une femme masculine ne sera bien chérie d'un homme ; il croirait pécher avec elle comme avec son semblable, et il éprouve presque le même genre de répugnance' (*F*, 194).[34] Autrement dit, la femme masculine remet la virilité de son amant en question parce que ce dernier serait attiré par les caractéristiques de son propre sexe et serait donc soupçonné d'homosexualité, un risque qu'aucun homme ne peut se permettre de prendre, comme nous le verrons plus loin.

La femme masculine peut elle-même être perçue comme lesbienne, ou tribade, terme plus courant au début du dix-neuvième siècle, que le *Dictionnaire de l'Académie française* définit pudiquement comme 'femme qui abuse de son sexe avec une autre femme' en précisant 'terme qu'on évite d'employer'.[35] Les références aux tribades sont cependant rares dans les écrits scientifiques du début du dix-neuvième siècle — Éric Bordas parle '[d']invisibilité lesbienne' au

---

33 *Dictionnaire de l'Académie française* (1835), II, p. 940.

34 Voir aussi Menville de Ponsan, *Histoire médicale et philosophique de la femme*, I, p. 39.

35 *Dictionnaire de l'Académie française*, II, p. 882.

dix-neuvième siècle — pour plusieurs raisons.[36] Le saphisme n'est pas perçu comme une relation purement sexuelle, contrairement à l'homosexualité masculine liée à la sodomie. Or, les médecins de cette époque ne s'intéressent encore qu'aux problèmes physiques causés par les relations homosexuelles (contrairement aux Français Jean-Martin Charcot et Valentin Magnan, et surtout à l'Allemand Richard Krafft-Ebing et l'Anglais Havelock Ellis qui auront une approche plus psychologique de l'homosexualité) et examinent les traces physiques causées par les relations homosexuelles sur le corps humain.[37] De plus, les savants ont des préjugés moins prononcés envers le lesbianisme, bien qu'il défie le modèle patriarcal de la société, en raison de l'attrait voyeuriste des relations entre femmes pour les hommes hétérosexuels.[38]

Moreau de la Sarthe mentionne néanmoins cette 'aberration de l'amour' qu'est le saphisme et s'inquiète de ses 'suites funestes', sans pour autant les détailler.[39] Il recommande dès lors aux mères et aux institutrices de surveiller de près les petites filles afin d'éviter de tels écarts de conduite. Les fillettes apparaissent donc dans son texte comme de petits êtres pervers 'naturellement' enclins aux débordements licencieux (homosexuels mais aussi autoérotiques) si on ne les en empêche pas. Il est donc manifeste dans le texte de Moreau de la Sarthe comme chez d'autres auteurs que les observations à propos des lesbiennes sont surtout d'ordre sociologique. Pour Alexandre Parent-Duchâtelet, auteur d'une célèbre enquête sur la prostitution à Paris, le lesbianisme est un phénomène courant parmi les prostituées et les détenues, mais il ne décrit pas leur apparence.[40] Comme les prostituées sont jugées hommasses, on peut en inférer que les lesbiennes le sont tout autant.

Masculinité féminine et lesbianisme sont également associés dans le texte de Virey. Le lesbianisme semble alors être la conséquence de la virilité des

---

36 Éric Bordas, 'Introduction : Comment en parlait-on ?', *Romantisme* 159 (2013), 3–17 (p. 15).

37 Louis Crompton, *Homosexuality and Civilization* (Cambridge, MA : Harvard University Press, 2003), pp. 472–73 ; Alain Corbin, 'La Rencontre des corps', dans *Histoire du corps : de la Révolution à la Grande Guerre*, éd. par Alain Corbin (Paris : Seuil, 'Points', 2005), II, pp. 151–219 (pp. 207–08).

38 Leslie Choquette, 'Homosexuals in the City : Representations of Lesbian and Gay Space in Nineteenth-Century Paris', *Homosexuality in French History and Culture*, éd. par Jeffrey Merrick et Michael Sibalis (New York : Harrington Park Press, 2001), pp. 149–63 (p. 149).

39 Moreau de la Sarthe, *Histoire naturelle de la femme*, II, p. 270.

40 Alexandre Parent-Duchâtelet, *De la prostitution dans la ville de Paris, considérée sous le rapport de l'hygiène publique, de la morale et de l'administration : ouvrage appuyé de documents statistiques puisés dans les archives de la Préfecture de police*, 2 vols (Paris : Baillière, 1836), I, pp. 161–65.

femmes. Virey remarque que 'la femme hommasse, ayant trop de qualités masculines, tend à se rejeter sur son sexe, comme pour s'efféminer, et afin de retrouver ses qualités naturelles' (*F*, 198). Son commentaire soulève plusieurs questions. D'abord, qu'advient-il de la partenaire de la femme hommasse ? Se virilise-t-elle à son tour ? Ensuite, la femme hommasse parvient-elle à éradiquer sa masculinité par le lesbianisme ? Autrement dit, les relations entre femmes sont-elles prescrites pour 'soigner' la masculinité ? On voit ici que le savant n'a pas approfondi sa réflexion sur le saphisme — sans doute parce qu'elle l'entraînerait à défendre des principes en désaccord avec le modèle patriarcal.

Explications psychologiques de la masculinité féminine

Paradoxalement, la femme masculine n'est pas qu'une femme ayant reçu trop de sperme ; elle peut être aussi être une femme qui n'en a jamais reçu, autrement dit une vieille fille, car '[l]a continence [...] est un état contre nature'.[41] Si la femme âgée est condamnée à la virilisation de ses traits — et à devenir barbue, tout comme l'étaient les vivandières et les paysannes — il en va *a fortiori* de même pour la vieille fille.[42] Alors qu'ils recommandent l'abstinence avant le mariage et la modération pendant le mariage, nombreux sont les savants du dix-neuvième siècle, dont Virey fait partie (*F*, 169–70), qui considèrent que, passé un certain âge, la chasteté peut générer des maladies telles que l'anémie, l'absence de règles, l'hystérie et différentes formes de cancers. De telles maladies ne peuvent être guéries que par le mariage. Adoptant une morale résolument laïque, les savants dénoncent les pratiques de l'Église catholique qui impose le célibat aux religieuses.[43]

Ainsi, le principe biologique de masculinisation de la femme en raison de l'absorption d'une quantité excessive de sperme cède la place à des explications psychologiques et comportementales de la masculinité féminine. Est dès lors également rangée dans la catégorie de femme masculine la femme pédante, l'intellectuelle, le *bas-bleu*, voire la femme auteur. Cette dernière enfreint la séparation des sexes en s'appropriant l'activité supposée virile de l'écriture et menace ainsi sa santé.[44] Si une femme peut se faire remarquer par son esprit et

---

41 Menville, *Histoire médicale et philosophique de la femme*, III, p. 165.

42 Moreau de la Sarthe, *Histoire naturelle de la femme*, I, p. 404.

43 Ibid., II, p. 274 ; Virey, *De la Femme*, pp. 82–83.

44 Sandra M. Gilbert et Susan Gubar, *The Madwoman in the Attic : The Woman Writer and the Nineteenth-Century Literary Imagination*, 2e éd. (New Haven : Yale University Press, 2000

par sa capacité d'observation, les activités intellectuelles lui sont en revanche déconseillées parce qu'elles sont jugées peu compatibles avec sa constitution délicate ; elles dégradent sa beauté, entraînent la stérilité et causent des dysfonctionnements de l'utérus. Virey déclare en effet : 'la grande fécondité de l'esprit de la femme produit presque toujours la stérilité corporelle, ou du moins des dérangements vicieux dans les fonctions de l'utérus' (*F*, 171), tandis que Moreau de la Sarthe affirme :

> Le développement immodéré des facultés intellectuelles, les études abstraites, la contention d'esprit, et des méditations qui semblent concentrer toutes les puissances de la vie dans l'organe de la pensée, ne seraient pas moins préjudiciables [que les excès de passion], surtout dans l'âge que la nature consacre à d'autres fonctions, et pendant lequel un semblable travail ne pourrait perfectionner l'esprit sans porter atteintes aux grâces et à la beauté.[45]

Cependant, insiste Cabanis, peu de femmes sont de véritables intellectuelles ; leur concentration est limitée, leurs connaissances sont superficielles et leurs raisonnements sont peu convaincants.[46]

En revanche, les femmes avec de réelles dispositions intellectuelles voient leur existence certes reconnue, mais leur situation est reléguée par Moreau de la Sarthe au rang des 'cas extraordinaires' et des 'phénomènes, desquels on ne peut rien conclure, sinon que la nature réalise tous les possibles'.[47] Bref, la femme intellectuelle ne peut être tolérée qu'à condition de représenter l'exception qui confirme la règle de la médiocrité de l'esprit féminin. En raison de son statut d'*accident* de la nature[48] — nous ne sommes pas loin du concept aristotélicien du monstre comme erreur de la nature[49] — cette femme n'est pas critiquée mais prise en pitié, car elle n'appartient à aucune catégorie : 'Dans la jeunesse, dans l'âge mûr, dans la vieillesse, quelle sera la place de ces êtres incertains, qui ne sont, à proprement parler, d'aucun sexe ?', s'inquiète Cabanis.[50] La

[1979]), pp. 3–11 ; Diana Holmes, *French Women's Writing : 1848–1994* (Londres : Athlone, 1996), p. 30.

45 Moreau de la Sarthe, *Histoire naturelle de la femme*, II, p. 403.

46 Cabanis, *Rapports du physique et du moral de l'homme*, I, pp. 362–63.

47 Moreau de la Sarthe, *Histoire naturelle de la femme*, I, p. 119.

48 Ibid.

49 Jean Céard, 'Monstres et monstruosités à la Renaissance', dans *Monstre et imaginaire social*, éd. par Anna Caiozzo et Anne-Emmanuelle Demartini (Paris : Creaphis, 2008), pp. 203–19 (p. 204).

50 Cabanis, *Rapports du physique et du moral de l'homme*, I, p. 363.

question rhétorique est un procédé discursif qui permet aux savants d'affirmer des vérités réputées générales (ici, que les êtres au genre incertain n'ont pas leur place dans la société) tout en laissant affleurer les doutes des auteurs et leur inquiétude quant à leur incapacité à contrôler certains facteurs sociaux (ici, que les êtres incertains bouleversent les catégories socio-sexuelles qu'ils ont établies).[51] La question oratoire de Cabanis souligne donc l'ancrage sociologique et plus seulement biologique ou médical de la réflexion des savants, en laissant entendre que les femmes masculines n'ont pas leur place dans la société française. Leur masculinité, qu'elle soit physique ou intellectuelle, les empêche d'exercer leurs fonctions sociales. Comme elles manquent de délicatesse féminine, elles sont incapables de remplir leurs devoirs domestiques :

> Par quel attrait peuvent-elles fixer le jeune homme qui cherche une compagne ? Quels secours peuvent en attendre des parents infirmes ou vieux ? Quelles douceurs répandront-elles sur la vie d'un mari ? Les verra-t-on descendre du haut de leur génie, pour veiller à leurs enfants, à leur ménage ? Tous ces rapports si délicats qui font le charme et qui assurent le bonheur de la femme, n'existent plus alors : en voulant étendre son empire, elle le détruit.[52]

Ici, les fonctions d'une femme se limitent à la sphère domestique et aux interactions avec d'autres membres de la famille. À l'opposé, la femme intellectuelle fuit ses devoirs conjugaux et maternels et est donc considérée comme une aberration. Il en va de même pour la vieille fille. Cette dernière échappe au système social esquissé par le Code civil instauré en 1804 selon lequel les femmes sont légalement reléguées au rang de mineures et soumises à l'autorité d'un mari ou à celle d'un père.[53] En effet, la femme célibataire ne dépend ni de l'un ni de l'autre ; elle peut jouir d'une certaine autonomie financière et son statut est pour le moins ambigu.[54] De manière presque revancharde, et comme

---

51 Dans *De la Femme*, après avoir décrit le cas des courtisanes et vivandières hommasses, Virey s'interroge de la même manière : 'Après avoir outrepassé les bornes de l'honneur, quelles seront les limites du vice chez elle [la fille qui a perdu la pudicité] ? Avec son caractère extrême en tout, impétueux dans ses amours comme dans ses haines, où s'arrêtera-t-elle ?' (*F*, 86–87).

52 Cabanis, *Rapports du physique et du moral de l'homme*, I, p. 363.

53 *Code civil*, art. 212–26.

54 Voir Claudia Moscovici, Claudia, 'Gendered Spheres in Balzac's *La Cousine Bette*', *International Journal of Politics, Culture and Society*, 10, 3 (1997), 469–96 (pp. 469–70, 478–79).

pour renforcer l'autorité du cadre légal, les savants la condamnent au vieillissement prématuré, au cancer et à la stérilité.[55]

La domestication de la femme masculine

Le malaise des savants face aux femmes masculines est ici perceptible. Il ne fait aucun doute pour eux que la femme est par principe un être mystérieux pour l'homme, à la fois 'abîmes impénétrables' et 'inextricable labyrinthe' (*F*, 213). La femme masculine l'est encore plus, car elle échappe à toutes les catégories méticuleusement définies par la science. Menville de Ponsan refuse à la femme 'cette hardiesse, cette fermeté de caractère qui doit être l'attribut de notre sexe' ; alors qu'il affirme vouloir écrire également pour les femmes, c'est l'entre-soi masculin qui l'emporte.[56] De plus, il ne met en évidence comme qualités féminines que les lieux communs d'intuition, de générosité, de sensibilité et d'ardeur affective, tous ces traits étant rehaussés par le charme féminin.[57] Il affirme ainsi avec véhémence : 'tout doit être féminin dans la femme'.[58] En refusant de se marier, en ayant des relations saphiques, en exerçant des activités physiques ou intellectuelles réservées aux hommes ou en recevant un excès de semence masculine, ces femmes masculines défient l'organisation patriarcale de la société et remettent en question la sacro-sainte séparation des sexes. Avec les femmes auteurs, ces femmes qui osent prendre la plume comme des hommes, c'est tout l'ordre social qui s'effondre, car, comme le remarque Christine Planté : 'elles font usage de capacités intellectuelles et humaines qui prouvent qu'elles ne sont pas par nature inférieures aux hommes, et posent donc de ce fait la question de l'égalité et celle du rapport entre ordre de la nature et lois humaines'.[59]

Ce qui est en jeu ici, finalement, c'est le pouvoir. La masculinité de ces femmes choque moins que leur prétention au pouvoir, c'est-à-dire leur

---

55 Virey, par exemple, affirme : 'Lorsqu'elles arrivent à l'âge critique où le flux menstruel cesse, l'utérus et les mamelles n'ayant pas rempli les fonctions auxquelles la nature a destiné ces organes, ils peuvent conserver soit une sensibilité surabondante, soit des restes de l'humeur non évacuée, et qui deviennent les causes fréquentes de squirrhes, d'indurations, de cancers, de polypes, etc.' (*F*, 83).

56 Menville, *Histoire médicale et philosophique de la femme*, I, xiv-xv, xxxii.

57 Ibid., I, xv.

58 Ibid., I, xiv.

59 Christine Planté, *La Petite Sœur de Balzac : essai sur la femme auteur* (Paris : Seuil, 1989), p. 57.

usurpation potentielle de prérogatives réputées masculines.[60] Comme l'indique Halberstam : '[m]asculinity in this society inevitably conjures up notions of power and legitimacy and privilege'.[61] Reconnaître les capacités physiques et intellectuelles des femmes masculines revient implicitement à admettre l'infériorité des hommes ou, du moins, la possibilité qu'ils ne constituent pas l'unique pôle du pouvoir. La femme masculine qui fait son apparition dans les traités scientifiques représente en quelque sorte les signes avant-coureurs de changements sociaux majeurs. Non seulement elle s'inscrit dans la droite ligne des femmes auteurs, pour lesquelles la monarchie de Juillet constitue un 'véritable âge d'or', nous rappelle Planté,[62] mais elle préfigure également certains mouvements féministes tels que le saint-simonisme et le fouriérisme, qui revendiquent l'émancipation de la femme.[63] Elle évoque encore les intervenantes du journal féministe *La Tribune des femmes* sous la monarchie de Juillet, qui prennent la plume sous leur prénom plutôt que leur nom de famille pour effacer toute trace patriarcale, revendiquent leurs droits et pratiquent même l'union libre.[64] En d'autres termes, la femme masculine des traités scientifiques fait écho à une prise de conscience, certes limitée, mais réelle, d'une possible autonomisation de la femme.

---

60 Lillian Faderman, *Surpassing the Love of Men : Romantic Friendship and Love between Women from the Renaissance to the Present* (Londres : The Women's Press, 1985), p. 17.

61 Halberstam, *Female Masculinity*, p. 2.

62 Planté, *La Petite Sœur de Balzac*, p. 43.

63 Claire Goldberg Moses, *French Feminism in the Nineteenth Century* (Albany : State University of New York Press, 1984), pp. 41–59, 90–98.

64 Ibid., pp. 61–87. Nombreux également sont les personnages de femmes masculines qui apparaissent dans les romans français des années 1830 et 1840. La Lélia du roman éponyme de George Sand (Paris : Gallimard, 'Folio Classique', 2003 [1833]) fait figure d'intellectuelle, voire de philosophe, tandis que sa sœur, la courtisane Pulchérie, compare le mariage à la prostitution : 'être amante, courtisane et mère, trois conditions de la destinée de la femme auxquelles nulle femme n'échappe, soit qu'elle se vende par un marché de prostitution ou par un contrat de mariage' (p. 153). Mademoiselle de Maupin, l'héroïne du roman éponyme de Gautier (Paris : Gallimard, 'Folio Classique', 1973 [1835]), est un véritable garçon manqué qui se revendique d'un troisième sexe (pp. 393–94). Lisbeth Fischer incarne dans *La Cousine Bette* de Balzac (Paris : Librairie Générale Française, 'Le Livre de Poche Classiques', 2000 [1846]) la vieille fille par excellence, qui associe à des anomalies physiques, telles que le teint basané, la maigreur et la sécheresse, des 'qualités d'homme' (p. 59). Félicité des Touches, autre héroïne de Balzac, est une écrivaine et une compositrice qui a reçu dans *Béatrix* (Paris : Librairie Générale Française, 'Le Livre de Poche Classiques', 2012 [1839–1845]) une éducation masculine, conjuguant lecture intensive et activités de plein air, et qui rejette 'les premières malices du mariage', c'est-à-dire 'l'enfant, les couches, et ce trafic de maternité qu['elle] n'aime point' (p. 178).

Ainsi, aussi peu nombreuses soient-elles, les femmes masculines menacent le système patriarcal. Elles ne sont d'ailleurs pas les seules. Les traités scientifiques de la première moitié du dix-neuvième siècle sont hantés par d'autres figures qui, par leur simple existence, défient la dichotomie sexuelle. Ce sont les eunuques, les homosexuels et les hermaphrodites. Tout comme les femmes masculines, ces individus semblent appartenir aux deux sexes en raison de leurs caractéristiques physiques et/ou comportementales ambiguës. Virey assimile les eunuques aux femmes, car ils ne semblent pas jouir des bienfaits du sperme (*F*, 180). Le médecin du bagne de Toulon Hubert Lauvergne voit en un forçat homosexuel 'un homme douteux' et 'une erreur de la nature'.[65] Plus encore que les femmes masculines, les hermaphrodites, les homosexuels ou les eunuques sont perçus comme bisexués. Les savants tentent dès lors de déterminer un sexe prédominant afin de les associer à une catégorie sexuelle définie.[66]

Dans tous les cas, il faut faire rentrer ces individus qui contestent la séparation des sexes dans les rangs du pouvoir masculin. En un mot, il faut domestiquer ces êtres par essence rebelles. Pour ce faire, les savants leur dénigrent le statut d'êtres humains. Les hermaphrodites sont assimilés à des monstres étant donné qu'ils sont confinés aux traités de tératologie comme celui d'Isidore Geoffroy Saint-Hilaire (1832–1837), pourtant novateur dans sa volonté d'expliquer les monstruosités par les lois de la nature qui gouvernent également l'organisation des êtres 'normaux'. Les organes génitaux des homosexuels sont assimilés à ceux des animaux ou à des objets (pénis en forme de tire-bouchon et anus en forme d'entonnoir).[67] Quant aux femmes masculines, même si elles ne subissent pas de traitements aussi radicaux que ceux-là,

---

65 Hubert Lauvergne, *Les Forçats considérés sous le rapport physiologique, moral et intellectuel, observés au bagne de Toulon* (Paris : Baillière, 1841), p. 293.

66 Marc, 'Hermaphrodite,' *Dictionnaire des sciences médicales par une société de médecins et de chirurgiens*, éd. par Nicolas-Philibert Adelon et al., 60 vols (Paris : Panckoucke, 1812–1822), XXI (1817), pp. 86–121 (p. 115) ; Isidore Geoffroy Saint-Hilaire, *Histoire générale et particulière des anomalies de l'organisation chez l'homme et les animaux* [...], *ou Traité de tératologie*, 4 vols (Paris : Baillière, 1832–1837), III, p. 577. Sur le corps des homosexuels et des hermaphrodites dans les traités savants de la première moitié du dix-neuvième siècle, voir notre article : 'Valorising Genitalia : Homosexuality and Hermaphroditism in French Scientific Writings in the Nineteenth Century', *Harts & Minds*, 1, 2 (automne 2013) <http ://www.harts-minds.co.uk/#!space-place/c1zt6>.

67 C'est particulièrement frappant dans l'*Étude médico-légale sur les attentats aux mœurs*, 2e éd. (Paris : Baillière, 1858 [1857]) du médecin légiste Ambroise Tardieu (voir pp. 135–37, 145–47), véritable *best-seller* de la médecine légale du Second Empire, mais ce type de propos se retrouve chez ses prédécesseurs.

elles voient leurs qualités intrinsèques niées par l'usage de termes injurieux, tels que *virago* et *hommasse*. De plus, leurs aptitudes intellectuelles et sociales ainsi que leur séduction sont dénigrées par les savants, qui les jugent laides, incapables de soutenir un raisonnement complexe ni d'assurer leurs fonctions domestiques. Elles sont en outre assimilées, sinon à des monstres, du moins à des accidents de la nature et à des êtres surnaturels, ou plutôt extra-naturels, puisque, comme l'affirme Virey, '[l]a femme qui se fait homme [est] hors de la nature' (*F*, 214). Enfin, tout comme les homosexuels, elles apparaissent comme des corps anormaux et sont inexorablement condamnées par les médecins, avec une pointe de satisfaction, au cancer et à la stérilité. Ces derniers ne reculent d'ailleurs jamais devant les raisonnements les plus confus — ceux-là même qui semblaient être le propre des pseudo-intellectuelles masculines — pour étayer leurs propos. Ainsi, ils n'hésitent pas à soutenir que la masculinisation d'une femme est à la fois due à l'excès de sperme et à l'absence de sperme.

Les multiples contradictions dans le discours des savants cherchent en quelque sorte à calfeutrer les fissures dans la dichotomie sexuelle. C'est au prix de ces ajustements discursifs que le modèle de la différence des sexes peut et doit continuer à exister. Si le corps humain ne détermine plus la différence entre masculinité et féminité, si ces caractéristiques ne sont plus biologiques, cela signifie que la féminité d'une femme et la masculinité d'un homme dépendent d'autres facteurs tels que l'éducation et l'environnement. En un mot, elles ne sont pas 'naturelles'. Rien, dès lors, ne s'oppose à l'épanouissement intellectuel d'une femme ni à la sollicitude parentale d'un homme. Alors que la science refuse d'entrevoir les possibilités d'une remise en question de la dichotomie sexuelle en d'autres termes que ceux de la 'déviance' ou de l'anecdote, la littérature du début des années 1830, avec des œuvres telles que *Fragoletta* de Latouche (1829), *Sarrasine* de Balzac (1831) ou *Mademoiselle de Maupin* de Gautier (1835), explore les ambiguïtés sexuelles et de genre en critiquant parfois les fondements de la dichotomie sexuelle. Pour les savants du dix-neuvième siècle, il demeure impossible de considérer la femme masculine autrement que comme un paradoxe inexplicable, et par là effrayant.

Conclusion

Référons-nous pour conclure à Virey qui, comme Cabanis, considère que les femmes ne sont pas censées exercer une activité intellectuelle approfondie. Si elles en sont capables, c'est que ce sont des femmes masculines et qu'elles représentent des exceptions à la norme ; en un mot, c'est qu'elles ne sont pas entièrement des femmes :

> Jamais femme ne s'est élevée, par la culture de son intelligence, à ces hautes conceptions du génie dans les sciences et la littérature, qui semblent être la plus sublime conquête de l'esprit humain. Celles qui se sont le plus distinguées dans cette carrière ont souvent mérité l'épithète *mascula* qu'Horace donnait à Sapho [...]. (*F*, 5–6)

Virey affirme qu'il y a un ordre naturel, que les distinctions sociales entre hommes et femmes sont dues à des différences physiologiques. Lutter contre la nature est vain et nuit même à la santé. Au contraire, les femmes qui se soumettent à 'une douce sujétion' (*F*, 88) ou à 'un doux esclavage' (*F*, 254) (c'est-à-dire celles qui se soumettent aux hommes, qui prennent soin de leurs enfants, qui ne quittent pas la sphère privée et qui évitent les activités physiques et intellectuelles peu compatibles avec leur constitution délicate) ont plus de chance de vivre heureuses que celles qui recherchent 'une domination pour laquelle elles ne sont pas nées' (*F*, 88). L'argument consiste à invoquer une domestication de la femme pour son propre bien. Cependant, on peut entrevoir derrière cette volonté prétendument altruiste non seulement la figure du médecin paternaliste qui sait mieux que quiconque — et en particulier mieux que sa patiente — ce qui convient à sa patiente, mais surtout celle de l'homme angoissé à l'idée que la femme soit effectivement capable, physiquement, psychologiquement et intellectuellement, d'exercer des activités viriles. Car, si tel est le cas, *quid* de la supériorité masculine ? La femme masculine n'est donc pas qu'une simple anecdote dans les ouvrages savants du début du dix-neuvième siècle, malgré son manque de visibilité, car elle symbolise une idée effrayante pour la gent masculine : celle du remplacement de la relation de complémentarité entre l'homme et la femme par celle d'égalité pure et simple.

Bibliographie

Balzac, Honoré de, *Béatrix*, éd. par Michel Lichtlé (Paris : Librairie Générale Française, 'Le Livre de Poche Classiques', 2012)

——, *La Cousine Bette*, éd. par Roger Pierrot (Paris : Librairie Générale Française, 'Le Livre de Poche Classiques', 2000)

Bertaud, Jean-Paul, 'L'Armée et le brevet de virilité', dans *Histoire de la virilité : le triomphe de la virilité. Le XIXe siècle*, éd. par Alain Corbin (Paris : Seuil, 2011), II, pp. 63–79

Bordas, Éric, 'Introduction : Comment en parlait-on ?', *Romantisme* 159 (2013), 3–17

Bourdieu, Pierre, *La Domination masculine* (Paris : Seuil, 'Points/Essais', 2002 [1998])

Butler, Judith, *Gender Trouble : Feminism and the Subversion of Identity* (New York : Routledge, 1990)

Cabanis, Pierre-Jean-Georges, *Rapports du physique et du moral de l'homme*, 2 vols (Paris : Crapart, Caille et Ravier, 1802)

Céard, Jean, 'Monstres et monstruosités à la Renaissance', dans *Monstre et imaginaire social : approches historiques*, éd. par Anna Caiozzo et Anne-Emmanuelle Demartini (Paris : Creaphis, 2008), pp. 203–19

Choquette, Leslie, 'Homosexuals in the City : Representations of Lesbian and Gay Space in Nineteenth-Century Paris', *Homosexuality in French History and Culture*, éd. par Jeffrey Merrick et Michael Sibalis (New York : Harrington Park Press, 2001), pp. 149–63

Code civil des Français, édition originale et seule officielle (Paris : Imprimerie de la République, 1804)

Corbin, Alain, 'La Rencontre des corps', dans *Histoire du corps, II : de la Révolution à la Grande Guerre*, éd. par Alain Corbin (Paris : Seuil, 'Points', 2005), pp. 151–219

Crahay, Géraldine, 'Valorising Genitalia : Homosexuality and Hermaphroditism in French Scientific Writings in the Nineteenth Century', *Harts & Minds*, 1, 2 (automne 2013) < http ://www.harts-minds.co.uk/#!space-place/c1zt6 >

Crompton, Louis, *Dictionnaire de l'Académie française*, 6e éd., 2 vols (Paris : Firmin-Didot, 1835)

——, *Homosexuality and Civilization* (Cambridge, MA : Harvard University Press, 2003)

Faderman, Lillian, *Surpassing the Love of Men : Romantic Friendship and Love between Women from the Renaissance to the Present* (Londres : The Women's Press, 1985)

Foucault, Michel, *Histoire de la sexualité, I : la volonté de savoir* (Paris : Gallimard, 1976)

Gautier, Théophile, *Mademoiselle de Maupin*, éd. par Michel Crouzet (Paris : Gallimard, 'Folio Classique', 1973)

Geoffroy Saint-Hilaire, Isidore, *Histoire générale et particulière des anomalies de l'organisation chez l'homme et les animaux, ouvrage comprenant des recherches sur les caractères, la classification, l'influence physiologique et pathologique, les rapports généraux, les lois et les causes des monstruosités, variétés et vices de conformation, ou Traité de tératologie*, 4 vols (Paris : Baillière, 1832–1837)

Gilbert, Sandra M. et Susan Gubar, *The Madwoman in the Attic : The Woman Writer and the Nineteenth-Century Literary Imagination*, 2e éd. (New Haven : Yale University Press, 2000 [1979])

Halberstam, Judith, *Female Masculinity* (Durham, NC : Duke University Press, 1998)

Holmes, Diana, *French Women's Writing : 1848–1994* (Londres : Athlone, 1996)

Laqueur, Thomas, *Making Sex : Body and Gender from the Greeks to Freud* (Cambridge, MA : Harvard University Press, 1990)

——, 'Orgasm, Generation, and the Politics of Reproductive Biology', dans *The Making of the Modern Body : Sexuality and Society in the Nineteenth Century*, éd. par Catherine Gallagher et Thomas Laqueur (Berkeley : University of California Press, 1987), pp. 1–41

Lauvergne, Hubert, *Les Forçats considérés sous le rapport physiologique, moral et intellectuel, observés au bagne de Toulon* (Paris : Baillière, 1841)

Marc, 'Hermaphrodite', dans *Dictionnaire des sciences médicales par une société de médecins et de chirurgiens*, éd. par Nicolas-Philibert Adelon et al., 60 vols (Paris : Panckoucke, 1812–1822), vol. XXI (1817), pp. 86–121

Menville de Ponsan, Charles François, *Histoire médicale et philosophique de la femme considérée dans toutes les époques principales de sa vie avec tous les changements qui surviennent dans son physique et son moral avec l'hygiène applicable à son sexe et toutes les maladies qui peuvent l'atteindre aux différents âges*, 3 vols (Paris : Amyot-Labé, 1845)

Moreau de la Sarthe, Jacques Louis, *Histoire naturelle de la femme suivie d'un traité d'hygiène appliquée à son régime physique et moral aux différentes époques de la vie*, 2 vols (Paris : Duprat, 1803)

Moscovici, Claudia, 'Gendered Spheres in Balzac's *La Cousine Bette*', *International Journal of Politics, Culture and Society*, 10, 3 (1997), 469–96

Moses, Claire Goldberg, *French Feminism in the Nineteenth Century* (Albany : State University of New York Press, 1984)

Nye, Robert A., *Masculinity and Male Codes of Honor in Modern France* (Berkeley : University of California Press, 1998)

Parent-Duchâtelet, Alexandre-Jean-Baptiste, *De la prostitution dans la ville de Paris, considérée sous le rapport de l'hygiène publique, de la morale et de l'administration : ouvrage appuyé de documents statistiques puisés dans les archives de la Préfecture de police*, 2 vols (Paris : Baillière, 1836)

Planté, Christine, *La Petite Sœur de Balzac : essai sur la femme auteur* (Paris : Seuil, 1989)

Roberts, Mary, *Intimate Outsiders : The Harem in Ottoman and Orientalist Art and Travel Literature* (Durham, NC, et Londres : Duke University Press, 2007)

Rousseau, Jean-Jacques, *Émile ou de l'éducation*, éd. par André Charrak (Paris : Garnier-Flammarion, 2009)

Sand, George, *Lélia*, éd. par Pierre Reboul (Paris : Gallimard, 'Folio Classique', 2003 [Garnier, 1960])

Said, Edward W., *Orientalism* : *Western Conceptions of the Orient* (Londres : Penguin Books, 1995)

Tardieu, Ambroise, *Étude médico-légale sur les attentats aux mœurs*, 2e éd. (Paris : Baillière, 1858 [1857])

Virey, Julien-Joseph, *De la Femme, sous ses rapports physiologique, moral et littéraire*, 2e éd. (Paris : Crochard Libraire, 1825 [1823])

Yeğenoğlu, Meyda, *Colonial Fantasies : Towards a Feminist Reading of Orientalism* (Cambridge : Cambridge University Press, 1998)

CHAPTER 2

Genre Trouble on the Battlefield: Pharmaceutical, Medical, and Literary Accounts of Napoleonic Campaigns

Larry Duffy

The nineteenth century sees a proliferation of medical narratives, made possible at least in part by the same technological developments that enable the wide dissemination of literary narratives. These medical and literary narratives in fact share many stylistic features, in particular their privileging of dispassionate observation. In this sense, the realist novel — the 'clinical' aspects of which are frequently highlighted by critics — is, along with the medical treatise containing case studies, the archetype of objective, detached narrative.[1] It is thus unsurprising, for example, that an archetype of realist literary discourse such as *Madame Bovary* should have strongly medical themes, or rather, engage with medical discourse, borrowing from contemporary medical treatises and more generally articulating the discursive development of health professions in the nineteenth century. Flaubert's novel — this chapter's key point of canonical literary reference — collapses distinctions between literary and other discourses, including medicine and, notably, pharmacy. At the same time, *Madame Bovary* practises what might be termed a 'pharmaceutical' operation in orchestrating this collapse. While medicine and pharmacy become professionally aligned in the early nineteenth century, pharmacy is distinctive in its representativity of expanding disciplines precisely because of its disciplinarily hybrid nature. Moreover, whereas medical narratives might well be objective, clinical, and dispassionate, pharmaceutical narratives are in many ways reflective of the polyvalency of pharmacy. One of pharmacy's key professional and discursive concerns is to express that polyvalency.[2] A significant context for its expression is an area of nineteenth-century life represented

1 See, for example, Mary Donaldson-Evans, *Medical Examinations: Dissecting the Doctor in French Narrative Prose, 1857–1894* (Lincoln: University of Nebraska Press, 2000); Lilian R. Furst, 'Realism and Hypertrophy: A Study of Three Medico-Historical "Cases"', *Nineteenth-Century French Studies*, 22. 1–2 (1993), 29–47.

2 See Larry Duffy, '*Madame Bovary* and the Institutional Transformation of Pharmacy', *Dix-neuf*, 15, 1 (2011), 70–82 (p. 71, pp. 74–75).

 | DOI:10.1163/9789004368019_004

variously in literary, medical, and pharmaceutical narratives: the military campaign.

This chapter argues that there is a clear distinction between pharmaceutical and medical narratives of war, and that the former participate wholeheartedly in pharmacy's wider assertion of its discursive polyvalency. While medical memoirs contain gruesome details of battlefield injuries and treatments, their pharmaceutical counterparts do not dwell excessively on horror and suffering, instead taking the form of eclectic *récits de voyage* by learned men of leisure, rather than purely of *récits de guerre* by the high-ranking soldiers that the *pharmaciens de l'Empereur* effectively were.[3] The distinction between what are effectively two genres may be seen in accounts of the Napoleonic campaigns by a senior military surgeon, Dominique de Larrey, and two senior military pharmacists: Charles-Louis Cadet de Gassicourt and Pierre-Irénée Jacob. The medical, or rather more specifically surgical, accounts are *mémoires* in a double sense. They contain some, albeit minimal, elements of the travel diary and provide a record of major events in Napoleon's campaigns. These, however, are mere intercalations in what consist largely of documentary and didactic *mémoires chirurgicales*: Dominique de Larrey's account of his campaign is to all intents and purposes a compendium of medical case histories and recommended treatments — usually amputation — derived from the theatre of war as an ideal ground for experimentation. Larrey's intended audience consists of medical students and practitioners, specialist rather than general readers: as he states in a preface, he has been 'sollicité par des chirurgiens militaires' to provide accounts of the campaigns, and has set himself a 'but', 'celui de contribuer à l'instruction de jeunes chirurgiens'.[4] The *mémoires* of the pharmacists, on the other hand, rather than simply being the jottings of detached, or at least semi-detached, *dilettantes*, while on the surface resembling contemporary travel narratives, are at the same time very much in keeping with what might be termed a contemporary ideology of pharmacy.

L'idéologie pharmaceutique française

This ideology is shaped by institutional changes early in the Empire (including an alignment of pharmaceutical and medical training), and by pharmacy's

3 Larry Duffy, *Flaubert, Zola and the Incorporation of Disciplinary Knowledge* (Basingstoke: Palgrave, 2015), pp. 39–40; 47–48.

4 Dominique Jean Larrey, *Mémoires de chirurgie militaire, et campagnes*, 4 vols (Paris: Smith, 1812–17), I (1812), v–vi.

professional reassertion of itself after having been relegated to a position of artisanal subordination to chemistry. It affirms the properly scientific status of pharmacy (presented as being synonymous with chemistry), the equivalence of its professional status to that of medicine, and, on account of that, the self-evident right of pharmacy to involve itself in multiple fields.[5] Pharmacy thus asserts a polyvalency that finds — along with other elements of contemporary pharmaceutical propaganda — its most effective literary expression in *Madame Bovary*, through the pronouncements of the *apothicaire*, Homais, such as that uttered to Mme Lefrançois the innkeeper on the occasion of the Comices Agricoles:

> [J]e suis pharmacien, c'est-à-dire chimiste! Et la chimie, ayant pour objet la connaissance de l'action réciproque et moléculaire de tous les corps de la nature, il s'ensuit que l'agriculture se trouve comprise dans son domaine. Et, en effet, composition des engrais, fermentation des liquides, analyse des gaz et influence des miasmes, qu'est-ce que tout cela, je vous le demande, si ce n'est de la chimie pure et simple?[6]

The definition of chemistry from which Homais makes his agricultural extrapolation is strikingly similar to that presented in an 1813 article on 'Chimie' in the *Dictionnaire des sciences médicales*, by Charles-Louis Cadet de Gassicourt, namechecked by Homais while Emma lies dying as 'une de nos sommités pharmaceutiques, un de nos maîtres' (*OC*, I, 683). Cadet was indeed 'une sommité pharmaceutique', not only because he was *pharmacien de l'Empereur*, but also on account of the key role he played in the professional reorientation of pharmacy in the early nineteenth century, a reorientation subtly articulated in *Madame Bovary* as part of a more generalized destabilization of disciplinary boundaries and discursive categories, including that of the boundary between the literary and the 'non-literary'. Cadet de Gassicourt, founding editor in 1809 of the *Bulletin de Pharmacie*, was the greatest propagandist of pharmacy's properly scientific status as chemistry, and thereby of the expansion of its disciplinary remit to various fields. If Homais — 'à qui les titres ne manquaient point' — relentlessly exploits his discipline's connections with chemistry and medicine to enhance his stranglehold over 'cidre', 'le puceron laniger', 'statistique', 'moralisation des classes pauvres' (*OC*, I, 691), his practice reflects what

---

5 Duffy, '*Madame Bovary* and the Institutional Transformation of Pharmacy', p. 72.

6 Gustave Flaubert, *Œuvres complètes*, ed. by Bernard Masson, 2 vols (Paris: Seuil, 1964), I, 619. Subsequent references to *Madame Bovary* are to this edition, which is abbreviated as *OC*, I, followed by the page number.

was happening at provincial and national levels. Indeed, the polyvalency of pharmacy had been evident since the early Empire in the highest echelons of the state, and notably, the army. Like Homais, and real-life pharmacists, the great pharmacists were also agriculturalists, and, significantly, many of them were military men. Cadet and Parmentier — both distinguished in agriculture as well as pharmacy — are buried alongside one another in Père-Lachaise, among the tombs of the heroes of Napoleon's armies, including the surgeon Dominique de Larrey. On Parmentier's tombstone is an illustration of the fruitful combination of chemistry and agriculture — the chemist's *alambic*, and a basket of the potatoes of which he is the celebrated importer — and on the other side, the cannon symbolizing his military career.

Madame Bovary, as well as articulating the hybridity of pharmacy and its corresponding applicability to other fields, links this hybridity to the Napoleonic era and its military adventures through traces of, and allusions to, pharmacists and other health professionals working in specifically military contexts.[7] Charles Bovary's father, for example, an 'ancien aide-chirurgien-major' (*OC*, I, 576), would doubtless have been present at numerous amputations, given that amputation was a key activity of *chirurgiens-major* in Napoleon's armies. Similarly, the potato-growing gravedigger Lestiboudois (*OC*, I, 599) — the namesake of another great military pharmacist and agriculturalist — holds Hippolyte's leg as Dr Canivet ampututates it 'en philosophe', having heard Homais compare 'le sang-froid d'un chirurgien à celui d'un général' (*OC*, I, 636).

A generalized allusion in such traces to the persistence of the repercussions of the Napoleonic campaigns in the social reality of the July Monarchy is thus combined with expression of the professional and discursive polyvalency of pharmacy. Pharmacy might in fact itself be seen as emblematic of a recalibration of disciplinary limits pursued by professions in the nineteenth century, and of a destabilization of the limits whereby fields of discourse — scientific, medical, pharmaceutical, literary — are circumscribed. Pharmacy may well be the ideal vehicle allowing an author such as Flaubert to challenge the notion of a pure scientific or professional discourse, and thus implicitly of a pure literary, mimetic, realist discourse uncontaminated by others. However, a challenge — albeit a possibly unwitting one — to discursive purity arguably exists already in the work of author-pharmacists, of whom the signal example is Cadet de Gassicourt.

It is important to consider this *sommité pharmaceutique et militaire* as a writer when examining his *écrits de guerre*. He was an individual of extreme

7 Duffy, '*Madame Bovary* and the Institutional Transformation of Pharmacy', p. 75.

versatility: pharmacist, chemist, soldier, quasi-diplomat, socialite, agriculturalist, but above all a writer, an author of works on numerous subjects in various fields and across diverse genres. Cadet authored biographies both historical and professional (the Comte de Mirabeau, Parmentier), scathing parodies of Chateaubriand, texts on freemasonry and electoral statistics, political pamphlets, and a proposition for an 'Institut nomade' consisting of experts who would travel around the national territory educating the public in fields of knowledge and practice usually only accessible to inhabitants of major urban centres.[8] In Cadet's more properly pharmaceutical writings, he produced *mémoires* on tea and coffee, denunciations of charlatanism and of the 'inconcevable' menace presented by the availability of 'Spencer's preservatives' or 'capotes de santé', which risked giving the impression that 'officines' were in fact 'archives de prostitution'.[9] In the latter text Cadet retains a droll style and sensibility while at the same time presenting an earnest defence of what he sees as the integrity of his profession. This again is testimony to the essential hybridity of his writings: there is no purely pharmaceutical discourse. In the most esoterically literary area of his activity as a writer, Cadet was author of a *Traité sur l'élognostie ou l'esprit des sots* (1813), containing an 'Éloge de la bêtise', and a compendium of lipogrammatic texts.[10] Cadet dabbled in travel writing, authoring a quasi-philosophical epistolary travelogue explicitly emulating works by Sterne and other travel writers and recounting — in the person of Charles writing to his mistress Eugénie — a journey through Normandy, featuring a visit to Rouen cathedral, where the narrator is accosted by a

8 C. L. F. Cadet de Gassicourt, *Essai sur la vie privée d'Honoré-Gabrielle Riquetti, Comte de Mirabeau* (Paris: Droits de l'Homme, An VIII [1800]); Cadet de Gassicourt, *Éloge d'A.-A. Parmentier* (Paris: Fain, 1814); Cadet de Gassicourt, *St. Géran, ou la nouvelle langue française, anecdote récente; suivie de l'itinéraire de Lutèce au Mont Valérien, en suivant le fleuve Sequanien et revenant par le Mont des Martyrs; petite parodie d'un grand voyage* (Brussels: Weissenbruch, 1812); Cadet de Gassicourt, *Le Tombeau de Jacques Molai, ou histoire secrète et abrégée des initiés, anciens et modernes, des templiers, franc-maçons illuminés, etc.* (Paris: Desenne, An V [1797]); Cadet de Gassicourt, *Projet d'Institut nomade* (Paris: Baudouin, 1820).

9 Cadet de Gassicourt, *Le Thé est-il plus nuisible qu'utile? ou histoire analytique de cette plante et moyens de la remplacer avec avantage* (Paris: Colas, 1808); Cadet de Gassicourt, 'Sur les cafés indigènes', *Bulletin de Pharmacie*, 5 (1813), 501–58; Cadet de Gassicourt, 'Charlatanisme', *Dictionnaire des sciences médicales*, IV (1812), 543–55; Cadet de Gassicourt, 'Note sur un article inséré dans le *Dictionnaire des sciences médicales*', *Journal de pharmacie et des sciences accessoires*, 7 (1821), 29–30.

10 Cadet de Gassicourt, *Traité de l'élognostie, ou l'esprit des sots* (Paris: chez tous les marchands de nouveautés, 1813).

limbless beggar and by a *bedeau* (or 'porte-baguette') anxious to instruct him on the curiosities of the 'vaste et gothique édifice', in particular on its bells.[11] It is clear, therefore, that Cadet was a polyvalent *savant* and *littérateur* with interests befitting the polyvalency of his profession. It is in that light that his supremely eclectic war writings are most productively seen. Thus we return to that *année de merveilles*, 1809, year of the launch of the *Bulletin de pharmacie*, and also of Cadet's departure on Napoleon's Austrian campaign.

Pharmacists at War

The first thing to remark upon in relation to Cadet's war memoir is the complexity of discursive status implied by its title: *Voyage en Autriche, en Moravie et en Bavière fait à la suite de l'armée française, pendant la campagne de 1809* (1818). Is it a scholarly work, as the listing of Cadet's scientific titles might suggest? Is it a *récit de guerre* or a *récit de voyage*? In his preface, Cadet admits that he is not even sure himself:

> Il m'était impossible de rédiger un voyage régulier ou de tracer l'histoire de la guerre. [L']épouvante qui précède une armée, la dévastation qui la suit, ne me laissaient pas les moyens d'étudier les mœurs de nos ennemis, les productions naturelles et industrielles de leur pays.[12]

There is already a suggestion here that this is an anthropological travel narrative inconveniently intruded on by war, a travelogue which, in spite of itself, becomes a generically hybrid narrative of war, travel, and useful knowledge. Cadet's method is chosen accordingly:

> Recueillir des renseignements imparfaits, peindre des scènes isolées, conserver des aperçus fugitifs, jeter sur le papier des notes incohérentes; mais ces notes, ces aperçus, ces scènes fourniront peut-être des matériaux à l'histoire. [...] Dans un style négligé, dans un désordre apparent, je serai plus rapide et je paraîtrai du moins original. (*V*, 6)

---

11 Cadet de Gassicourt, *Mon Voyage, ou lettres sur la ci-devant province de Normandie, suivie de quelques pièces fugitives* (Paris: Desenne, An VII [1799]), pp. 35–38.

12 Cadet de Gassicourt, *Voyage en Autriche, en Moravie et en Bavière fait à la suite de l'armée française pendant la campagne de 1809* (Paris: L'Huillier, 1818), p. 6. Hereinafter referred to as *V*, followed by the page number.

It thus purports to be a literary rather than an historical text, an eyewitness record subordinated to an aesthetic of disorder. But this very disorder ensures a great variety of subjects of varying relevance to war, and a great variety of discursive forms.

The same can be said of the *carnets de guerre* of another military pharmacist, Pierre-Irénée Jacob, documenting Napoleon's German and Austrian campaign of 1805–06, the Spanish campaign of 1809–12, and the Russian and German campaigns of 1812–13. Jacob's writings, like Cadet's, contain occasional references to the horrors of war: corpse-strewn roads or amputations of limbs.[13] In the case of senior officers, amputated limbs were embalmed and sent back to Paris by the pharmacist. A representative passage presenting such appalling spectacles can be found in Jacob's account of the 1806 campaign:

> J'ai aidé Vanderback à faire des pansements; j'ai tenu des membres qu'il amputait. En peu d'instants, je vis là un échantillon de ce que la guerre offre de plus horrible. Le plancher de la chambre de la ferme fut bientôt couvert de sang, et l'on jetait derrière la porte, les membres amputés comme les abats des animaux à la boucherie. Quel spectacle! Les cris des malheureux opérés me portaient au cœur. Je ne sais si sur le champ de bataille l'animation, le danger, l'entraînement, le bruit des instruments guerriers peuvent donner à l'homme qui pense, à l'homme doué de quelque sensibilité, les qualités d'un héros, mais il me semble qu'il suffit d'avoir passé par les ambulances d'armée pour prendre la guerre en horreur.[14]

Despite the compelling awfulness of such episodes, Jacob's memoirs, however, consist primarily of topographical accounts of cities, biographical and character studies of surgeons and other pharmacists, and evaluations of their poetry and writing. The pharmacist Boisard, for example, is depicted as the 'pharmacien principal du corps d'armée', 'qui fait avec facilité des vers très agréables', and has 'quelque chose de la physionomie de Bernardin de St-Pierre'. Jacob includes details of visits to local *sociétés savantes* and *académies*, guarded criticisms of Napoleon's character based on close observation, the observation of *curiosités d'histoire naturelle*, and anthropological and physiological

13 Pierre-Irénée Jacob, 'Journal et itinéraire de dix années de campagne', *Revue d'histoire de la pharmacie*, 54, (1966), pp. 81–96; 187–204; 249–64. See also François Stupp, *Les Carnets de route de Pierre-Irénée Jacob: pharmacien dans la Grande Armée, 1805–1814* (Polignac: Éditions du Roure, 2005).

14 Jacob, 'Journal', p. 190.

observations of local populations.[15] In his diary of the Spanish campaign of 1809–12, for example, Jacob recounts visits to theatres and libraries; documents geographical features, urban topography, and the architectural grandeurs of Spain (the specifically 'mauresque' qualities of which are foregrounded); and presents lurid and exoticizing accounts of vendettas 'd'une atrocité révoltante' carried out by *guerrilleros* which would not be out of place in the works of, say, Mérimée. One of these anecdotal stories — a tale of a Spanish monk-turned-*josefino* punished for his treachery by having each of his dismembered limbs displayed at a corner of the city of Segovia, and his head placed in a sack outside the governor's palace — leads Jacob to conclude that 'l'Espagne n'a rien d'européen; c'est une Afrique, une Arabie baptisée et se croyant chrétienne'.[16] This quasi-academic travelogue is of a kind later finding literary expression in such works as Mérimée's *Carmen* (1845–47). Mérimée's frame narrator is a traveling scholar inspecting archaeological sites in Spain, recounting, as light relief from his serious academic work, a series of suitably exotic events in a setting presented for French bourgeois readers as irredeemably Other.[17] Interestingly, the eponymous anti-heroine's skills at tending to wounds are qualified by their recipient, Don José, as being on a par with those of a 'chirurgien-major', seemingly the gold standard of medical care within the cultural context represented by Mérimée's *nouvelle*, and which its readers would recognize.[18]

What appears to characterize the pharmaceutical war diary, then, is its polyvalency: it contains an eclectic mix of anecdote, *couleur locale*, knowledge, and accounts of learned activities, complemented by occasional scenes of devastation or amputation. Importantly, it has elements that are either in and of themselves literary, or are reformulated by literary discourse as representative of an archetypal academic or disciplinary discourse as it expresses itself in the form of the travel narrative. Flaubert's mid-century choice of pharmacy as representative archetype of professional discipline may well be a masterstroke, facilitating the problematization of disciplinary knowledge and of the

15 Jacob, 'Journal', pp. 88, 190, 194, 260.

16 Ibid., p. 195.

17 Prosper Mérimée, *Carmen*, in *Romans et nouvelles*, ed. by Maurice Parturier, 2 vols (Paris: Garnier, 1967), II, pp. 337–409; Larry Duffy, '*Perdue en traduction*: Translation, Betrayal and Death in Mérimée's *Carmen*', in *Birth and Death in Nineteenth-Century French Culture*, ed. by Lisa Downing, Nigel Harkness, Tim Unwin and Sonya Stephens (Amsterdam: Rodopi, 2007), pp. 49–61.

18 Mérimée, *Carmen*, p. 383. Don José, the soldier-turned-bandit corrupted by Carmen, relates his tragic story to Mérimée's archaeologist frame narrator.

relationships between discourses (literary and extraliterary; pharmaceutical and medical, and so on). However, early in the century, long before Homais's demonstrations of his erudition, pharmaceutical discourse already lends itself very well to the scholarly (or pseudoscholarly) exposition of eclectic knowledge characteristic of literary travel narratives such as Mérimée's.

Cadet's campaign narrative is similar to Jacob's in this respect. Before encountering the reality of war, Cadet adopts the hybrid tone of the travel narrative combined with the statistical manual. 'Une des plus belles routes de France est celle qui conduit à Strasbourg'. And then:

> La quantité énorme d'engrais qu'amassent les agriculteurs prouve l'abondance, et assure la fécondité de ces pays: aussi les Champenois et les Lorrains sont-ils sains, vigoureux et assez bien vêtus; mais leurs chevaux, leurs bœufs et leurs vaches ne sont pas d'une belle espèce. (*V*, 1)

This is truly a pharmacist writing, in that the contemporary disciplinary parameters of pharmacy which Cadet was in the process of producing extend to the expression of expert opinion on agricultural matters. Arriving in Strasbourg, noting the coming and going of troops, generals and *aides-de camp*, and reverentially observing that '*Le Maître n'est pas loin*' (*V*, 7, emphasis in original), Cadet adopts a tone later to characterize '*les ouvrages qui traitent de la cathédrale*' vaunted by the Suisse in *Madame Bovary* (*OC*, I, 656).[19] He recounts:

> J'ai monté ce matin sur la flèche du Munster (la cathédrale). Sa hauteur est à peu près double de celle des tours de Notre-Dame: on compte six cent cinquante-huit marches, qui équivalent environ à cinq cent soixante-quatorze pieds. (*V*, 8)

At the Société des Sciences de Strasbourg, Cadet reads 'un mémoire sur la fabrication du tabac et ses falsifications', reproduced in the first edition of the *Bulletin de Pharmacie*, visits 'le cabinet de minéralogie de M. Mathieu, banquier', and collects carps, of which he sends samples back to Paris (*V*, 12–13).[20] He offers observations on the conduct of Strasbourg's 'prêtresses de Vénus' (*V*, 14), and, some days later, on the 'police des filles publiques' in 'Stuttgard' (*V*, 37). Stendhal, following the same itinerary as Cadet at exactly the same time,

---

19 See also Théodore Licquet, *Rouen; précis de son histoire, son commerce, son industrie, ses manufactures, ses monumens; guide nécessaire pour bien connaître cette capitale de la Normandie*, etc., 2nd edn (Rouen: Frère, 1831), pp. 58–59.

20 *Bulletin de pharmacie*, I (1809), p. 263.

makes rather similar observations in his *Journal*, in particular on local geography, local women, and local potatoes.[21] As in the case of Mérimée's account of Spain, a manifestly 'literary' account of travel displays similar preoccupations and stylistic expression to those of the pharmaceutical *récit de voyage*, which in Cadet's case nevertheless contains enough 'scientific' detail to retain its disciplinary credentials as the *mémoire* of a man of science.

Cadet, like Stendhal, intercalates his highly personal impressions with character studies of his travelling companions, and news of Napoleon's victories. Delays in the journey are exploited for the collection of information. 'La ville d'Augsbourg est fort agréable', he remarks some days before reaching the front line. He continues:

> Malgré le désir que j'avais de rejoindre promptement l'Empereur, le manque de chevaux m'obligea de rester quelques heures dans cette ville d'Auguste. J'en profitai pour prendre sur elle quelques informations, et voir plusieurs édifices curieux. (*V*, 45)

But soon, the shifting focus of the polyvalent narrative alights on a much more sombre object of interest. Cadet begins, like Jacob before him, to witness the concrete and altogether human effects of war, even if he is not involved in the fighting. In Schwarbhausen:

> J'ai passé au milieu des camps que les Autrichiens avaient occupés la veille. Les feux fumaient encore. J'ai vu pour la première fois les restes d'un champ de bataille: des morts, des blessés tout le long de la route, des débris de toutes espèces, des champs dévastés des découvertes et des fermes pillées. Ce spectacle nouveau pour moi affaiblit bien dans mon opinion le prestige de la gloire militaire. (*V*, 53)

From this point on, the narrative is concerned with the devastating effects and contingencies of war such as looting, the mistreatment of civilians in whose homes French soldiers are billeted, and the scorched earth of the retreating Austrians. In Ebersburg:

> Le tableau qu'offrait cette malheureuse ville, quelques heures après le combat, réunissait tous les genres d'horreurs; le pont couvert de morts et

---

21 Stendhal, *Journal*, 12–18 avril 1809, *Œuvres complètes*, 3 vols (Paris: Champion, 1969), II, 318–19.

> de blessés; la rivière remplie de cadavres et de débris; toutes les maisons écroulées et fumantes, les rues jonchées de corps mutilés et brûlés, conservant encore après la mort l'attitude et l'expression de la plus horrible douleur; des femmes, de malheureux enfants consumés dans les bras l'un de l'autre; et, dans ce désastre général, une armée traversant ce théâtre de destruction au bruit d'une musique guerrière, les voitures roulant sur quinze cents morts, brisant leurs crânes et emportant les lambeaux de leur dépouille. (*V*, 72)

The shocking yet compassionate accounts of these disturbing sights, also discussed in similarly despairing terms — in this specific location of Ebersburg — by Stendhal and Larrey, stand in stark contrast to the levity of Cadet's anecdotes on military manners and the life accompanying a military campaign. These include, for example, the relation of an encounter with a *vivandière* who, with her children, has been following her husband for several campaigns:

> Voilà huit campagnes que je fais, et celle-ci est la plus belle. J'ai suivi le régiment, parce que j'aimais un sergent. Il a été blessé, je l'ai soigné; il m'a fait un enfant; je l'ai mis au monde à l'ambulance. Je suis toujours restée dans le corps, et ces marmots faits au bivouacs et baptisés sous notre aigle, seront un jour, j'espère, de bons grenadiers. Le métier que j'ai commencé par fantaisie, je l'ai continué par habitude, et je le fais aujourd'hui par intérêt. Tout ce qui compose mon bagage et mes provisions ne m'a pas coûté un sou. (*V*, 75)

This kind of reportage, given the practical constraints involved, doubtless requires a certain amount of literary invention. And it is indeed the kind of anecdotal character sketch that is found in literary discourse: for instance, a similar encounter between Stendhal's hero Fabrice and a similarly spirited *vivandière* near Waterloo is recounted in *La Chartreuse de Parme*.[22]

Cadet shifts away, then, from the horrors of war to anecdote and local colour, on the battlefield and off. The taking of Vienna, for instance, is related not from a military point of view but in terms of an opportunity to enumerate the qualities of the Schoenbrunn palace, of Marie-Thérèse's *chaise volante*, and of the botanical and zoological gardens (*V*, 90–94). Indeed, Cadet remains in Vienna for some time, and becomes a *de facto* courtier, which possibly accounts for the

---

22 Stendhal, *La Chartreuse de Parme* (Paris: Flammarion, 2000), pp. 99–105, p. 124.

considerable amount of Napoleonic hagiography present in the work, such as in the following decidedly non-hellish military scene:

> Le soldat boit, rit, chante et adore son chef. L'Empereur se porte comme sa gloire; il étonne tous les jours ses généraux même, par l'activité de son génie qui suffit à tous les détails: il a fait beaucoup de promotions, d'une manière touchante, neuve et digne des beaux temps de Rome et de la Grèce. (*V*, 100)

Praising the collective bravery occasioned by the battle of Essling, Cadet does not neglect to foreground Napoleon: '— Que de traits d'héroïsme la journée d'Essling a produits! L'Empereur s'est constamment exposé comme un sous-lieutenant' (*V*, 116). But the hagiography is not unqualified. Cadet specifies in his preface that it was only in 1818 that he dared publish his war memoirs, which in fact contain numerous indirect criticisms of Napoleon (*V*, viii). Cadet adopts the strategy of having Napoleon criticized by others, such as the Duc de Montebello, dying after losing his legs on the island of Lobau near Vienna. Cadet presents Napoleon's visit to his wounded comrade as 'une scène attendrissante, et digne du pinceau de Gérard', which had 'ranimé le courage des malheureux blessés qui, se soulevant sur le sable, ont crié: Vive l'Empéreur' (*V*, 117). Cadet then reports the words of Montebello himself, who, *sommité militaire* about to die, has greater impunity in criticizing his prince:

> Ton ambition insatiable te perdra; tu sacrifies sans nécessité, sans ménagement, sans regrets, les hommes qui te servent le mieux. Ton ingratitude éloigne de toi ceux-mêmes qui t'admirent; tu n'as plus autour de toi ceux-mêmes qui t'admirent; tu n'as plus autour de toi que des flatteurs; je ne vois pas un ami qui ose te dire la vérité. On te trahira, on t'abandonnera; hâte-toi de terminer cette guerre: c'est le vœu de tes généraux; c'est sans doute celui de ton peuple. Tu ne seras jamais plus puissant, tu peux être bien plus aimé! Pardonne à un mourant ces vérités, ce mourant te chérit… (*V*, 127)

It is at this point that Cadet relates what appears to be his only truly 'pharmaceutical' exploit in this affair, that is, his embalming of Montebello's body:

> [L]e maréchal était en pleine putréfaction, et cette opération qui a duré trois jours a été pénible et dangereuse. Les lotions d'acide muriatique, les fumigations, guytonniennes, les cassolettes de benjoin, etc., ne pouvaient corriger l'odeur horrible de ce cadavre. (*V*, 128)

Embalming is very much the preserve of pharmacists during the Napoleonic campaigns (as in the case of Jacob's *confrère* mentioned above), and is moreover a feature of pharmacy more generally, given the unique access of pharmacists to the ingredients required for concocting embalming fluid.[23] The officer overseeing the enbalming of Montebello's body is not however a pharmacist but a surgeon, Dominique Larrey, who had amputated the Duke's leg.

Le médecin de campagne: Larrey's clinical accounts

Larrey's *Mémoires de chirurgie médicale et de campagne*, published between 1812 and 1817, deal with twenty years of soldiering and battlefield surgery, and are of a quite different order and scale from the pharmaceutical *journal de campagne*. If the pharmaceutical memoir, accessible to a general readership, is impressionistic, eclectic, and adopts a variety of discursive styles, the medical memoir is totalizing, clinical, objective, all-seeing, and, while not lacking in compassion, is not primarily concerned with the feelings of patients. This is presumably due at least in part to the fact that the medical memoir's readership consists primarily of medical professionals and students; it is necessarily expository and didactic, with very occasional anecdotal digression.

Larrey's work — a textbook on surgery much more than the memoir of a surgeon, despite its title, which arguably implies 'memoranda', that is, case studies rather than reminiscences — exposes how medical provision is organized on a military campaign. Going into close detail, it provides a properly historical as well as medical record. It does — in its occasional descriptions of locations and their inhabitants — have elements of the travelogue, but these are minor by comparison with Cadet's and Jacob's works, and are predominantly concerned with matters that may be construed as medical. For example, in his account of the Spanish campaign, Larrey comments on Spanish women, but primarily in terms of their physiological features, such as their height and the quality of their teeth.[24] He also discusses injuries resulting from social practices in exotic locations, such as bullfighting, or cretinism among Pyrenean peasants, 'disgraciés par la nature' (*M*, 113), or the prevalence of syphilis amongst Spanish prostitutes ('il paraît que les Espagnols l'ont reçue primitivement des Arabes', *M*, 228–29), or the anti-scientific superstition and obscurantism prevailing in

23 Consider, for example, 'les fœtus du pharmacien', embalmed and put on display by Homais in *Madame Bovary* (OC, I, 599).

24 Larrey, *Mémoires*, III (1812), pp. 112–13. All future references to Larrey's *Mémoires* are abbreviated as *M*, followed by the page number in the text.

Spain where he visits the torture chambers of the Inquisition (*M*, 240–41). So, if there is some of the exoticism of the travelogue, particularly the Spanish travelogue, there is very much less of it, and where it does exist it is cloaked in the objective language of medical discourse and of the Enlightenment reason which the Napoleonic project will bring to a hitherto benighted people. For the most part, though, Larrey's *mémoires* consist of case histories, relating *ouvertures de cadavres*, autopsies (*M*, 177), dog-poisoning experiments (*M*, 180–81), descriptions of pathologies — 'telle est la marche de cette maladie', 'le travail pénible de la nature' (*M*, 168) — along with discrete *mémoires* on topics such as gangrene, syphilis, the dangers of onanism or elephantiasis. Above all, however, they contain numerous accounts of amputation, of which Larrey is a pioneering and enthusiastic practitioner. Hundreds of pages are given over to individual case histories of battlefield injuries (mostly caused by cannonballs or kicks from horses) incurred by soldiers of all ranks requiring amputation, detailed narratives of the kinds of amputation necessitated and carried out, of post-operative treatment and rehabilitation, and of the conclusions to be drawn from the dissection of amputated members (before they are embalmed by the pharmacists).

Larrey has two major contributions to make to the practice of amputation: first, the privileging of a new technique of amputation through joints rather than on either side of them, where possible; and, second, the need to carry out immediate amputation on the battlefield. The expression 'nécessité d'amputer sur-le-champ', where 'le champ' is literally and explicitly the *champ de bataille*, is reiterated in multiple cases.[25] In this, Larrey is going against an established consensus among *confrères*, who have traditionally held to the view that amputations should be carried out in hospitals removed from the battlefield, out of sight of other soldiers. Larrey's view is that immediate battlefield amputation is reassuring, rather than fear inducing. He approvingly quotes another famous military surgeon, 'Dufouard' [sic], affirming that 'l'amputation chirurgicale d'un membre est l'œuvre la plus philosophique de toutes les sciences humaines' (*M*, 353).[26] Indeed, continues Larrey, 'il doit appartenir à l'homme véritablement sensible, courageux et expérimenté, de connaître et de savoir apprécier les merveilleux effets de l'amputation', as its principal effect is the saving of soldiers' lives (*M*, 352–53). Another key advantage of the practice

25 Ibid., pp. 247, 278, 350, 352, 380.

26 Pierre Dufouart (1737–1813), whose surname is misspelt by Larrey, was a military surgeon and author of a work — presumably the one Larrey quotes — entitled *Analyse des blessures d'armes à feu et de leur traitement* (Paris: Pougens, 1801).

is that '[l']amputation détruit d'abord la contagion' (*M*, 154). Contagion has been a key military health issue during the Napoleonic campaigns, and the source of much controversy: Cadet reports, but then refutes, the allegation that Napoleon had 500 military patients poisoned by a pharmacist in Jaffa to head off the risk of contagion (*V*, 386–95). In a sense, Larrey, in promoting amputation, is implementing a Napoleonic imperative beginning at the level of the individual body.

The most prominent case history in Larrey's *Mémoires*, in the sense that it is not just a case history but part of his narrative of the Austrian campaign is that involving the mortally wounded duc de Montebello. This episode, as we have seen, is also related in Cadet's *Voyage*. Whilst Cadet recounts the personal drama and meeting with Napoleon occasioned by Montebello's mortal injuries, Larrey recounts what has befallen the Maréchal with clinical precision:

> Un boulet de gros calibre, après avoir fait un premier ricochet dans le fort de sa course, rencontra le genou gauche du maréchal, le traversa dans son épaisseur, et, changeant de direction, sans perdre de sa force, effleura la cuisse droite, dont il coupa les tégumens et une portion du muscle vaste interne, au lieu le plus saillant, et très-près de l'articulation du genou, laquelle, fort heureusement, n'avait pas été entamée. Le duc fut renversé sur le coup, en éprouvant une violente commotion au cerveau, et un très-grand ébranlement dans tous les organes. (*M*, 278)

Montebello's death is then recounted in lengthy clinical terms. This is at odds with Cadet's account of the episode, which although it does mention Montebello, relates primarily the experience of amputation among the common soldiery, and moreover in a melodramatic rather than clinical manner:

> [Les blessés], rangés sur la terre dans l'île Lobau, ne pouvaient être opérés que les uns après les autres: ils voyaient approcher les chirurgiens comme des bienfaiteurs. Lorsqu'on paraissait en négliger un, il les appelait: *C'est à moi*, disait-il, *c'est mon tour. Messieurs, venez me couper la jambe, mon voisin peut attendre* ... (*V*, 118)

Again there is a striking contrast between the clinical account of the military surgeon (Larrey), and the very human and compassionate account of the military pharmacist (Cadet). This contrast is hardly surprising, however, if the status of the pharmaceutical memoir as compendium of all kinds of human activity is taken into consideration. This eclectic status is evidenced in Cadet's table of contents (*V*, 420–38), which again stands in contrast to Larrey's. For Cadet, A is for 'l'Amour chez les Viennoises', 'Antiques', 'Arbres rares', and so on. 'Amputations' does appear, but the reference is to a discussion of comparative custom and etiquette in different cultures, rather than on actual clinical practice. In Larrey's index, it is a matter of 'aneurysmes', 'anasarque', and of course 'amputations', in all their variety. It would be easy to mistake it for a medical dictionary with no obvious military connection.[27]

Conclusion

If Larrey's work appears to be a medical treatise based on professional experience of war, Cadet's is almost impossible to categorize. Scarcely is combat interrupted than Cadet resumes his observations on the *mœurs* of defeated provinces: love, prostitution, agriculture, statistics, costumes, learned culture. The chapter following the one recounting the disaster of Lobau is entitled 'Détails statistiques sur l'Autriche. Ses productions, ses institutions savantes'. We learn that 'quant aux bestiaux, il y a environ 1 661 900 bœufs et vaches, 5 803 240 moutons, et 834 000 chevaux' (*V*, 138). These observations are followed by ruminations on 'Vienne — Ses monuments, ses promenades, ses théâtres', and then on the differences between the operations of learned societies in France and in Vienna, where the lack of an *académie* ensures that learned societies lack a coherent organizing principle, and that savants 'sont privés de ces communications utiles qui établissent des rapports entre les sciences' (*V*, 144). This again is arguably emblematic of a particular attitude towards the organization of knowledge, which allows for a certain eclecticism, and also for the possibility of transcending disciplinary boundaries. This attitude — a firm belief in the desirability of relationships between various fields of knowledge — is in fact at the heart of the revolution in pharmacy's relationship with other disciplines and professions that is being promoted at the very same moment by Cadet in the pages of *Le Bulletin de pharmacie*.

This interdisciplinary imperative finds expression precisely in the intergeneric quality of Cadet's war memoir. Cadet's *Voyage* is a hybrid work, neither a *récit de guerre*, nor a *récit de voyage*. It nevertheless remains a diverting account of events, local colour, social practices and comparative cultures of knowledge, and learned activity. Cadet's text is not strictly speaking a pharmaceutical one. It can be regarded, however, as being consistent with contemporary

27 Larrey, *Mémoires*, IV (1817), pp. 485–500.

pharmaceutical discourse, of which Cadet is a representative *sommité*, in that pharmacy is still defining itself in relation to medicine, chemistry, and other fields in which pharmacy may have practical applications. That is, the multifarious nature of a revitalized and professionally emboldened pharmacy seeking uncharted territories in which to extend its disciplinary tentacles is incorporated stylistically within the writings of its practitioners. Cadet's memoir, like Jacob's, is the opus of a pharmacist who is imposing his professional and discursive purview on numerous fields, including battlefields, and it is an opus containing elements clearly identifiable as literary.

Both pharmacy and medicine undergo major institutional developments from the Napoleonic period, and are shaped at least in part by their military associations. This chapter has identified a distinction between two tendencies in nineteenth-century narrative discourse: the 'clinical/surgical', frequently associated with objective mimetic discourse, and the 'pharmaceutical', characterized by its stylistically and generically eclectic presentation of information. Although the latter more overtly contains elements of the exoticizing travelogue, the former's clinical objectivity provides a smokescreen for essentializing discourses. Pharmaceutical discourse — as can be seen in the writings of actual pharmacists, and in the utterances of Flaubert's fictional pharmacist — ostentatiously puts its finger in every pie.[28] The narrative hybridity of pharmaceutical discourse draws attention to the discipline's instability and insecurity, as well as to the complex relationship between pharmacy, chemistry, and medicine in the early nineteenth century. Medical discourse, on the other hand, downplays its polyvalency, to present an ostensibly objective account. If the pharmaceutical works (and Flaubert) demonstrate the versatility of pharmacy within various contemporary discursive idioms, the medical work comprehensively asserts the all-seeing nature of the medical gaze.

Bibliography

Cadet de Gassicourt, Charles-Louis, 'Charlatanisme', *Dictionnaire des sciences médicales*, IV (1812), 543–55

——, *Éloge d'A.-A. Parmentier* (Paris: Fain, 1814)

——, *Essai sur la vie privée d'Honoré-Gabrielle Riquetti, Comte de Mirabeau* (Paris: Droits de l'Homme, An VIII [1800])

28 On pharmacy's changing status in early nineteenth-century France, particularly vis-à-vis chemistry, see Jonathan Simon, *Chemistry, Pharmacy and Revolution in France, 1777–1809* (Aldershot: Ashgate, 2005).

——, *Le Thé est-il plus nuisible qu'utile? ou histoire analytique de cette plante et moyens de la remplacer avec avantage* (Paris: Colas, 1808)

——, *Le Tombeau de Jacques Molai, ou histoire secrète et abrégée des initiés, anciens et modernes, des templiers, franc-maçons illuminés, etc.* (Paris: Desenne, An V [1797])

——, *Mon Voyage, ou lettres sur la ci-devant province de Normandie, suivie de quelques pièces fugitives* (Paris: Desenne, An VII [1799])

——, 'Note sur un article inséré dans le *Dictionnaire des sciences médicales*', *Journal de pharmacie et des sciences accessoires*, 7 (1821), 29–30

——, *Projet d'Institut nomade* (Paris: Baudouin, 1820)

——, *St. Géran, ou la nouvelle langue française, anecdote récente; suivie de l'itinéraire de Lutèce au Mont Valérien, en suivant le fleuve Sequanien et revenant par le Mont des Martyrs; petite parodie d'un grand voyage* (Brussels: Weissenbruch, 1812)

——, 'Sur les cafés indigènes', *Bulletin de Pharmacie*, 5 (1813), 501–58

——, *Traité de l'élognostie, ou l'esprit des sots* (Paris: chez tous les marchands de nouveautés, 1813)

——, *Voyage en Autriche, en Moravie et en Bavière fait à la suite de l'armée française pendant la campagne de 1809* (Paris: L'Huillier, 1818)

Donaldson-Evans, Mary, *Medical Examinations: Dissecting the Doctor in French Narrative Prose, 1857–1894* (Lincoln: University of Nebraska Press, 2000)

Duffy, Larry, '*Perdue en traduction*: Translation, Betrayal and Death in Mérimée's *Carmen*', in *Birth and Death in Nineteenth-Century French Culture*, ed. by Lisa Downing, Nigel Harkness, Tim Unwin and Sonya Stephens (Amsterdam: Rodopi, 2007), pp. 49–61

——, '*Madame Bovary* and the Institutional Transformation of Pharmacy', *Dix-neuf*, 15, 1 (2011), 70–82

Dufouart, Pierre, *Analyse des blessures d'armes à feu et de leur traitement* (Paris: Pougens, 1801)

Flaubert, Gustave, *Œuvres complètes*, ed. by Bernard Masson, 2 vols (Paris: Seuil, 1964)

Furst, Lilian R., 'Realism and Hypertrophy: A Study of Three Medico-Historical "Cases"', *Nineteenth-Century French Studies*, 22, 1–2 (1993), 29–47

Jacob, Pierre-Irénée, 'Journal et itinéraire de dix années de campagne', *Revue d'histoire de la pharmacie*, 54 (1966), 81–96

——, 'Journal et itinéraire de dix années de campagne (suite)', *Revue d'histoire de la pharmacie*, 54 (1966), 187–204

——, 'Journal et itinéraire de dix années de campagne (suite et fin)', *Revue d'histoire de la pharmacie*, 54 (1966), 249–64

Larrey, Dominique Jean, *Mémoires de chirurgie militaire, et campagnes*, 4 vols (Paris: Smith, 1812–17)

Licquet, Théodore, *Rouen; précis de son histoire, son commerce, son industrie, ses manufactures, ses monumens; guide nécessaire pour bien connaître cette capitale de la Normandie*, etc., 2nd edn (Rouen: Frère, 1831)
Mérimée, Prosper, *Carmen*, in *Romans et nouvelles*, ed. by Maurice Parturier, 2 vols (Paris: Garnier, 1967), II, 337–409
Stendhal, pseud. Henri Beyle, *Œuvres complètes*, 3 vols (Paris: Champion, 1969)
——, *La Chartreuse de Parme* (Paris: Flammarion, 2000)
Simon, Jonathan, *Chemistry, Pharmacy and Revolution in France, 1777–1809* (Aldershot: Ashgate, 2005)
Stupp, François, *Les Carnets de route de Pierre-Irénée Jacob: pharmacien dans la Grande Armée, 1805–1814* (Polignac: Éditions du Roure, 2005)

CHAPTER 3

Alcoolisme et acédie : le monstre alcoolique dans la pensée clinique du XIXe siècle

Julie Müller

Le concept d'alcoolisme naît au milieu du XIXe siècle. C'est en 1848 que le médecin suédois Magnus Huss invente ce néologisme heureux afin de désigner ce qui apparaît alors aux cliniciens comme une pathologie nouvelle. En effet, le mal des buveurs d'eaux-de-vie et autres boissons industrielles ne semble plus répondre à l'ancienne définition de l'ivrogne et de l'ivrognerie qu'avait transmise l'Antiquité. Les cliniciens ne localisent plus le mal du buveur au niveau des organes digestifs mais cherchent désormais sa source du côté des parties cérébrales, comme semble l'indiquer l'aggravation des pathologies nerveuses et des symptômes psychosomatiques aigues liés à la consommation d'alcool durant tout le siècle. Dans le même temps, la médecine clinique, influencée par le courant hygiéniste, reste fidèle à l'ancienne conception du buveur véhiculée par la tradition. Depuis l'Antiquité, le phénomène de trop boire est associé à un vice. Médecins, philosophes, et moralistes considèrent ce trouble comme le signe visible d'une faute, celle d'un buveur qui se laisse aller à l'excès de plaisir.

Mais de quel vice parle-t-on ici exactement ? S'agit-il toujours, au XIXe siècle, de la *gula* comme le voulait jusqu'ici la tradition chrétienne, qui associait depuis des siècles le péché d'ivrognerie à l'organe du glouton, aux excès de ventre du bon vivant ? Ou y a-t-il eu un déplacement de signification ? L'appréhension de la faute est-elle toujours la même à une époque où le regard médical connaît une véritable révolution et où l'ivrognerie elle aussi change de forme ?

Pour répondre à ces questions, il nous faut d'abord revenir à la source du problème : remonter à l'acte de naissance de l'alcoolisme et à ce qui va alors différencier, à partir du milieu du XIXe siècle, l'ivrogne traditionnel d'une nouvelle forme de buveur qu'on nomme désormais alcoolique.

Ivresse, ivrognerie, et alcoolisme

Au XIXe siècle, l'abus d'alcool n'est pas un phénomène nouveau. Les médecins qui, depuis l'Antiquité, préconisent son emploi comme tonique ou

 | DOI:10.1163/9789004368019_005

thérapeutique, notent dans le même temps les troubles que cause son usage abusif. Hippocrate, Galien, Théophraste relèvent dans leurs écrits les symptômes caractéristiques que provoque la maladie du trop boire : tremblements, vomissements, troubles de la vue et de la motricité, abattement psychique, engourdissement, infertilité, accès de folie, débauche : le 'problème XXX' attribué au XVIe siècle à Aristote résume par exemple l'état de ces connaissances.[1] Dès ses débuts, le discours médical entretient une image à la fois double et contradictoire de l'ivresse : d'un côté, il vante les bienfaits d'un usage hygiénique des boissons enivrantes, qui serait le fait d'un buveur raisonnable respectant les préceptes de la science ; de l'autre côté, il condamne la mauvaise ivresse de ceux qui se laissent aller à l'abus de boisson. Pour les Anciens, l'abus d'alcool est donc avant tout lié à une forme d'inconduite. L'ivrognerie résulte d'une faiblesse morale du buveur. Elle trahit son manque de volonté et surtout son incapacité à bien vouloir maîtriser son plaisir. Dès l'ère chrétienne, l'ivrognerie est associée par les pères de l'Église à la démesure d'un estomac glouton. Dans le catalogue traditionnel des vices, l'ivrognerie correspond au péché charnel de gourmandise, péché véniel mais aussi capital, puisqu'il conditionne à lui seul l'apparition de nombreux vices comme le rappellent, par exemple, les sermons sur l'ivrognerie de Jean Chrysostome ou de Basile-le-Grand.[2] Au XIIIe siècle, Saint-Thomas d'Aquin précise cet enseignement. Dans la *Somme Théologique*, Saint-Thomas insiste en particulier sur la dimension volontaire de l'abus. Celui qui s'adonne de manière répétée à la boisson, c'est-à-dire l'ivrogne, connaît, selon lui, l'origine de son vice puisqu'il a généralement déjà éprouvé les troubles de l'ivresse. Il connaît son mal, mais cela n'empêche pas ce-dernier de récidiver. Selon Saint-Thomas, l'ivrogne choisit donc de manière consciente de céder — ou non — à la tentation. Le péché d'ivrognerie est en cela considéré comme un péché mortel, car il implique une faute répétée du buveur qui engage sa pleine responsabilité :

> Il peut arriver que l'on sache bien que l'on boit immodérément et qu'on va s'enivrer, mais qu'on aime mieux être dans l'ivresse que de s'abstenir de boire, et c'est à proprement parler ce qu'on entend par un homme ivre […]. En ce cas l'ivresse est un péché mortel, parce que l'homme se

1 Aristote, *L'Homme de génie et la mélancolie, Problème XXX*, vol. 1 (Paris : Payot & Rivages, 2006).

2 Jean Chrysostome, *Homélies sur la Résurrection, l'Ascension et la Pentecôte*, 1 (Paris : Cerf, 2013) ; Basile de Césaré, *Homélies, discours, lettres choisies de Saint Basile-le-Grand* (Lyon : Francois Guyot, 1827). Sur le péché de gourmandise voir Florent Quellier, *Gourmandise : histoire d'un péché capital* (Paris : Armand Colin, 2010).

> prive volontairement et sciemment de l'usage de la raison qui le fait agir conformément à la vertu et l'éloigne du péché. Par conséquent il pèche mortellement en s'exposant au danger de pécher.[3]

Jusqu'à l'époque moderne, médecins et moralistes font ainsi état d'une manière de 'mal boire' qui est le fait de celui qui boit trop, de celui qui, ne respecte pas les règles de la convenance, c'est-à-dire l'ivrogne. Cette manière de 'mal boire' s'oppose toutefois à une manière de 'bien boire' incarnée par l'image d'un 'honnête buveur' qui reste au fil des siècles profondément ancrée dans les mentalités françaises. En effet, une longue culture de l'ivresse et de l'enivrement promeut en France, au moins jusqu'à la fin de l'Ancien Régime, une image très fortement positive de l'alcool. Il s'agit de celle d'un buveur bon-vivant qui fait un usage modéré mais régulier de l'alcool, l'utilisant soit comme tonique soit comme thérapeutique.[4] Jusqu'au XVIIIe siècle, un discours répressif sur l'alcool a donc encore bien du mal à s'imposer en France.[5] Ivresse et ivrognerie se définissent avant tout comme un problème d'ordre quantitatif qui relève essentiellement de la morale individuelle. Selon les médecins, il s'agit donc d'un simple phénomène de débordement que l'ivrogne devrait pouvoir juguler, à condition de bien le vouloir.

Sur le plan physiologique, l'ivrognerie est traditionnellement diagnostiquée comme un phénomène de trop plein qui vient troubler le flux digestif. Les vapeurs nutritives qui, selon l'ancienne théorie des humeurs, servent à constituer le sang et la bile jaune (ces liquides nécessaires au bon fonctionnement de l'organisme) dégagent aussi, lors de la digestion, des vapeurs résiduelles, des sortes de déchets organiques qui prennent la forme d'un gaz ou d'un liquide toxique appelé par les médecins bile noire ou mélancolie (du grec *mêlas* : noir et *kholê* : bile). L'excès de bile noire, provoqué par exemple par un surplus de vin, encombre l'économie de l'organisme. Ces vapeurs digestives se frayent alors un chemin et remontent par la voie du sang jusqu'aux parties cérébrales où elles paralysent les sens et troublent la raison humaine.[6] À travers l'exemple de certains patriarches, le texte biblique met déjà en garde contre l'abus des boissons alcooliques qui provoque le délire et la déraison : dans le récit de la Genèse, Noé comme Lot se laissent aller à la débauche

3 Thomas d'Aquin, *Somme théologique II : la tempérance* (Paris : Cerf, 1999), p. 891.

4 Matthieu Lecoutre, *Ivresse et ivrognerie dans la France moderne* (Rennes : PUFR, 2011), pp. 31–53.

5 Ibid., pp. 47–53.

6 Sur la pathologie antique de la mélancolie voir Hélène Prigent, *Mélancolie : les métamorphoses de la dépression* (Paris : Gallimard, 2005), pp. 14–18.

suite à un excès de vin.[7] Toutefois, les troubles que provoque chez eux l'abus d'alcool sont représentés dans le récit biblique sous la forme d'un acte involontaire, d'une folie irresponsable. Le délire auquel ils s'adonnent se déroule, en effet, dans un état de complète inconscience, une absence de soi que rend manifeste le sommeil lourd de l'ivrogne. En outre, dans ces récits, la faute, l'outrage est d'abord provoqué par un tiers qui tire parti de l'absence à la fois physique et psychologique du buveur assommé d'ivresse. Une fois le trop-plein d'alcool évacué, il semble toutefois que le délire disparaisse et que le buveur, temporairement déviant, réintègre le groupe. Donc, si la figure de l'ivrogne est traditionnellement associée à celle du fou, cela ne se fait pas — encore — au sens pathologique du terme. Comme le rappelle Lecoutre, l'ivrogne est jusqu'à l'époque moderne perçu dans les mentalités comme une figure bouffonne et dérisoire, un sot que l'on rapproche du côté de l'animalité de la figure du 'singe' ou du 'pourceau', ou encore que l'on compare à un trou sans fond, symbole de ce corps qui a visiblement perdu toute maîtrise de ses flux.[8] Donc, à l'aube du XIXe siècle, l'ivrogne n'est pas encore à proprement parler un sujet médical.

Aux alentours de 1820, l'ivresse jusqu'ici tolérée à demi-mot prend cependant une forme nouvelle. Avec l'arrivée de nouvelles boissons distillées issues de la fabrication industrielle, de nouveaux alcools (absinthes, eaux-de-vie, et liqueurs vendues à bas prix) envahissent le marché. Comme le souligne Didier Nourrisson dans son étude centrale sur *Le Buveur du XIXe siècle*, c'est au milieu de ce siècle que l'ivresse alcoolique se démocratise.[9] Le loisir de s'alcooliser est mis à la portée de tous. Cafés, cabarets, estaminets pullulent et quadrillent rapidement l'espace français. Homme ou femme, du nourrisson à la bourgeoise, du Nord au Sud de l'hexagone, tout le monde boit, et ce dans des quantités aujourd'hui difficilement concevables. Sur la période qui nous intéresse, il faut donc se représenter une France littéralement imbibée d'alcool, un alcool qui, de surcroît, s'avère le plus souvent extrêmement toxique et se présente aux consommateurs sous la forme de gaz frelatés : le 'rouge' comme la 'blanche' vendus à l'ouvrier à quelques sous le verre dans les cabarets populaires sont généralement coupés ou bien entièrement élaborés à l'aide d'additifs chimiques (comme de l'arsenic ou de l'acide sulfurique) afin d'accélérer la production, d'optimiser le goût ou encore la couleur du produit. Ces alcools

7 Gn 9, *20–21* et Gn 19, *31–36*. Suite à un excès de vin, Noé se retrouve nu sous sa tente. Cham, l'un de ses fils, va profiter de la situation pour l'outrager. Lot est, lui, ennivré par ses filles pour qu'elles puissent avoir une relation incestueuse avec leur père.

8 Lecoutre, *Ivresse et ivrognerie*, pp. 110–20.

9 Didier Nourrisson, *Le Buveur du XIXe siècle* (Paris : Albin Michel, 1990), pp. 63–108.

et vins frelatés causent des troubles nerveux et psychiques graves chez les buveurs. La traditionnelle folie des ivrognes change radicalement de forme. Sa symptomatologie (troubles physiques, psychiques et comportementaux : tremblements, paralysie, délires, hallucinations, accès de violence) s'aggrave et développe désormais des formes chroniques. La nouvelle science psychiatrique qui se constitue à cette époque sous le nom d'aliénisme va alors faire du gros buveur un de ses objets d'étude privilégiés.

Au sein de l'ancien concept d'ivrognerie qui restait inchangé depuis des siècles, une distinction semble maintenant devenue nécessaire : l'ivresse traditionnellement 'gaie' et passagère du bon vivant (certes moralement répréhensible mais finalement plutôt inoffensive) laisse place de plus en plus souvent à un délire violent causé par l'abus du vin et des liqueurs spiritueuses. Dès les années 1820, dans les premiers services psychiatriques, les cliniciens repèrent la montée fulgurante de ces cas. À la fin du siècle, Pierre Garnier, médecin en chef des hôpitaux de Paris, résume en ces termes ce changement :

> Il semble bien que, de nos jours, grâce à la toxicité beaucoup plus grande des boissons alcooliques en usage, l'ivresse est à la fois plus prompte à se produire et surtout s'accompagne de troubles mentaux plus profonds et plus durables qu'autrefois. L'individu qui, après quelques manifestations bruyantes dues à de copieuses libations, allait coucher au violon et se réveillait, le lendemain, dégrisé et confus de son aventure, tend, de plus en plus, à céder la place à un ébrieux autrement plus violent et infiniment plus troublé. La symptomatologie et l'évolution de l'ivresse ont changé avec la nature des boissons enivrantes. Celle que nous voyons maintenant est aussi lente à se dissiper qu'elle est prompte à se produire : l'obnubilation psychique, les divagations se poursuivent pendant quarante-huit heures et plus [...]. Entre de tels dehors et ceux de l'aliénation mentale, les analogies ont paru assez grandes pour motiver un examen à l'infirmerie spéciale.[10]

C'est sur le terrain de l'aliénisme que la médecine moderne va donc immédiatement appréhender la déviance du gros buveur, et son image restera pour longtemps dépendante de cette approche psychiatrique. La figure de l'ivrogne perd alors ses allures bouffonnes et se confond désormais avec l'image du dégénéré et du criminel. Du coup, c'est aussi son acception dans le catalogue des vices qui va changer : l'ivrogne ne sera plus du côté des 'copieuses libations'

---

10 Dr Pierre Garnier, *La Folie à Paris : étude statistique, clinique et médico-légale* (Paris : Baillière, 1995), p. 13.

et de la *gula* qui menace le bon vivant ; c'est désormais du côté de l'acédie, de la psyché, et de la tête qu'il faudra aller le chercher. Car les premiers aliénistes attestent, à l'image d'Esquirol dans son *Traité des maladies mentales* publié en 1838, qu'il existe une corrélation évidente entre ivrognerie et folie psychiatrique. L'alcool rend fou, l'observation clinique le prouve. Mais les cliniciens du début de ce siècle ne peuvent pas encore expliquer son mécanisme. La pathogénie reste encore à trouver.

C'est le concept de maladie alcoolique avancé par le médecin suédois Magnus Huss peu avant 1850 qui va relancer le débat. À travers ce néologisme, Huss va pour la première fois proposer un fonctionnement précis de la maladie.[11]

Le monstre alcoolique

Ce qui fonde le nouveau concept d'alcoolisme introduit par les travaux de Huss en Europe vers le milieu du siècle, c'est avant tout l'idée d'un processus d'empoisonnement. L'alcoolisme se définit comme une intoxication chronique de tout l'organisme suite à la consommation de liquides alcooliques. Cette notion sera reprise et développée en France à partir des années 1860 à travers la théorie de l'auto-intoxication de Charles Bouchard,[12] qui va servir de clé

11 Magnus Huss fait paraître pour la première fois en 1849 une étude sur 'l'alcoolisme chronique'. La nouvelle théorie de Huss concernant la maladie alcoolique est très largement reprise en France, et ce dès le début des années 1860. Toutefois, la diffusion de ce nouveau concept ne se fait pas sous la forme d'une traduction intégrale de son œuvre, mais exclusivement sous la forme d'articles résumés, comme celui d'Étienne Lancereaux paru dans *Le Dictionnaire des sciences médicales* en 1865, et qui simplifient, atténuent en grande part l'orientation très fortement neurologique qu'Huss avait donnée initialement à ses recherches. Avec le nouveau concept d'alcoolisme Huss avait, en effet, pour la première fois, voulu instaurer une distinction très nette, établissant ainsi une frontière séparant le problème fort ancien de l'ivrognerie relevant de la morale, d'un écart de conduite, une manière de 'mal boire' d'un côté, d'un nouvel objet scientifique, de l'autre : l'alcoolisme, qui relève, quant à lui, désormais du domaine médical. Les synthèses qui font connaître en France le travail de Huss gomment en grande partie cette distinction essentielle que Huss avait souhaité établir. La vulgarisation de sa pensée scientifique conduit en France à une sorte de confusion, à une 'démédicalisation' de ses théories qui visaient pourtant, justement, à isoler une nouvelle pathologie, à identifier une pathogénie précise pour la maladie du trop boire afin de faire passer l'image du traditionnel buveur débauché du côté du malade nécessitant des soins.

12 Charles Bouchard (1837–1915) fût médecin et professeur de pathologie générale à la Faculté de médecine de Paris. Ami de Charcot et Brissaud, il publie en 1887 ses *Leçons*

d'explication essentielle jusqu'à la fin du siècle pour éclairer l'origine de pathologies nerveuses encore mal définies et qui posent problème à l'œil du clinicien. L'alcoolisme, comme nombre de pathologies nerveuses, est en effet considéré pour l'heure comme une maladie *sine materia*. C'est-à-dire que la démarche anatomo-clinique n'arrive pas encore à déterminer la cause organique précise qui permettrait de retracer de manière visible l'origine lésionnelle ou bien encore le cheminement de la maladie à l'intérieur du corps. La théorie de l'auto-intoxication de Bouchard affirme, quant à elle, que des résidus gazeux issus de la digestion seraient capables d'empoisonner le corps, ce qui provoquerait et expliquerait l'apparition de maladies. Sans la nommer, la théorie de l'auto-intoxication de Charles Bouchard revitalise en fait, en plein XIXe siècle, l'action de la bile noire tirée de l'ancien système humoral dans l'imaginaire d'une science médicale qui se veut pourtant résolument positiviste.

La notion d'auto-intoxication sur laquelle se fonde le nouveau concept d'alcoolisme nécessite aussi de penser désormais une dimension évolutive au sein même de l'histoire de la maladie : le concept d'alcoolisme introduit en ce sens un point de bascule dans l'ancienne pathogénie du trop boire, il implique un moment de rupture à partir duquel l'ivrogne traditionnel se transformerait en alcoolique. C'est sur ces bases et en particulier grâce à la nouvelle notion de métamorphose introduite par la théorie de Huss que les autorités vont alors pouvoir débattre à nouveau de la question de la faute et qu'elles vont pouvoir redéfinir la responsabilité juridique du buveur. Cette question se fait de plus en plus pressante tout au long de la seconde moitié du XIXe siècle face à la montée fulgurante des cas de folies alcooliques généralement associés à des crimes et délits graves. Dans ses écrits consacrés à la naissance du système psychiatrique en France, Michel Foucault a parfaitement rappelé combien cette nouvelle branche du savoir clinique s'est formée à ses débuts sur la base d'une pensée très fortement pénaliste et moralisante, en grande partie en raison d'un système juridique qui restait jusqu'ici déficient quand il s'agissait de juger les actes criminels de malades déments.[13] L'article 64 du Code Pénal (qui date de 1810 et qui ne sera abrogé qu'en 1992 !) affirme en effet qu'il n'y a ni crime ni délit, lorsque le prévenu

---

sur les auto-intoxications dans les maladies (Paris : Savy, 1887). Face à un premier courant de pensée qui, durant la seconde moitié du XIXe siècle pense dans le champs de la médecine que le corps sain tombe malade suite à l'agression d'un élément étranger extérieur (bactérie, virus), la théorie de l'auto-intoxication de Charles Bouchard défend au contraire l'idée que le corps sain peut lui-même secréter des substances toxiques dans son milieu intérieur qu'il arrive à éliminer à l'état dit 'normal' de santé, impliquant ainsi l'individu tout entier dans le processus d'éclosion de sa maladie.

13 Voir Michel Foucault, *Les Anormaux* (Paris : Gallimard/Seuil, 1999), p. 107.

était en état de démence au temps de l'action ou lorsqu'il a été contraint par une force à laquelle il n'a pu résister. Alors, comme le souligne Foucault, pour combler ce vide juridique, face à la montée inexorable des cas d'aliénation alcoolique qui nécessitent généralement l'internement de malades de plus en plus violents, la nouvelle science psychiatrique a dû rapidement rationaliser, responsabiliser la folie du buveur :

> Avant d'être une spécialité de la médecine, la psychiatrie s'est institutionnalisée comme domaine particulier de la protection sociale. [...] la psychiatrie, pour pouvoir exister comme institution de savoir, c'est-à-dire comme savoir médical fondé et justifiable, a dû procéder à deux codages simultanés. Il a fallu en effet, d'une part, coder la folie comme maladie ; il a fallu pathologiser les désordres, les erreurs, les illusions de la folie ; il a fallu procéder à des analyses (symptomatologie, nosographie, pronostics, observations, dossiers cliniques, etc. [...]. Il a fallu en même temps coder la folie comme danger, c'est à dire qu'il a fallu faire apparaître la folie comme porteuse de périls.[14]

Aimé Riant consacre en 1886 une grande partie de son mémoire intitulé *Les Irresponsables devant la justice* aux criminels alcooliques. Il constate :

> Devant l'alcoolisme envahissant, généralisé, dans des conditions toutes nouvelles et de plus en plus fatales, le médecin expert peut-il méconnaître la cause du mal, laisser frapper impitoyablement un malade ? N'est-il pas exposé, d'autre part, à faire absoudre un criminel, parce qu'il a trouvé en lui des traces d'alcoolisme ?
>
> Jamais la science n'a poussé ni si loin ni si haut ses recherches. L'hérédité, l'atavisme constatés, est-ce assez pour conclure à l'atténuation, à la suppression de la responsabilité ?
>
> Ainsi, de 1826 à 1830, la moyenne annuelle est de 129 accusés. De 1876 à 1880, la moyenne annuelle est de 809 accusés. Des recherches récentes, faites sur les crimes contre les personnes, tant en France qu'à l'étranger, on peut conclure que les crimes commis sous l'influence de l'alcool représentent à peu près 60.[15]

Grâce au nouveau concept d'alcoolisme, la médecine clinique va donc pouvoir dédoubler, complexifier la figure unique, traditionnelle de l'ivrogne. Loin de relever d'une dichotomie, le couple ivrogne-alcoolique qui s'impose à partir

---

14 Ibid., pp. 109–10.

15 Aimé Riant, *Les Irresponsables devant la justice* (Paris : Baillière, 1888), pp. 100–02.

des années 1850, suite à la naissance de ce nouveau concept, est en réalité fondé sur une figure du double dans laquelle s'oppose celui qui boit parce qu'il le veut bien (l'ivrogne) à celui qui boit mais pour qui la question du vouloir finalement ne se pose plus (l'alcoolique). Car la théorie de Huss et la pathogénie qui l'accompagne inscrivent irrémédiablement le vice de l'ivrogne dans la chair même du buveur. L'alcoolique et l'alcoolisme relèvent alors en quelque sorte, selon les médecins, d'une forme de distorsion pathologique, d'un vice de forme de l'ivrognerie et par là-même du monstrueux.

Le monstre alcoolique

Dans ses écrits, Huss définit l'alcoolisme comme 'un processus d'empoisonnement chronique, tant par l'effet direct de l'alcool sur le sang que par la modification de la composition du sang'.[16] Le changement de paradigme est décisif. C'est la longue tradition d'un corps machine, capable d'assimiler et d'évacuer les substances ingérées qui est maintenant remise en cause. C'est aussi une conception plus fortement chimiste du corps qui s'impose et qui visualise la possibilité de transformations intracellulaires capables de modifier sur le long terme l'état général du malade. Ce qui fonde le concept d'alcoolisme, c'est donc à l'origine l'idée d'une métamorphose radicale et, d'une certaine manière, irrémédiable de l'ivrogne puisque celle-ci engage une modification profonde de son métabolisme. Dans les années suivantes, la sémiologie médicale affine encore son diagnostic : l'empoisonnement du buveur se manifeste par exemple de manière visible, à l'examen clinique, à travers un abaissement significatif de la température du malade. Ce refroidissement trahit alors à la surface du corps un processus avancé de décomposition, 'de cadavérisation' selon l'expression d'Ernest Monin, qui agit d'abord de manière souterraine, invisible, à l'intérieur de l'organisme :

> L'alcoolique subit, peu à peu, une asphyxie lente, il devient un animal à sang froid. Le sang, mêlé de particules graisseuses, subit, en même temps qu'un abaissement de chaleur, une déformation de ses globules. D'où, l'anémie du buveur et son état de faiblesse générale, ses hémorragies

16 D'après la traduction de Renaudin, 'De l'Alcoolisme chronique par M. le Docteur Magnus Huss', *Annales médico-psychologiques*, vol. 5 (1853), pp. 60–88. L'œuvre de Huss sera diffusée en France sur la base de cet article résumant en français le contenu de sa nouvelle théorie.

> faciles (taches scorbutiques, purpura) et enfin le hideux cortège de maux qui vient assaillir tout son organisme.[17]

Désormais, la référence à l'animalité du buveur n'est donc plus à chercher du côté du singe ou du pourceau mais bien du côté du serpent tentateur de la Bible. Cette figure diabolique, revivifiée au goût du jour par l'imaginaire médical du XIXe siècle, est reprise dans de nombreux récits littéraires : au sein du courant naturaliste bien sûr, mais pas seulement, car la plaie sociale de l'alcoolisme occupe tous les genres (poésie, théâtre, romans …) et tous les courants littéraires des années 1850–1900.[18] Citons ici en particulier la figure omniprésente du serveur, du tenancier ou du buveur alcoolique en littérature, généralement représentés comme des tentateurs qui essayent d'entrainer d'autres buveurs vers le péché capital de l'alcoolisme auquel ils se sont voués.

Dans les récits de cas cliniques ou littéraires, l'alcoolique est caractérisé par son allure spectrale. Ce-dernier entretient un lien tout à fait particulier avec la mort car son corps s'apparente dans l'imaginaire médical de l'époque à l'image d'une charogne en état de putréfaction qui corrompt et contamine ses contemporains. Ce processus de décomposition interne caractéristique de la maladie alcoolique repose, selon les médecins, sur un double mécanisme. Il s'agit de deux principes parfois quasi concomitants : d'abord un principe de dilatation graisseuse suivi ensuite d'une asphyxie des organes due à cette hypertrophie qui amollit et sclérose rapidement les différents tissus. De là découlent les stigmates extérieurs, visibles, de la maladie du buveur (paralysie générale, anémie …). Les planches anatomiques élaborés pour l'enseignement antialcoolique dans les écoles primaires vers la fin du siècle exposent clairement ce principe. Marcel Pagnol évoque par exemple dans ses *Souvenirs d'enfance* qui remontent au début des années 1900 :

> ces tableaux effrayants qui tapissaient les murs des classes. On y voyait des foies rougeâtres et si parfaitement méconnaissables, à cause de leurs *boursouflures vertes*, et de *leurs étranglements violacés* qui leur donnaient la forme d'un topinambour : mais pour éclairer ce désastre, l'artiste avait peint, au beau milieu du tableau, le foie appétissant du bon citoyen, dont

17 Ernest Monin, *L'Alcoolisme : étude médico-sociale* (Paris : Doin, 1889), p. 50.

18 Citons ici, à titre d'exemple, en poésie : le cycle sur le Vin de Charles Baudelaire dans *Les Fleurs du mal* ainsi que le poème 'Aumône' de Mallarmé qui mettent en scène des personnages de buveurs déviants, et, au théâtre : le Vaudeville *L'Affaire de la rue Lourcine* d'Eugène Labiche qui, dès la fin des années 1850, à travers le personnage de Lenglumé, dresse le portrait d'un bourgeois oisif aux penchants alcooliques.

> la masse harmonieuse et le rouge triomphal permettaient de mesurer la gravité des catastrophes circonscrites.[19]

L'empâtement du buveur bon-vivant, si louable jusqu'ici dans la tradition de l'ivresse, devient donc, dans le nouveau concept d'empoisonnement alcoolique, un signe extérieur visible de maladie. La décomposition interne du buveur, masquée d'abord sous ces signes apparents — mais trompeurs — de bonne santé, s'affirme par la suite sous la forme d'une déliquescence, d'un amollissement général qui affecte non seulement l'apparence physique mais aussi toute la personnalité du buveur. Car le liquide alcoolique s'infiltre et imbibe les tissus, il humecte le corps jusqu'à la fibre nerveuse. Or c'est elle qui soutenait et assurait jusqu'ici la fermeté et le tonus de tout l'organisme. La nouvelle théorie de l'empoisonnement par l'alcool annule donc et retourne ce mécanisme. Sous l'effet de l'alcool, le corps de l'ivrogne devient humide et froid. Le tonus de la fibre se dérègle, les tissus se ramollissent, la mécanique du corps humain se détraque. En particulier sa volonté, sa moralité s'étiolent.

L'alcool déshumanise l'homme, médecins et moralistes sont là-dessus unanimes depuis des siècles. Mais le discours a changé sous le coup des nouvelles lois de l'évolution et de la biologie. La bestialité de l'homme ivre est devenue visible, concrète, incarnée dans sa chair. L'alcoolique se distingue à travers une pilosité marquée, signe, bien sûr, de sa négligence, mais aussi et surtout de sa chute sur l'échelle de l'évolution à la fois biologique et morale de l'humanité. Les propos moralisateurs des médecins hygiénistes et des théoriciens de la dégénérescence se fondent sur une parole religieuse fort ancienne qui définissait communément l'enivré comme un être 'au-dessous de la bête', comme le précise ici l'homélie contre l'ivrognerie de Basile-le-Grand au IVᵉ siècle :

> Celui qui par ivresse éteint les lumières de son intelligence se rend semblable aux bêtes de somme, et se ravale jusqu'à elles (Ps. 48.13). Que dis-je ne se met-il pas même plus bas que les animaux qui broutent ? […] Celui qui boit avec excès altère l'usage de ses sens, et se met encore par là au-dessous de la bête.[20]

Mais, si la rhétorique chrétienne insistait jusqu'ici pour renvoyer l'ivrogne dans un 'en-deça' des lois naturelles qui le déréalisait et en faisait ainsi une simple

19 Marcel Pagnol, *Souvenirs d'enfance : la gloire de mon père*, dans *Œuvres complètes* III (Paris : Fallois, 1857), p. 19, je souligne.

20 Basile le Grand, *Homélie contre l'ivrognerie* (Lyon : François Guyot, 1827), p. 172.

aberration de l'entendement, les nouvelles lois de l'évolution et de la biologie, au contraire, redonnent, elles, corps à la bête. Elles relocalisent le buveur dans une pensée de l'involution pathologique mais aussi de l'involution morale et civilisationnelle qui le fait accéder désormais au rang de monstre, au sens cette fois pleinement étymologique du terme. Ce changement dans le discours répressif sur l'alcool est tout particulièrement sensible dans le livre d'antialcoolisme destiné à l'enseignement scolaire. Vers la fin du siècle, on enseigne en effet dans les écoles primaires que l'ivresse rabaisse l'homme 'au rang de la bête'. Reclassé dans un 'en-deça' désormais bien visible — grâce aux nouvelles lois de l'évolution — de l'involution pathologique, le corps de l'alcoolique dès lors fait signe. À travers ses symptômes, il affiche la preuve tangible d'une sclérose généralisée, d'un principe de dégénérescence qui touche à la fois le corps organique de l'individu malade mais qui contamine aussi, à une autre échelle, l'ensemble de la société.

Aux yeux de cette nouvelle pathogénie et de la symptomatologie nerveuse qui caractérise l'alcoolisme, le lien entre alcoolisme et dégénérescence est en effet vite établi. Durant la seconde moitié du siècle, Bénédicte-Augustin Morel (1857), Valentin Magnan (1874, 1893) et Marcel Legrain (1889) fondent le concept de dégénérescence en rapport étroit avec le nouveau concept d'alcoolisme.[21] D'après la perspective fortement religieuse et eschatologique choisie par Morel, le 'rabougrissement', l'affaiblissement progressif de l'espèce humaine seraient dus à des facteurs à la fois environnementaux et héréditaires parmi lesquels l'alcoolisme apparaît comme le plus important. Relevant à la fois d'une influence du milieu et du terrain biologique, l'alcoolisme est perçu par les spécalistes comme une force dégénérative hors-norme qui s'autopotentialise.[22] Le corps du buveur est perçu comme le lieu de germination et de prolifération sans fin des plus grandes maladies de ce siècle : pneumonie, tuberculose, choléra, paralysie générale, fièvre typhoide, épilepsie, hystérie,

---

21 Voir Morel, *Traité des dégénérescences* (Paris : Baillière, 1857) ; *Traité des maladies mentales* (Paris : Masson, 1860) ; Dr Magnan, *De l'Alcoolisme et des diverses formes du délire alcoolique* (Paris : Delahaye, 1874), *L'Alcoolisme, folie des héréditaires dégénérés* (Paris : Masson, 1893) ; Legrain, *Hérédité et alcoolisme : étude psychologique et clinique sur les dégénérés buveurs et familles d'ivrognes* (Paris : Doin, 1889).

22 Cf. Legrain, *Du délire chez les dégénérés : observations prises à l'asile Saint-Anne, 1885–1886* (Paris : Delahaye et Lecrosnier, 1886) : 'L'alcoolisme est une des causes les plus puissantes de la dégénérescence mentale, en d'autres termes les fils d'alcooliques sont des dégénérés. Les rapports qui existent entre l'alcoolisme et la dégénérescence mentale se résument donc dans ce terrible cercle vicieux qui trouve sa confirmation aujourd'hui dans une infinité d'observations médicales les plus éloquentes' (pp. 251–52).

syphilis. Toutes ces pathologies sont, d'après les médecins, favorisées par le terrain alcoolique.

Alcoolisme et acédie

Ce qui dans le grand tableau nosographique de la dégénérescence distingue cependant l'alcoolique des autres malades, c'est qu'à l'origine l'alcoolique a, selon les médecins, et ce malgré l'atavisme, le choix de céder ou non à son vice. L'alcoolique est donc perçu comme un dégénéré hors-norme. Les études sur l'alcoolisme de la fin du XIXe siècle reprennent encore de manière quasi unanime la position de Saint-Thomas et affirment : 'à moins d'être produite accidentellement ou à l'insu du sujet, chose assez rare, l'ivresse est un état imputable entièrement à la volonté'.[23] Le penchant premier de l'ivrogne pour la boisson, qui le pousse vers l'alcoolisme, continue donc d'être perçu comme un problème relevant essentiellement de la morale et de la volonté individuelle. L'éducation des masses devient alors pour les médecins une priorité. Ils se transforment en véritables prosélytes et prêchent la bonne parole antialcoolique jusque sur les bancs des écoles.

Pour lutter efficacement contre l'alcoolisme, la clinique moderne met en place une rhétorique qui se réapproprie l'ancien catalogue des vices diffusé par la morale chrétienne. Mais le savoir scientifique y opère toutefois un réajustement décisif : la cartographie des péchés s'y retrouve très nettement redéfinie et vient désormais se concentrer autour d'un seul péché capital dont semblent découler tous les autres : il s'agit du péché d'acédie, un péché fort ancien mais jusqu'ici très largement tombé dans l'oubli.

Étymologiquement, l'acédie chrétienne est tirée du mot grec *akèdia* qui signifie de manière générale le manque de soin, l'indifférence et l'irrespect vis-à-vis des lois et de l'obligation morale, une négligence envers soi et les autres. Cette notion est reprise du monde grec par l'Église chrétienne au IVe siècle et introduite dans le système des péchés sous la forme d'une lassitude, d'une torpeur mélancolique et dangereuse qui pousse le croyant à se détourner de Dieu. Cette paresse dépressive généralement accompagnée d'instabilité et d'accès de colère, est le signe d'une attaque du démon et la preuve d'une tentation qu'il faut apprendre à surmonter. Si acédie et mélancolie sont des notions qui renvoient, l'une, au domaine du vice, l'autre, à la maladie, ces deux types de désordre (moral ou organique) représentent en fait dès l'Antiquité un doublet, deux dimensions complémentaires attribuées à un même mal qui se

23 Monin, *L'Alcoolisme : étude médico-sociale*, p. 133.

manifeste sous la forme d'une paresse excessive, un abattement physique et mental menant généralement à la folie, à la mort, ou au suicide.[24]

Il faut noter que, jusqu'au XVIIIe siècle, la paresse ne constitue pas vraiment un trait consubstantiel du buveur. L'endormissement et la fatigue sont pour le moment des conséquences physiques de l'abus, des troubles passagers liés à la boisson et non au caractère inné du malade. Ce sera la grande nouveauté du XIXe siècle. Le regard clinique va rapidement faire de la paresse et de cet abattement physique et psychique caractéristique du buveur, un élément central du mal alcoolique. D'abord, parce que les lois de la nouvelle chimie organique, énoncées dans les années 1850–60 par Liebig ou Pasteur, affirment que les nouvelles boissons alcooliques élaborées généralement à partir de grains, du sucre de la betterave ou de la pomme de terre alourdissent et perturbent l'économie de l'organisme. En raison de leur base amylacée ou sucrée, elles provoquent, à court terme, la somnolence et l'apathie du buveur, à long terme, des dilatations graisseuses, une hypertrophie des organes, un embonpoint trompeur qui en réalité étouffe l'être, sclérose les tissus, et provoque leur étranglement.[25] L'iconographie de la seconde moitié du XIXe siècle représente systématiquement le buveur la tête lourde de pensées déviantes, et, de manière récurrente, met en scène l'alcoolique dans la pose caractéristique de la mélancolie.[26] Ce mal antique, rappelé à la science par le savant anglais Robert Burton au XVIIe siècle et qui perdure par la suite dans la pensée médicale à travers la théorie des esprits animaux, va être rationalisé et pathologisé au sein de la nouvelle approche psychiatrique de la maladie alcoolique. Dès les années 1820, sous l'influence du courant hygiéniste, la mélancolie, ce délire causé par des gaz nutritifs extrêmement corrosifs et trompeurs corrompant les sens et l'esprit, va être de nouveau intimement liée à l'ancien concept d'acédie sous l'aspect d'une force débilitante et d'une passion oppressive.

Maîtrise et hygiène du corps sont devenues au XIXe siècle les nouvelles valeurs d'une société dominée par un modernisme galopant. Alors, si tonus et fermeté sont signes de bonne santé, mollesse et relâchement signalent au

---

24 À propos de la parenté entre acédie et mélancolie, voir Yves Hersant, *Mélancolies de l'antiquité au XXe siècle* (Paris : Robert Laffon, 2005), pp. 775–82 ; Bernard Forthomme, *Émergence et résurgence de l'acédie*, dans *Tristesse, acédie et médecine des âmes*, éd. par Nathalie Nabert (Paris : Beauschesne, 2005), pp. 15–35.

25 Justus Liebig, *Nouvelles lettres sur la chimie* (Paris : Charpentier, 1852), pp. 134–37.

26 Citons ici à titre d'exemple pour les années 1880–1900 : *La Prune* de Manet (1878), *Les Buveurs d'absinthe ou les déclassés* de Jean-Francois Rafaelli (1881), *La Buveuse* de Toulouse Lautrec (1887–88), *Le Buveur d'absinthe* de viktor Oliva (1889–1901), *Femme au café* de Pablo Picasso (1901–1902), *Les Buveurs d'absinthe* de Jean Béraud (1908).

contraire une distorsion morale de l'être, comme on peut par exemple le lire dans le livre de morale destiné à l'enseignement scolaire (1895) :

> Le travail est à la fois une nécessité et un devoir pour l'homme. Il lui permet de subvenir à ses besoins et à ceux de sa famille, lui donne plaisir et santé et ennoblit son existence. L'oisiveté, au contraire, engendre la misère et est la mère de tous les vices. *Celui qui ne fait rien n'est pas loin de mal faire.*[27]

L'apathie du buveur, c'est le mal qui couve en lui et qui le rend sensible à la tentation comme le souligne Bergeron :

> L'alcool fait de l'ouvrier laborieux un paresseux et un envieux, un voleur et souvent pis encore, mais à coup sûr une recrue toute prête pour l'émeute, à laquelle le poussera tôt ou tard un autre buveur, un lettré celui-là, grand faiseur de promesses, qui, n'ayant jamais su se gouverner lui-même, aspire à gouverner les peuples par la plume ou par la parole.[28]

Lors de l'anamnèse, oisiveté, et paresse sont souvent diagnostiquées par les médecins comme causes premières et conséquences directes de l'ivrognerie. Dans l'article de synthèse que Lancereaux rédige en 1865 dans le *Dictionnaire encyclopédique des sciences médicales à propos de la nouvelle notion d'alcoolisme*, on peut lire :

> Parmi les causes morales propres à engendrer l'intempérance, on doit placer avant tout l'oisiveté. [...] Le goût de la dissipation, la légèreté de caractère, les causes tant excitantes que déprimantes sont encore autant de circonstances qui favorisent le vice de l'ivrognerie.[29]

L'oisiveté pousse à boire celui qui ne boit pas, tandis que la paresse enferme le malade dans son vice. Vers la fin des années 1880, le manque de volonté morale s'imposent aux cliniciens comme un des plus grands fléaux de cette fin

---

27 Louis Boyer, *Livre de morale des écoles primaires*, p. 187.

28 Bergeron, *Rapport sur la répression de l'alcoolisme*. Académie de médecine, séance du 5 décembre 1871. Cité par Nourrisson, *Le Buveur du XIXe siècle*, p. 196.

29 Lancereaux, *Alcoolisme*, p. 690.

de siècle. Et la faiblesse du vouloir semble alors à leurs yeux expliquer l'origine d'un très grand nombre de maladies mentales.[30]

Apathie, inactivité et langueur mélancolique sont le ressort récurrent de nombreux récits littéraires qui traitent à cette époque de l'alcoolisme. Voici, par exemple, le portrait que Huysmans fait de son héroïne Marthe dans le roman éponyme intitulé aussi *Histoire d'une fille*, qui paraît pour la première fois en 1876 :

> C'était, au reste, une singulière fille. Des ardeurs étranges, un dégoût de métier, une haine de misère, une aspiration maladive d'inconnu, une désespérance non résignée [...]
>
> Une appétence de bien-être et d'éclat, un alanguissement morbide, une disposition à la névrose qu'elle tenait de son père, une certaine paresse instinctive qu'elle tenait de sa mère, si brave dans les moments pénibles, si lâche quand la nécessite ne la tenaillait point, fourmillaient et bouillonnaient furieusement en elle.
>
> L'atelier n'était malheureusement pas fait pour raffermir son courage à bout de force, pour relever sa vertu aux abois.[31]

Mais la paresse n'est pas l'apanage du prolétariat ouvrier. Il est intéressant de relever que la littérature permet là de dépasser certains tabous de l'epistémè scientifique, en particulier en ce qui concerne l'alcoolisme dans la classe aisée. À travers la figure du flâneur, la littérature évoque très souvent le personnage d'un rentier plongé dans l'inertie et qui est, aux yeux des médecins, l'incarnation même de cet alcoolique oisif qui peuple très largement les rangs de la bonne société mais que la science a bien du mal à interroger. Le vaudeville *L'Affaire de la rue de Lourcine* d'Eugène Labiche (1857) qui met en scène les instincts criminels de gros buveurs de la haute société est, en ce sens, à la date où il paraît, véritablement révolutionnaire. Quelques années plus tard, le personnage du flâneur oisif tenté par l'alcoolisme se retrouve aussi chez Hector Malot à travers le personnage de Maurice dans la trilogie intitulée *Victimes d'amour* (1862) ou encore chez Maupassant dans la nouvelle 'Garçon un Bock !' qui paraît pour la première fois dans *Gil Blas* en 1884. Dans ce texte, Maupassant semble avoir

---

30 Voir les travaux de Théodule Ribot, *Les Maladies de la volonté* (Paris : Felix Alcan, 1888) ; Jules Dejerine, *L'Hérédité dans les maladies du système nerveux* (Paris : Asselin et Houzeau, 1886) ; Paul-Emile Lévy, *L'Éducation rationnelle de la volonté. Son emploi thérapeutique* (Paris : Felix Alcan 1899).

31 Joris-Karl Huysmans, *Marthe : histoire d'une fille* (Paris : Galaade, 2010), pp. 22–23.

parfaitement relevé le mécanisme déclencheur de l'alcoolisme tel que le relaie le discours hygiéniste de l'époque, qui établit un lien direct entre les notions de paresse et d'oisiveté et cette nouvelle pathologie. La nouvelle s'ouvre sur ces mots du narrateur qui, en véritable flâneur, se laisse attirer dans une brasserie :

> Pourquoi suis-je entré, ce soir-là dans cette brasserie ? Je n'en sais rien. Il faisait froid. Une fine pluie, une poussière d'eau voltigeait, [...]. Je n'allais nulle part. Je marchais un peu après dîner. Je passai le Crédit Lyonnais, la rue Vivienne, d'autres rues encore. J'aperçus soudain une grande brasserie à moitié pleine. J'entrai, sans aucune raison. Je n'avais pas soif.[32]

Il reconnaît alors un bockeur (c'est-à-dire un buveur de bière) qui s'avère être le comte Jean des Barrets, un ancien camarade de collège. À la vague question : 'qu'est-ce que tu fais ?', le comte répond par une diatribe contre le travail qu'il rythme à coups de bocks de bière :

> « À quoi bon travailler ?
> [...]
> moi, je ne fais rien, je me laisse aller, je vieillis. En mourant je ne regretterai rien. Je n'aurai pas d'autre souvenir que cette brasserie. Pas de femme, pas d'enfants, pas de soucis, pas de chagrins, rien. Ça vaut mieux.
> [...]
> Je me lève à midi, je viens ici, je déjeune, je bois des bocks, j'attends la nuit, je dîne, je bois des bocks ; puis, vers une heure et demie du matin, je retourne me coucher, parce qu'on ferme. C'est ce qui m'embête le plus. Depuis dix ans, j'ai passé six années sur cette banquette, dans mon coin ; et le reste dans mon lit, jamais ailleurs. »
> [...]
> Je le regardais bien en face. Sa figure ridée, mal soignée, semblait presque celle d'un vieillard. Sur le sommet du crâne, quelques longs cheveux voltigeaient au-dessus de la peau d'une propreté douteuse. Il avait des sourcils énormes, une forte moustache et une barbe épaisse. J'eus brusquement, je ne sais pourquoi, la vision d'une cuvette d'eau noirâtre, l'eau où aurait été lavé tout ce poil.[33]

32 Guy de Maupassant, 'Garçon, un bock !', dans *Contes et nouvelles* (Paris : Gallimard, 2014), p. 818.

33 Ibid., pp. 819–20.

De l'eau donc, pour laver le vice, pour purger la bête, mais de l'eau dans laquelle le corps du buveur en même temps disparaît et s'efface. Sur le plan physiologique, l'alcoolique se liquéfie. Son corps est mou, flasque, informe. La déliquescence des organes étant ainsi en quelque sorte le prolongement logique, l'aboutissement d'une mollesse morale qui commence avec l'oisiveté. Dans *L'Assommoir* (1876), Gervaise prend conscience de cette altérité effrayante en voyant son ombre roulée sur les grands boulevards :

> Et brusquement, elle aperçut son ombre par terre. Quand elle approchait d'un bec de gaz, l'ombre vague se ramassait et se précisait, *une ombre énorme, trapue, grotesque tant elle était ronde. Cela s'étalait, le ventre, la gorge, les hanches, coulant et flottant ensemble.* Elle louchait si fort de la jambe, que, sur le sol, l'ombre faisait la culbute à chaque pas ; un vrai guignol ! Puis, lorsqu'elle s'éloignait, le guignol grandissait, devenait géant, emplissait le boulevard, avec des révérences qui lui cassaient le nez contre les arbres et contre les maisons. Mon Dieu ! qu'elle était drôle et effrayante ! *Jamais elle n'avait si bien compris son avachissement.*[34]

Conclusion

La fusion qui s'opère dans la seconde moitié du XIXe siècle entre l'ancienne figure de l'ivrogne et la nouvelle figure de l'alcoolique, autour de ce noyau d'explication essentiel qu'est devenue l'acédie alcoolique dans la pensée médicale moderne, est particulièrement repérable si l'on s'intéresse à l'iconographie que diffuse la propagande antialcoolique à cette époque. C'est cette donnée essentielle, réactualisée par la science et la morale bourgeoise axée sur le progrès et le travail, qui va permettre aux cliniciens d'identifier enfin l'origine du mal et d'établir pour cette maladie une étiologie claire autour de laquelle l'histoire du buveur va pouvoir se tisser, le ramenant ainsi de manière implacable à son vice.

Une première image est une carte postale éditée aux alentours de 1900 (Fig. 3.1). Elle représente un buveur qui n'a pas encore sombré dans l'alcoolisme : ses vêtements sont bien tenus. Cet homme se fait servir par un garçon qui représente une allégorie de la mort. Le geste de boire de cet ivrogne n'est pas encore intériorisé. Il nécessite un intermédiaire et pose ainsi la question du choix volontaire de céder — ou non — à la tentation du démon de l'alcoolisme. Mais la figure du garçon de café annonce aussi à l'observateur le sort

---

34 Émile Zola, *L'Assommoir* (Paris : Gallimard, 1978), pp. 447–48. Je souligne.

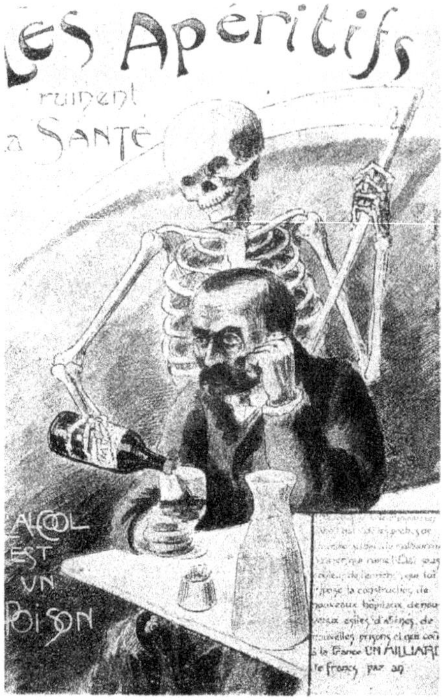

FIGURE 3.1
'Les Apéritifs ruinent la santé', carte postale, vers 1900 (coll. particulière).

réservé à cet alcoolique en devenir. L'ivrogne prend la pose caractéristique de la mélancolie : ses yeux sont ouverts, le regard est fixe et son front proéminent indique — d'après les lois de la craniométrie en vogue à l'époque — un net penchant pour le crime. Si ce buveur n'est pas encore un alcoolique au sens médical du terme, il n'est plus cette figure d'ivrogne risible, de noceur ridicule que véhiculait la tradition. Avec la naissance du concept d'alcoolisme, l'ivrogne est lui aussi devenu un personnage en rupture totale avec les lois sociales de son époque. La table marque d'ailleurs une opposition très nette entre l'observateur extérieur que nous sommes (et que la fonction didactique de l'image souhaite inscrire visiblement, à l'opposé du buveur, du côté du bien, de la santé, de la morale bourgeoise), tandis que l'ivrogne se retrouve, lui, rejeté de l'autre côté de cet espace, déclassé dans un monde à part, qui est celui de la marginalité malsaine. Car l'ivrogne-malade s'y confond déjà en arrière-plan avec l'avenir de sa maladie : le démon de l'alcoolisme, symbole de mort et de corruption.

Concluons sur cette dernière image (Fig. 3.2) : un tableau mural élaboré par Legrain pour l'enseignement scolaire vers la fin du siècle. Il représente un alcoolique qu'on reconnaît tout de suite à son aspect négligé et à son

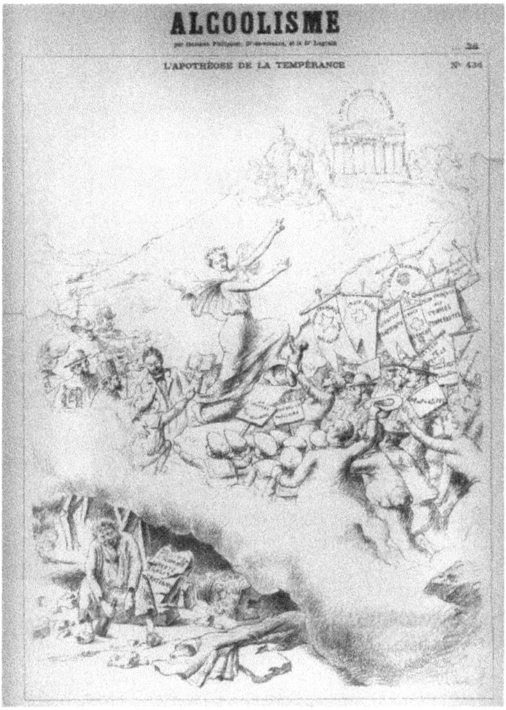

FIGURE 3.2
'L'Alcoolisme : L'apothéose de la tempérance', tableau mural (coll. Émile Deyrolle, planche n°434).

avachissement significatif. L'alcoolique est enfermé dans un en deçà de la civilisation symbolisé par une grotte qui pourrait aussi être l'antre de l'enfer. Lourd et hébété d'ivresse, le corps de l'alcoolique semble attiré vers le sol. Sa chute est symbolisée à deux niveaux : une double dégradation, à la fois biologique et morale, sur le plan de l'évolution humaine. L'alcoolique est relégué au rang de la bête, retombé dans une pré-histoire de l'humanité. Des ordures jonchent le sol, les tables de la loi républicaine sont brisées derrière lui et, à ses côtés, un poignard démontre sa volonté criminelle. Enfermé dans cet espace d'une inhumanité hors-norme, la rupture entre l'alcoolique et la société est totale : tout l'oppose à l'au-delà de la morale bourgeoise dont il s'est visiblement détourné et dans lequel, la Bible à la main, des représentants des ligues de tempérance, des enfants et des pères de famille, travailleurs abstinents, gravissent l'olympe de la civilisation bourgeoise.

La pensée scientifique du XIXe siècle revivifie au goût du jour un péché chrétien tombé dans l'oubli. C'est la notion ancienne d'acédie, en lien avec la notion de mélancolie antique, qui va permettre à l'imaginaire de la science positiviste de transformer de manière radicale — et ce pour longtemps — l'image traditionnelle du gros buveur en faisant passer ce malade du côté de l'alcoolisme, c'est-à-dire du malsain. En réactualisant certains mythes de l'ancienne médecine humorale, ce nouveau concept arrive à préfigurer dès la fin du XIXe siècle les grands traits de l'anxio-dépression moderne.

Bibliographie

Aquin, Thomas d', *Somme théologique II* (Paris : Cerf, 1999)

Aristote, *L'Homme de génie et la mélancolie*, trad. de J. Pigeaud (Paris : Payot & Rivages, 2006)

Bouchard, Charles, *Leçons sur les auto-intoxications dans les maladies* (Paris : Savy, 1887)

Boyer, Louis, *Le Livre de la morale des écoles primaires et des cours d'adultes* (Paris : Éditions des équateurs, 2011)

Bouchard, Charles, *Leçons sur les auto-intoxications dans les maladies* (Paris : Savy, 1887)

Burton, Robert, *Anatomie de la mélancolie* (Paris : Gallimard, 2005)

Césaré, Basile de, *Homélies, discours, lettres choisis de Saint Basile-le-Grand*, trad. par M. l'Abbé Auger (Lyon : Francois Guyot, 1827)

Chrysostome, Jean, *Homélies sur la Résurrection, l'Ascenscion et la Pentecôte*, tome 1 (Paris : Cerf, 2013)

Dejerine, Jules, *L'Hérédité dans les maladies du système nerveux* (Paris : Asselin et Houzeau, 1886)

Deyrolle, Émile, *Leçons de choses* (Paris : Michel Lafon, 2010)

Forthomme, Bernard, *Émergence et résurgence de l'acédie*, dans *Tristesse, acédie et médecine des âmes : anthologie de textes rares et inédits* (*XIII*^e^*–XX*^e^ *siècle*), éd. par Nathalie Nabert (Paris : Beauschesne, 2005), pp. 15–35

Foucault, Michel, *Les Anormaux. Cours au Collège de France, 1974–1975* (Paris : Gallimard/Seuil, 1999)

Garnier, Pierre, *La Folie à Paris* (Paris : Baillières et fils, 1890)

Hersant, Yves, *Mélancolies de l'Antiquité au XX*^e^ *siècle* (Paris : Robert Laffont, 2005)

Huysmans, Joris-Karl, *Marthe : histoire d'une fille* (Paris : Galaade, 2010)

Klibansky, Raymond, Erwin Panofsky, et Fritz Saxl (éds), *Saturne et la mélancolie* (Paris : Gallimard, 1989)

Labiche, Eugène, *L'Affaire de la rue de Lourcine*, dans *Théâtre I* (Paris : Robert Laffont, 1857), pp. 477–507

Lancereaux, Étienne, 'Alcoolisme', dans *Dictionnaire encyclopédique des sciences médicales*, ed. par A. Deschambres (Paris : Masson et fils, 1865), pp. 615–703

Lecoutre, Matthieu, *Ivresse et ivrognerie dans la France moderne* (Rennes : PUFR, 2011)

Legrain, Paul-Maurice, *Du Délire chez les dégénérés : observations prises à l'asile Saint-Anne, 1885–1886* (Paris : Delahaye et Lecrosnier, 1886)
——, *Hérédité et alcoolisme : étude psychologique et clinique sur les dégénérés buveurs et familles d'ivrognes* (Paris : Doin, 1889)
Lévy, Paul-Émile, *L'Éducation rationnelle de la volonté : son emploi thérapeutique* (Paris : Felix Alcan, 1899
Liebig, Justus, *Nouvelles lettres sur la chimie* (Paris : Charpentier, 1852)
Magnan, Valentin, *De l'Alcoolisme et des diverses formes du délire alcoolique* (Paris : Delahaye, 1874)
——, *L'Alcoolisme, folie des héréditaires dégénérés* (Paris : Masson, 1893)
Malot, Hector, *Les Victimes d'amour* (Paris : Marpon et Flammarion, 1862)
Maupassant, Guy de, 'Garçon, un bock !', dans *Contes et nouvelles* (Paris : Gallimard, 2014), pp. 818–22
Monin, Ernest, *L'Alcoolisme : étude médico-sociale* (Paris : Doin, 1889)
Morel, Bénédicte-Augustin, *Traité des dégénérescences* (Paris : Baillière, 1857)
——, *Traité des maladies mentales* (Paris : Masson, 1860)
Nabert, Nathalie, *Tristesse, acédie et médecine des âmes : anthologie de textes rares et inédits XIIIe–XXe siècle* (Paris : Beauschesne, 2005)
Nourrisson, Didier, *Le Buveur du XIXe siècle* (Paris : Albin Michel, 1990)
Ohnet, Georges, *Marchand de poisons* (Paris : P. Olendorff, 1903)
Pagnol, Marcel, *Souvenirs d'enfance : la gloire de mon père*, dans *Œuvres complètes III* (Paris : Fallois, 1957), pp. 9–152
Prigent, Hélène, *Mélancolie : les métamorphoses de la dépression* (Paris : Gallimard, 2005)
Quellier, Florent, *Gourmandise : histoire d'un péché capital* (Paris : Armand Colin, 2010)
Quétel, Claude, *Histoire de la folie* (Paris : Tallendier, 2012)
Renaudin, 'De l'Alcoolisme chronique par M. le Docteur Magnus Huss', *Annales médico-psychologiques* [no. 5] (1853), 60–88
Riant, Aimé, *Les Irresponsables devant la justice* (Paris : Baillière, 1888)
Ribot, Théodule, *Les Maladies de la volonté* (Paris : Felix Alcan, 1888)
Zola, Émile, *L'Assommoir* (Paris : Gallimard, 1978)

CHAPTER 4

Twice Shy: Two Accounts of Timidity in *fin-de-siècle* France

Philippa Lewis

In her cultural history of fear, Joanna Bourke refers to shyness, the 'mild apprehension of other people', as a 'commonplace' anxiety.[1] For Christopher Lane, it is a 'routine emotion', or 'ordinary trait'.[2] This assessment of shyness, or timidity, as a trivial affliction is not new. In his 1922 *Les Grands Timides*, for example, the philosopher and psychologist Ludovic Dugas described timidity as one of the 'menues questions de psychologie'.[3] But the apparently 'minor' status of shyness has not prevented it becoming a major research topic in the fields of psychology and psychiatry. Indeed, Dugas was one of the first thinkers to establish it as a sustained subject of scientific enquiry in France: in 1898, he published a monograph entitled *La Timidité: étude psychologique et morale*.[4] Then, in 1901, the psychiatric doctor Paul Hartenberg brought out *Les Timides et la timidité*,[5] responding to and nuancing Dugas's theories. Together, these two texts constitute a crucial, but frequently overlooked, moment in the history of shyness in France, and in particular the history of its medicalization.[6]

Neither Dugas's nor Hartenberg's turn-of-the-century texts is well known today, despite the fact that shyness is a thriving area of international research in disciplines ranging from developmental psychology and sociology to

1 Joanna Bourke, *Fear: A Cultural History* (London: Virago, 2006), p. 2.

2 Christopher Lane, *Shyness: How Normal Behavior Became a Sickness* (New Haven: Yale University Press, 2007), p. 12, p. 10.

3 Ludovic Dugas, *Les Grands Timides* (Paris: Félix Alcan, 1922), viii.

4 Ludovic Dugas, *La Timidité: étude psychologique et morale*, Bibliothèque philosophie contemporaine (Paris: Félix Alcan, 1898). All page references will be to this edition. Subsequent references to the work, abbreviated as *T*, are given in the text, followed by the page number.

5 Paul Hartenberg, *Les Timides et la timidité* (Paris: Félix Alcan, 1901). References to *Les Timides et la timidité* are abbreviated as *TT*, followed by the page number.

6 The research undertaken for this chapter is part of an ongoing project examining the history of shyness in modern France, generously supported by the Leverhulme Trust (Early Career Fellowship scheme).

 | DOI:10.1163/9789004368019_006

behavioural genetics and neurobiology.[7] In these disciplines, ordinary-language words like 'timidity' or, more commonly in Anglophone contexts, 'shyness',[8] are used alongside clinical terms such as 'social anxiety' or 'social phobia' (*la phobie sociale* in French) to discuss a condition which many consider to be on the rise.[9] Following the introduction of 'social phobia' as a diagnostic category in the American Psychiatric Association's *Diagnostic and Statistical Manual of Mental Disorders* in 1980, pharmacological research into social difficulties and their treatment has also increased.[10] Work in this area tends towards ahistoricism.[11] As this chapter will demonstrate, the medical history of shyness and its cognate terms predates the twentieth century, but this fact was almost entirely disregarded by mental health professionals until recently.[12]

---

7 See *Extreme Fear, Shyness, and Social Phobia: Origins, Biological Mechanisms, and Clinical Outcomes*, ed. by Louis A. Schmidt and Jay Schulkin (New York: Oxford University Press, 1999); W. Ray Crozier, *Understanding Shyness: Psychological Perspectives* (New York: Palgrave, 2001); Susie Scott, *Shyness and Society: The Illusion of Competence* (Basingstoke: Palgrave Macmillan, 2007); *The Psychological Significance of the Blush*, ed. by W. Ray Crozier and P. J. de Jong (Cambridge and New York: Cambridge University Press, 2012).

8 Definitions of 'shyness' vary widely, but the term can broadly be understood as the experience of fear and/or self-consciousness in social situations; 'timidity' refers to a more general lack of confidence or courage. In this chapter, I privilege the term 'timidity' given its etymological proximity to the French *timidité*, but the context is always that of social interaction, as it is in the work of Dugas and Hartenberg. Definitions will be discussed at greater length in the second and third parts of this chapter.

9 Philip Zimbardo and Lynne Henderson, 'Foreword', in *Shyness: Development, Consolidation and Change* (London: Routledge, 2000), xiii–xv.

10 Research in this area is, inevitably, controversial: scepticism about the transformation of so-called everyday emotions into medical disorders, making large profits for pharmaceutical companies in the process, has resulted in a number of critiques; see Lane, *Shyness* and Susan Cain, *Quiet: The Power of Introverts in a World That Can't Stop Talking* (London: Viking, 2012). For analyses of the specific controversies surrounding social phobia as a diagnostic category in contemporary French psychiatry, see Stephanie Lloyd, 'The Clinical Clash Over Social Phobia: The Americanization of French Experiences?', *BioSocieties*, 1, 2 (2006), 229–49, and Lloyd, 'Morals, Medicine and Change: Morality Brokers, Social Phobias, and French Psychiatry', *Culture, Medicine, and Psychiatry*, 32, 2 (2008), 279–97.

11 On the frequent neglect of history in psychology as a discipline, see Kurt Danziger, *Naming the Mind: How Psychology Found its Language* (London: Sage, 1997), pp. 9–14.

12 The relationship, and threshold, between shyness, social anxiety, and social phobia is heavily debated amongst psychologists and psychiatrists, and evidence remains inconclusive. Some argue that the terms are essentially synonymous; others, that they refer to qualitatively different phenomena. See Denise A. Chavira, Murray B. Stein and Vanessa L. Malcarne, 'Scrutinizing the Relationship Between Shyness and Social Phobia', *Journal of Anxiety Disorders*, 16, 6 (2002), 585–98; Nancy A. Heiser, Samuel M. Turner and Deborah C.

In 1996, for example, German E. Berrios remarked that 'the impression has recently been given that [social phobia] was only recognized in or defined in 1966'.[13] In more recent years, however, the role of the French psychiatrist Pierre Janet in the original naming of social phobia, in his 1903 *Les Obsessions et la psychasthénie*,[14] has begun to be acknowledged.[15] What have not been sufficiently explored, however, are the sources which Janet himself drew on in his study, which include work by Dugas and Hartenberg on timidity and the psychopathology of sociability.[16]

Why did Dugas's and Hartenberg's monographs on timidity appear, within a few years of each other, at the turn of the twentieth century? What sparked the writers' interest in this elusive experience, and what can their work tell us about *fin-de-siècle* French society more broadly? This chapter will use Dugas's and Hartenberg's monographs to expand the historical parameters of our contemporary understandings of shyness, but also to probe the ambivalence which marked — and still marks — much research into this particular form of social difficulty. Both Dugas and Hartenberg identified timidity as a problem with cultural and societal implications, and both drew on similar, often literary, sources to construct their theories of timidity. Nonetheless, fundamental differences of approach and opinion emerge from their texts. Is timidity always an obstacle to individual and collective wellbeing, as Hartenberg asserts? Or, as Dugas implies, can it on occasion be a healthy and even productive experience? In the context of *fin-de-siècle* France, such questions were shaped by

---

Beidel, 'Shyness: Relationship to Social Phobia and Other Psychiatric Disorders', *Behaviour Research and Therapy*, 41, 2 (2003), 209–21.

13 G. E. Berrios, *The History of Mental Symptoms: Descriptive Psychopathology Since the Nineteenth Century* (Cambridge and New York: Cambridge University Press, 1996), p. 272.

14 Janet refers to 'des *phobies sociales* ou des phobies de la société' in *Les Obsessions et la psychasthénie*, 2 vols (Paris: Félix Alcan, 1908), I, p. 217.

15 See, for example, Lloyd, 'The Clinical Clash over Social Phobia'; Lane, *Shyness*; Heather Buchanan and Neil Coulson, *Phobias* (Houndmills, Basingstoke, Hampshire: Palgrave Macmillan, 2012).

16 Scholars who have referred to Hartenberg include Berrios, *History of Mental Symptoms*; Bernard Jolibert, *L'Éducation d'une émotion: trac, timidité, intimidation dans la littérature* (Paris: Harmattan, 1997); Robert A. Nye, *Masculinity and Male Codes of Honor in Modern France* (Berkeley, CA: University of California Press, 1998); and Nichole Fairbrother, 'The Treatment of Social Phobia — 100 Years Ago', *Behaviour Research and Therapy*, 40, 11 (2002), 1291–304. Their references are generally cursory, however. Dugas's work on timidity has received even less attention; see Berrios, *History of Mental Symptoms*, pp. 272–73; Jolibert, *L'Éducation d'une émotion*, especially chapter 1, 'Le Trac: émotion primitive'; and Nye, *Masculinity and Male Codes of Honor*, p. 223, for some discussion.

restrictive understandings of bodily and mental health bound up with norms of gender, race, and class, and by a pervasive concern with national decline. Yet the questions still pertain to normative discussions surrounding shyness and sociability today. While the approach this chapter takes is historical, then, it is important to note the contemporary resonances of its analysis. More broadly, the two monographs under discussion move, whether implicitly or explicitly, between discourses and disciplines (between literature and medicine, for example, and between philosophy and psychology) and thus shed light on interdisciplinarity and the nineteenth-century construction of scientific knowledge.[17]

The Cultural Context

The preoccupation with timidity exemplified by Dugas's and Hartenberg's texts was not an isolated incident or ephemeral episode in French culture, but reflected ongoing forms of engagement with timidity as a puzzle and, often, a problem. We know that references to timidity as a moral flaw date back at least to the seventeenth century: in typically wily fashion, a maxim by La Rochefoucauld claims that 'La timidité est un défaut dont il est dangereux de reprendre les personnes qu'on en veut corriger'.[18] What emerges in the course of the nineteenth century, however — clearly drawing on and perpetuating much of the earlier moral discussion — is the sense of timidity as a medical disorder. And by the latter part of the century, we see a growing desire amongst psychopathologists to understand the mechanisms of this disorder in detail. As the study of mental disease, psychopathology encompasses the work of psychiatrists, psychologists, and, potentially, philosophers. In nineteenth-century France, the sciences of the mind were gradually taking shape and marking out their territory. Disciplinary boundaries were fluid, and shifting. In

---

17 For work on the interface between science, literature, and culture in the nineteenth century, see Sally Shuttleworth, *The Mind of the Child: Child Development in Literature, Science, and Medicine, 1840–1900* (Oxford: Oxford University Press, 2010); *Médecine, sciences de la vie et littérature en France et en Europe de la Révolution à nos jours*, ed. by Lise Dumasy-Queffélec and Hélène Spengler, 3 vols (Geneva: Droz, 2014); Miranda Gill, 'Self-Control and Uncontrollable Passion in Stendhal's Theory of Love', *French Studies*, 69, 4 (2015), 462–78.

18 François de La Rochefoucauld, *Maximes et réflexions morales du duc de La Rochefoucauld* (Paris: Lecointe, 1829), p. 102. La Rochefoucauld's elliptical allusions to the dangerously unpredictable, and highly sensitive, nature of the *timide* will later be taken up by *fin-de-siècle* thinkers.

Les Timides et la timidité, Hartenberg offers a particular perspective on these shifts when he evokes, with satisfaction, psychology's increasing distance from philosophy (and simultaneously affirms his own positivist, 'modern' position):

> Ce travail […] est un essai de psychologie positive et moderne, de psychologie scientifique en un mot. On sait que depuis une vingtaine d'années environ une évolution considérable s'est accomplie en matière de psychologie. Se dégageant peu à peu des nuages de la métaphysique et des abstractions de la méthode introspective pure, l'étude de la pensée humaine a bénéficié de la clarté et de la précision des méthodes scientifiques objectives, et la psychologie s'est déplacée progressivement pour passer du domaine de la philosophie sur le domaine de la science. (vi)

Here, Hartenberg is talking about psychology, but psychiatry — the specifically medical study and treatment of mental disorders — was also 'still in the making' in the nineteenth century.[19] From its initial association with the asylum and treatment of the 'insane' in the late eighteenth and early nineteenth century, as explored by Foucault,[20] the discipline broadened to include the treatment of outpatients with milder symptoms. The figure of the psychiatrist — or 'alienist', one of the terms most commonly used at the time — was becoming increasingly specialized, professionalized, and powerful.

It is against this background of transitioning disciplines and expanding professions that timidity became appropriated by psychopathological discourse and developed into a diagnostic category. As Jan Goldstein discusses,

---

19 Jan Ellen Goldstein, *Console and Classify: The French Psychiatric Profession in the Nineteenth Century* (Cambridge and New York: Cambridge University Press, 1987), p. 7. On the growth of French psychiatry in the nineteenth century and its reach beyond the asylum, see Goldstein, *Console and Classify*; Nye, *Crime, Madness, and Politics in Modern France*; Ian Robert Dowbiggin, *Inheriting Madness: Professionalization and Psychiatric Knowledge in Nineteenth-Century France* (Berkeley: University of California Press, 1991). For a study of the growth of psychiatry from an international perspective, see Edward Shorter, *A History of Psychiatry: From the Era of the Asylum to the Age of Prozac* (New York: John Wiley & Sons, 1997). On the emergence of psychology as an academic discipline in France, see Serge Nicolas and Agnès Charvillat, 'Introducing Psychology as an Academic Discipline in France: Théodule Ribot and the Collège de France (1888–1901)', *Journal of the History of the Behavioral Sciences*, 37, 2 (2001), 143–64. See also, *A Critical History and Philosophy of Psychology: Diversity of Context, Thought, and Practice*, ed. by Richard T. G. Walsh, Thomas Teo and Angelina Baydala (Cambridge: Cambridge University Press, 2014), pp. 207–08.

20 Michel Foucault, *Histoire de la folie à l'âge classique* (Paris: Gallimard, 2007).

the second half of the nineteenth century abounded with loosely defined, capacious terms for afflictions of the nervous system, including *névropathie, nervosisme*, and *neurasthénie*, which were falling increasingly under the dominion of the psychiatrist as opposed to the general practitioner.[21] The history of these nervous disorders is significant, not least as they shaped the environment in which, in Germany, Freud began to work. But for the purposes of this chapter, they are important as it was in part this focus on 'nervousness' which allowed timidity to become a scientific problem, and the object of medical enquiry. In *fin-de-siècle* scientific discourse, timidity as a concept was implicated in — indeed, only made sense within — the broader spectrum of interconnected psychopathologies and paradigms preoccupying mental health professionals at the time. These pathologies included obsessions, fears, and phobias as well as diseases of the will, like aboulia: conditions which, in the late nineteenth century, were often explained in terms of hereditary degeneration.[22] Timidity was also examined in the light of a range of popular methodologies and therapeutic practices, including physiognomy and hypnotism.[23]

Timidity was not only discussed within the domain of psychopathology, however. *Fin-de-siècle* French culture saw timidity treated in other scholarly disciplines, like sociology, and popular forms, such as journalism, indicative of the fluid relations and porous boundaries between disciplines, discourses, and media in the period. Eight years before timidity became a subject in its own right in Dugas's *La Timidité* (1898), for example, it was the object of sociological discussion in *Les Lois de l'imitation: étude sociologique*, by the criminal judge and sociologist Gabriel Tarde. Identifying the timid individual as one who resists, at least in part, what is called the universal social law of imitation, Tarde states that 'cette perturbation profonde de tout l'être et cette dépossession de soi qu'on appelle l'intimidation mériterait une étude à part'.[24] Timidity also became a recurrent theme in a series of *chroniques* published in the Parisian daily newspaper *Le Journal*, with a particular emphasis on stage-fright (*le trac*) as a debilitating condition abounding in the entertainment industry. These articles postdate Dugas's publication, and can thus be interpreted as evidence of its impact. Hartenberg, however, is able to draw on three of the *chroniques*

21 Goldstein, *Console and Classify*, pp. 331–38.

22 Aboulia was a popular term in the nineteenth century. It was defined in 1892 as 'a form of insanity characterized by inability to exert the will' (cited in Berrios, *History of Mental Symptoms*, p. 361).

23 Paolo Mantegazza, *La Physionomie et l'expression des sentiments* (Paris: Félix Alcan, 1885); Janet, *Les Obsessions*, I, p. 570.

24 Gabriel Tarde, *Les Lois de l'imitation: étude sociologique* (Paris: Félix Alcan, 1890), p. 95.

in his monograph: one by Hugues La Roux on 4 December 1898, one by Henry Bauër on 23 March 1899, and one by Jules Claretie on 5 July 1899.

These examples, drawn from a range of disciplines and discourses, hint at the way the concept of timidity — although discussed in France for centuries — resonated in the closing years of the nineteenth century. Dugas's and Hartenberg's studies further heightened the topicality of timidity at this time and established it as a scientific as much as a moral matter. Both writers pathologized shyness. Yet the following section will show that Dugas's approach, less affected by the ideologically charged, interventionist agenda present in Hartenberg's monograph, allows him to demonstrate a greater level of tolerance towards, and even appreciation of, temperamental and behavioural difference.

Dugas: *La Timidité: étude psychologique et morale* (1898)

Although he is not widely known today, a 14-line obituary published in *L'Année psychologique* in 1945 described Dugas as the 'doyen des psychologues français'.[25] Born in 1857, Dugas trained under Théodule Ribot and proceeded to publish widely on psychopathology, philosophy, and education.[26] The anonymous obituary characterizes Dugas as the author of 'une série d'ouvrages sur la timidité'; indeed, Dugas had identified a fertile line of enquiry in the study of timidity which, from his original monograph *La Timidité* of 1898, led to

---

25 Anon., 'Chronique', *L'Année psychologique*, 1945, 665.

26 M. Sierra and G. E. Berrios, 'Introduction to "A Case of Depersonalization"', *History of Psychiatry*, 7, 27 (1996), 451–54 (p. 452). Théodule Ribot was a major French psychologist and psychopathologist who contributed to the establishment of psychology as an autonomous academic discipline in France: see Nicolas and Charvillat, 'Introducing Psychology'; Vincent Guillin, 'Théodule Ribot's Ambiguous Positivism: Philosophical and Epistemological Strategies in the Founding of French Scientific Psychology', *Journal of the History of the Behavioral Sciences*, 40, 2 (2004), 165–81. Ribot's 'physiological' psychology emphasized the importance of affective over intellectual life. Significant publications include *Les Maladies de la volonté* (Paris: Félix Alcan, 1882) and *La Psychologie des sentiments* (Paris: Félix Alcan, 1896); in the latter, Ribot refers to timidity in his section on 'le moi et ses manifestations affectives' (p. 238). Ribot's influence on *La Timidité* is clear, although Dugas pays only cursory attention to the physiological dimension of shyness in his monograph, suggestive of some divergence from Ribot's approach. See Dugas's biographical study of Ribot: 'Un philosophe breton, Théodule Ribot (1839–1916)', *Annales de Bretagne*, 32, 2 (1917), 145–68.

Les Grands Timides in 1922, and *Les Timides dans la littérature et l'art* in 1925.[27] Together, these three titles testify to a shift in focus away from timidity as a concept, and towards some of the *timides* who, in Dugas's first study, feature in more intermittent fashion to exemplify specific points (these *timides* include celebrated writers such as Rousseau, Constant, and Stendhal).

The later texts are useful for what they tell us of Dugas's method. Berrios refers to Dugas's *La Timidité* as an 'introspective study, based on the classical psychology tradition',[28] but we have to wait until the later volumes to see Dugas himself articulate his approach in these terms. In *Les Grands Timides*, for example, Dugas explains that his research draws on a corpus of first-person testimonials written by self-confessedly timid individuals who have methodically observed and analysed their own experiences of shyness. The practice of psychological self-observation may be subjective, Dugas acknowledges, but 'l'observation psychologique proprement dite, l'*introspection* […] acquiert une valeur objective par la *comparaison* des résultats qu'elle donne chez les sujets différents'.[29] It is the job of the psychologist to amass these observations, compare them, and draw conclusions. Dugas's repeated insistence on this point in *Les Timides* is evidence of introspection's marginalization in psychology,[30] and the growing sense of it as a method unable to attain the kind of generality demanded by an increasingly scientific, empirically based, discipline.[31] Dugas also makes clear his commitment to philosophy in the later volumes, alluding, regretfully, to the disciplinary splits between philosophy and psychology which we have already seen Hartenberg endorse:

> Un peu de philosophie ne nuit pas à l'étude des menues questions de psychologie, comme est celle de la timidité; elle les relève, elle en montre la signification et la portée; elle aide même à les résoudre; il n'est pas nécessairement vrai qu'elle ne serve qu'à les compliquer et à les fausser.[32]

---

27 Anon., 'Chronique'. Dugas also published articles on timidity: Dugas, 'La Timidité', *Revue philosophique de la France et de l'étranger*, 1896; Dugas, 'La Timidité de Waldeck-Rousseau', *Annales de Bretagne*, 34, 1 (1919), 68–76.

28 Berrios, *History of Mental Symptoms*, p. 273.

29 Dugas, *Les Grands Timides*, iv.

30 Dugas, *Les Timides dans la littérature et l'art* (Paris: Félix Alcan, 1937), i.

31 For a study of introspection and its decline as a method in psychology and philosophy, see William Lyons, *The Disappearance of Introspection* (Cambridge, MA: MIT Press, 1986).

32 Dugas, *Les Grands Timides*, viii.

Timidity may be a minor malady, but, Dugas argues, if approached in the correct way, it can illuminate a host of related psychological problems. The structure of *La Timidité* reflects this potential reach: Chapter One provides definitions of timidity and explores both its individual and societal causes; Chapter Two describes the form of spontaneous or raw (*brut*) shyness exemplified by stage-fright; Chapter Three furthers this discussion in relation to the concepts of temperament and mood; and Chapters Four and Five focus on the processes by which the shy subject analyses, and seeks to justify, his timidity.[33] Chapter Six focuses on 'special cases' of timidity, namely practical, intellectual, and sentimental timidity, and Chapter Seven examines the moral aspect, offering conclusions about whether and, if so, how, timidity should be cured.

Although Dugas claims that his first prerogative in *La Timidité* is to define the concept of timidity clearly, the reality is that a chain of differently nuanced definitions unfurl from chapter to chapter; it is, therefore, through a combination of definitions that a sense of what Dugas means by timidity emerges. Despite its etymological origins in the Latin *timor*, timidity is neither fear nor a fearful disposition. It is similar to fear ('un sentiment voisin, mais différent de la crainte', *T*, 3), but while fear can only be caused by real and mortal danger (*T*, 2), timidity is the apprehension of discomfort in the company of others: unlike fear, timidity can only operate in society. In essence, Dugas states, this apprehension manifests itself as a temporary disorder of one or more of the three faculties constituting the mind in terms of nineteenth-century faculty psychology: the will, the intellect, and the emotions (*T*, 4).[34] We thus see that timidity is viewed from the outset in terms of a mental disorder, even mental illness — a term Dugas will explicitly employ in 1922 ('la timidité

33 It will become apparent to the reader that both Dugas and Hartenberg are principally concerned with the male *timide* in their studies. This is evidence of the way 'shyness norms' were constructed along gender lines in the period: shyness did not correspond to culturally determined ideals of masculinity and was thus problematic for men, but it could be read as a natural, and healthy, function of femininity. This asymmetry will be discussed further in relation to Hartenberg's monograph.

34 For a useful discussion of faculty psychology and key nineteenth-century psychological concepts more generally, see Berrios, *The History of Mental Symptoms*, pp. 17–19; 419–42. On the gradual decline of interest in the will in psychology and psychiatry, linked to the rise of experimentalism, behaviourism, and psychoanalysis, Berrios notes: 'The "will" no longer plays a role in psychiatry and psychology. A hundred years ago, however, it was an important descriptive and explanatory concept, naming the human "power, potency or faculty" to initiate action', p. 351.

est une des maladies mentales qui se prêtent le mieux à l'analyse').[35] The tripartite schema which Dugas adopts allows him to structure the first chapter by faculty, and thus explore timidity in its multiple modes. First, Dugas notes, the timid individual may be subject to disorders of the will which render him momentarily incapable of producing voluntary movements.[36] That this state is aligned by Dugas in *La Timidité* with aboulia, a diminished ability to initiate actions and thoughts, and even paraboulia — a state in which the will is perverted, which can lead to crime — is characteristic of the way timidity borders on the insane and the deviant throughout the text, whether by association or analogy (*T*, 4). For example, while timidity can present, unobtrusively, as the paralysis of the will — Dugas uses the example of a young man in a salon desiring, but unable, to leave (*T*, 4) — it can also result in a dysfunctional motor system which leaves the timid individual unable to temper his behaviour in line with convention: 'Quand il n'est pas anéanti ou stupide, le timide est comme agité ou fou. […] Comme on a retrouvé chez certains timides les traits du caractère de l'aboulique, on retrouverait chez d'autres les traits du caractère de l'hystérique' (*T*, 6).[37] By connecting seemingly antithetical characteristics, Dugas casts timidity as a shape-shifting condition which, whether through its gestural insufficiencies or excesses, has the potential for social disruption.

Paralysis does not only affect the will in Dugas's schema, but also cognition. Certain modes of timidity thus manifest themselves as stupidity, or intellectual stupor: 'ce qu'on nomme vulgairement l'absence' (*T*, 7). Dugas is clear that to be timid is not to be unintelligent; rather, the attacks of timidity he evokes result from fleeting failures or meltdowns of the intellectual function. This distinction hints, implicitly, at the potential illegibility — even duplicity — of the timid individual, a theme pursued in later chapters: shy people are rarely what they seem, resisting easy identification and interpretation. As an example, Dugas

35 *Les Grands Timides*, v. Dugas argues that those who are shy tend towards introspection and self-analysis, producing written testimony of great use to the psychologist seeking to understand their condition: '[…] ceux qui en sont atteints étant ou pouvant être des sujets extraordinairement lucides et de plus, étant tous naturellement enclins à l'observation attentive et minutieuse de leur cas' (v).

36 The categories of the voluntary and the involuntary underpinned much nineteenth-century psychological and psychiatric thought, see *Paradigmes de l'âme: littérature et aliénisme au XIXe siècle*, ed. by Jean-Louis Cabanès, Didier Philippot, and Paolo Tortonese (Paris: Presses Sorbonne Nouvelle, 2012), chapter 1, 'La Volonté et l'involontaire: l'exemple de l'automatisme', pp. 23–37; and Gill, 'Self-Control and Uncontrollable Passion', p. 464.

37 For a history of male hysteria of relevance to this chapter, see Mark S. Micale, *Hysterical Men: The Hidden History of Male Nervous Illness* (Cambridge, MA: Harvard University Press, 2008).

evokes a young boy, intimidated by his schoolmaster: 'Combien d'hommes, et non seulement d'écoliers, passent de même pour butors, et ne sont que timides!' (*T*, 7–8). In Dugas's tripartite model, the third type of timidity affects the emotions: again, 'la timidité affective' is translated either by a complete loss of feeling (*T*, 8), or by a 'chaos' of contradictory sentiments which overwhelm the sufferer (*T*, 12). Sentimental stupor, particularly of the first type, is again described as absence (*T*, 15), or annihilation (*T*, 14). Dugas is keen to stress that while timidity is certainly the effect of a volitional, intellectual, or sentimental malfunction, the sufferer must be fully conscious of this malfunction for such symptoms to amount to timidity. Timidity takes place as a subjective, *self-conscious* state of suffering: 'Être gauche sans savoir qu'on l'est, c'est n'être que lourd ou maladroit; être gauche et savoir qu'on l'est, et souffrir de l'être, c'est là ce qu'on appelle proprement timide' (*T*, 17). A certain level of self-awareness is thus necessary, Dugas asserts, for the production of 'true' timidity.

Alongside the tripartite structure of will, intellect, and emotion underpinning Dugas's *La Timidité*, a bipartite structure is also evident in the distinction between the momentary fit (*accès*) of timidity — *la timidité brute* — and the cumulative effect of repeated attacks which leads to a chronic state or diathesis (*T*, 24). Drawing on the concept of temperament widely used in the nineteenth century,[38] Dugas suggests that the timid individual is often an 'impressionable' for whom the universal need for understanding and respect is particularly acute (*T*, 52). Dugas describes the timid man as 'à la merci de ses nerfs. Il est avide de sympathie et douloureusement sensible à l'antipathie [...]. Sa volonté et son jugement sont sans prises sur ses sensations. Au point de vue affectif, il est un enfant' (*T*, 60). While those with an impressionable, nervous temperament often become *timides*, it is not inevitable that this will occur. Rather, persistent timidity is the result of repeated bouts of mental faculty dysfunction which, over time, either through the 'affective memory' of past attacks (here Dugas draws on Ribot's *Les Maladies de la mémoire* (1881)) or sustained reflection on these attacks, develop into a chronic condition (*T*, 24–26). Timidity tends to appear in highly sensitive, weak-willed individuals, akin to children, but 'il n'y a point proprement, à l'état naturel, de *timidité*, il n'y a que des accès *d'intimidation*' (*T*, 69).

From the point of view of French literary and cultural history, the notion of 'systematic' timidity elaborated in Chapters Four and Five of *La Timidité*

---

38 For a discussion of nineteenth-century views of the ancient concept of temperament, see Berrios, *The History of Mental Symptoms*, p. 420. Temperament is still a working concept in contemporary psychology, see Jerome Kagan, *Galen's Prophecy: Temperament in Human Nature* (New York: Westview Press, 1994).

provides one of the richest elements of the study. These two chapters are devoted to an exploration of the psychological mechanisms through which those who suffer from timidity analyse, justify, and complicate it. In these chapters, Dugas paints a highly ambivalent picture of an individual who makes a habit of his timidity and, by doing so, condemns himself to 'l'isolement moral' (*T*, 71). Living alone, the *timide* turns to self-analysis to compensate for the lack of satisfactory interpersonal interactions he is able to conduct in reality. Building on Adam Smith's conceptualization of reflection as the splitting of the self,[39] Dugas describes the *timide* as both the actor and spectator in the drama of his life (*T*, 72). This state certainly has negative effects: adopting the moralizing vocabulary announced in the title of his study, Dugas discusses the egotism (*T*, 72), anti-socialness (*T*, 76), and duplicity it can result in (*T*, 110–14). The timid individual develops two co-existing modes of existence: one sincere, but private, and another public, but false, developed from a reluctance, or inability, to reveal the former to others. Listing examples of the lies his research has uncovered, Dugas evokes the 'manie de simulation' the *timide* can develop (*T*, 12), and his propensity to wallow in 'le mensonge paradoxal et fou' (*T*, 113). Yet, in keeping with the curious blend of sympathy and stigmatization evident in *La Timidité*, Dugas is not uniformly critical of these ruses. Rather, they are framed as an understandable consequence of the underlying dissatisfaction with the material world felt by those who struggle to socialize. Dugas identifies what he calls the 'maladie de l'idéal' (*T*, 82) in many of the sufferers he studies. This is clearly considered a disease and a deviation from what it is to be healthy. Yet there is, nonetheless, a sense of empathy and even admiration present in the way Dugas describes those who withdraw from the disappointments of everyday life to exist in the better world of their imagination.[40]

La Timidité is presented as a work of psychology, but its findings derive from a select corpus of literary writings rather than from clinical or experimental

39 Dugas provides no reference here, but it is likely he is alluding to *The Theory of Moral Sentiments* in which Smith writes that 'when I examine my own conduct [...] it is evident that, in all such cases, I divide myself, as it were, into two persons', Adam Smith, *The Theory of Moral Sentiments* (Cambridge: Cambridge University Press, 2002 [1759]), p. 131.

40 This mixture of understanding and admiration is evident, for example, when Dugas writes that 'Le timide reste d'ailleurs en partie fidèle à son rêve d'une société idéale et d'une intimité entière. [...] Il est donc un utopiste en affection [...]. Si les affections réelles viennent à lui manquer, il se crée une société idéale, celles des livres' (*T*, 94–95), or, 'Le caractère timide ne peut être érigé sans doute en idéal moral; mais il a néanmoins sa moralité et ses vertus propres' (*T*, 146).

research.[41] Dugas's cultural references stretch back as far as Virgil and Horace, but his allusions are primarily to works from the eighteenth and nineteenth centuries. While there are exceptions, he draws principally on life-writing (diaries, correspondence) and Romantic or post-Romantic literary forms (lyric poetry, the *roman intime*), frequently interpreting the latter in an autobiographical light: the monograph thus interchangeably cites excerpts from Rousseau's *Confessions* (1782) and diaries by Alfred de Vigny, Henri-Frédéric Amiel, and Marie Bashkirtseff alongside extracts from Eugène Fromentin's *Dominique* (1862), Louise Ackermann's *Poésies philosophiques* (1874), and Paul Bourget's *Le Disciple* (1889). The autobiographical emphasis to the corpus and subsequent analysis suggests that Dugas is ultimately less interested in the literary qualities of the passages he cites, and more in what they might reveal of the lived, embodied, reality of shyness palpable beneath the surface of the text: working within a hermeneutic paradigm rendered increasingly problematic in the twentieth century, Dugas sees in the writing he selects a way to access, more or less directly, the timidity experienced by the writer. Early on in his monograph, for example, Dugas uses an extract from Constant's *Adolphe* (1816) to support his observation that shy individuals often suffer from an acute sense of physical malaise when subjected to another's gaze. Dugas insinuates that Constant must have been familiar with this sensation himself: 'Benjamin Constant prête à son Adolphe, qui est un type de timide, ce trait de caractère trop particulier, trop précis pour être inventé' (*T*, 33). By this logic, which downplays any imaginative capacity on Constant's part, the nervous agitation Adolphe experiences at the sight of the human form can legitimately serve as proof that shyness is an affliction with a significant, but not exclusive, physiological element (*T*, 33). Constant also features prominently in Dugas's later works on timidity. These heavily biographical studies, structured around individual personalities such as Chateaubriand, Stendhal, and Mérimée, attempt to fashion what — inspired by Sainte-Beuve's literary criticism — Dugas refers to as a '"collection" ou mieux une "famille naturelle" d'esprits, — les timides, — caracterisée par des individus de choix'.[42]

In *La Timidité*, Dugas reads the striking, and similar, depictions of shyness in his chosen writers' work as evidence of universal psychological phenomena.

---

41 Literary analysis was a common feature of psychiatric and psychological treatises in this period, in part due to the influence of Max Nordau's *Dégénérescence* (1894), which interpreted the preoccupations of certain *fin-de-siècle* European writers as manifestations of disease. For a recent study of the relationship between medicine, the life sciences, and literature in the modern era, see *Médecine, sciences de la vie et littérature*, ed. by Lise Dumasy-Queffélec and Hélène Spengler.

42 Dugas, *Les Grands Timides*, i–ii.

Today, we might critique his conclusions by emphasizing the way in which these depictions are mediated through shared, culturally and historically embedded, literary structures, or by underlining the unrepresentative nature of the sample he draws on: male writers significantly outnumber female writers in his corpus, for example. Moreover, by limiting himself to a group of highly literate individuals, Dugas neglects to examine the way timidity might manifest itself beyond the parameters of this privileged world. Yet the links Dugas identifies between shyness and literature are nonetheless significant in nuancing his assessment of the consequences of long-term timidity. Indeed, one constructive consequence of timidity, Dugas proposes, is its ability to facilitate literary or intellectual vocations (a circular argument, admittedly, in light of the methodological issues outlined above). Referencing Rousseau and Vigny, and drawing on the age-old — and androcentric — binary distinction between the 'man of action' and the 'man of contemplation',[43] Dugas suggests that timidity, 'qui est une inaptitude à la vie pratique, devient par là même une prédisposition à la vie imaginative et à l'art' (*T*, 143). Moreover, 'les défauts du timide, le souci de la perfection, la maladie de l'idéal, se transforment en qualités pour l'artiste' (*T*, 146).[44] Dugas's balanced approach to the benefits and obstacles timidity brings, however, does not preclude his ultimate conclusion that while timidity may be the trigger for an artistic vocation, it becomes useless once this trigger has taken effect.

The delineation of timidity's tipping-point reflects the ambivalence which lies at the heart of Dugas's assessment. As a momentary, fleeting attack, timidity is acceptable. Timidity can be compatible with healthy psychic functioning and, in specific contexts, even generate it: the gradual overcoming of timidity as a child, for example, helps to develop genuine confidence and ease as an adult as well as, in certain cases, a creative or intellectual impulse. Timidity also facilitates the development of modesty, and deepened and authentic knowledge of the self.[45] When considered in retrospect, the occasional attack of timidity is 'la crise normale par laquelle doit passer l'organisation des fonctions psychiques' (*T*, 141); 'la condition du perfectionnement individuel' (*T*, 142). But in contrast to this narrative of timidity as a productive rite of passage, Dugas also emphasizes its other: a chronic state of suffering which ultimately harms

43 Cain, *Quiet*, p. 269.

44 Gabriel Tarde also makes a connection between shyness and creativity, suggesting that the true innovator is essentially anti-social, or rather, 'supra-social' (Tarde, pp. 95–97).

45 As Dugas writes, 'enfin on pourrait faire honneur à la timidité de certaines qualités morales, [...] de la pudeur des sentiments, de la sincérité dans l'examen de soi-même' (*T*, 146).

even the artist.[46] The final section of *La Timidité* considers the methods through which education can prevent or cure this affliction. Two principal strategies emerge: first, what Dugas, after the eighteenth-century moralist Vauvenargues, calls familiarity (*T*, 152), and, second, a process of reasoning ('un traitement rationnel', *T*, 156). The first strategy, suited to simple forms of timidity, centres on spending time in society and gaining experience of it, based on the premise that 'la vie n'effraie que ceux qui l'ignorent' (*T*, 154).[47] For what is labelled the moral disease of chronic timidity, however, Dugas proposes a logical exploration of the condition: this will reveal to the sufferer that the excuses he has made for his timidity are, in reality, built on a series of irrational, chimerical arguments. An acknowledgement of this is the first step towards dislodging the timid individual's fixation on his own condition: 'On ne peut être logiquement timide. La raison fait donc évanouir la timidité, par cela seul qu'elle s'en rend compte' (*T*, 156). Much as the sufferer feels an absence of volition, intellect, or emotion during an attack of timidity, timidity is ultimately forced to absent *itself* in the final pages of the book — cure, disturbingly, by denial. Such a loss, Dugas suggests, adopting a lexicon of male sexual health, is compensated for 'par le gain des vertus viriles' (*T*, 160); the sufferer, 'que la timidité stérilise' (*T*, 160–61), is finally able to assume an active role in the functioning and, by implication, reproduction of society.

Dugas's use of the imagery of sexual health is not developed explicitly in his study; nor does he focus in any sustained way on the advantages of a society in which timidity is absent, choosing instead to emphasize the importance of confidence for individual flourishing. Yet Paul Hartenberg's more overtly normalizing *Les Timides et la timidité*, published three years later, stresses both these aspects. The third part of this chapter turns to this text.

---

46 The extremely shy artist will produce work too far removed from reality, too idiosyncratic, to be considered art in a meaningful way: 'Enfin la timidité exerce sur les conceptions de l'artiste une influence funeste: elle développe en lui, comme on l'a montré, le goût du romanesque, du subtil et du raffiné; elle l'éloigne donc du but véritable de l'art, si bien marqué par le mot profond de [Johann Heinrich] Merck sur Goethe: "Ta tendance, la voie dont tu ne saurais t'écarter consiste à donner au réel une forme poétique: les autres cherchent à réaliser ce qu'ils appellent le poétique et l'idéal, et ne font rien qui vaille"' (p. 149).

47 As Dugas summarizes, 'la familiarité dont parle Vauvenargues est ce contact direct des personnes et des choses qui remet nos jugements au point, qui dissipe les fantômes de notre imagination, et fait évanouir nos craintes folles' (*T*, 154).

Hartenberg: *Les Timides et la timidité* (1901)

Hartenberg was born in Wolxheim (Bas-Rhin) in 1871. He pursued his medical and psychiatric training at the Faculty of Nancy, and later established a medical practice in Paris, specializing in mental illnesses.[48] Hartenberg's exploration of timidity positions itself in relation, and in certain ways in *opposition*, to Dugas's 1898 study ('récente, mais bien incomplète et bien obscure').[49] Indeed, Hartenberg begins his 1901 monograph by explicitly outlining his distance from the faculty theory and 'méthode introspective pure' adopted by Dugas (*TT*, vi). Rejecting the dualism of classical philosophy palpable in Dugas's work, Hartenberg insists on a materialist view of mind and body, identifying the brain and nervous system, rather than the mind or soul, as the objects of his enquiry (*TT*, vii). For Hartenberg, explicitly adhering to the James-Lange theory of emotions, the physiological manifestations of timidity are inseparable from the psychological, and equally significant (*TT*, x). His study thus adopts a complex methodological approach, which marries clinical observation and examination ('par le palper, la percussion, l'auscultation', *TT*, xiii) with first-person case histories, surveys, literature reviews, and experimental research.

Yet while Hartenberg appears dismissive of Dugas's subjective methods and eloquent writing style (*TT*, xv), it would be wrong to suggest that he disregards the conclusions Dugas derives from his research. Hartenberg may actively seek to 'correct' Dugas's introspective study ('où la partie physiologique et clinique fait entièrement défaut', *TT*, xiv), but he does nonetheless draw on much of Dugas's material, to the extent of citing entire pages from *La Timidité* at a time. Like Dugas, he identifies literature as a fertile source of material for his scientific investigations (*TT*, xiv). As well as lifting literary examples directly from Dugas's study, Hartenberg broadens the range of writing and writers to be viewed through the prism of timidity, most distinctively by including works

48 Fairbrother, 'The Treatment of Social Phobia', p. 1292. For a history of psychiatry in France, see Shorter, *History of Psychiatry*, pp. 81–87. As Shorter notes, psychiatric training was conducted in asylums for most of the century in France; it was only in 1877 that a government decree announced that the four main medical faculties (the Sorbonne, Lyon, Nancy, and Marseille) would offer specialist psychiatric teaching (p. 84). For further biographical and bibliographical information about Hartenberg, see 'Paul Hartenberg', in *Dictionnaire de biographie française*, ed. by M. Prévost, Roman d'Amat, and Tribout de Morembert (Paris: Letouzy et Ané, 1986), XVII, 686. See also, Alain de Mijolla, *Freud et la France: 1885–1945* (Paris: Presses universitaires de France, 2010).

49 Paul Hartenberg, 'Bulletin: La Timidité', *Revue de psychologie clinique et thérapeutique*, 3, 2 (1899), 33–42 (p. 34).

with a decadent or proto-decadent aesthetic. Baudelaire's prose poem 'Le Mauvais Vitrier', from *Le Spleen de Paris* (1869), for example, is incorporated into a section on the 'décharges explosives' (*TT*, 93) from which shy individuals periodically suffer: the poet-narrator's musings on the strange surges of energy and recklessness which visit his otherwise shy friend ('timide [...] à ce point qu'il lui faut rassembler toute sa pauvre volonté pour entrer dans un café') merge with the voice of the medic who likens these surges to attacks of epilepsy or hysteria (*TT*, 93–94). Hartenberg singles out Philippe from Maurice Barrès's *Le Culte du moi* (1888–1891) as an inspirational example of an individual overcoming his timidity, claiming that 'les livres de Maurice Barrès, tant goutés par les jeunes gens, ne sont autre chose que des manuels d'autothérapie de la timidité' (*TT*, 225).[50] He even alludes to the recent publication of a novel of his own, *L'Attente* (1901), in which the thematic and stylistic traces of these works can be read (*TT*, 122). In this light, it is perhaps most accurate to consider Hartenberg's study as an amplification and a reemphasis of Dugas's findings. And this reemphasis, as we shall see, is more ideologically charged: anxious about the societal implications of the confidence — or lack of it — of French citizens, and infused with the spectre of degeneration and decadence haunting *fin-de-siècle* France.

Les Timides et la timidité is divided into six chapters. Chapter One focuses on definitions of timidity. While Dugas approached timidity as a faculty malfunction, Hartenberg treats it as an *emotion* composed of both psychic and somatic elements:

> L'émotion [de timidité] est un état complexe de trouble, de confusion, d'embarras, d'hésitation, de crainte, de scrupule, de pudeur, etc., qui [...] s'accompagne de manifestations plus ou moins marquées, telles que battements de cœur, angoisse, sueur froide, tremblement, rougeur du visage, etc.[51] (*TT*, 3)

---

50 It was Hartenberg's willingness to analyse fictional representations of timidity alongside autobiographical material — like Dugas — which earned him this rebuke from Alfred Binet: 'Jean-Jacques [Rousseau] a réellement vécu, et ce sont là des interprétations possibles; mais examiner avec le même sérieux le Julien de Bourget, attester d'un ton grave que ce personnage imaginaire qui n'a vécu que d'une vie de roman est "avant tout un neurasthénique constitutionnel", voilà des affirmations qui ne peuvent passer qu'avec un grain de sel, et notre auteur paraît tout à fait sérieux', in '*Hartenberg, Les Timides et la timidité* [compte rendu]', *L'Année psychologique*, 8, 1 (1901), 510–13 (pp. 512–13).

51 Hartenberg frequently refers to *angoisse*, or at times *anxiété*, as a symptom of shyness, indicative of his interest in Freud's early work on the anxiety neurosis (*angstneurose*). However, Hartenberg's initial enthusiasm for Freud's ideas will later transform into marked hostility towards psychoanalysis; see Mijolla, pp. 63, 119, 249–50.

At root, Hartenberg continues, this 'complexus émotionnel' is a combination of two more fundamental emotions: fear and shame (*TT*, 3). Adopting a distinction similar to that of Dugas, and one which will motivate the structure of the study as a whole, Hartenberg separates the isolated attack of timidity from the timid individual who is gradually shaped by the experience and memory of these attacks (*TT*, 8). While timidity is the emotion, the *timide* is the individual who is inclined to suffer this specific emotion in social situations, and whose 'interparoxystique' mental state is affected as a result (*TT*, 9). Chapter Two proceeds to analyse the fit of timidity in greater detail, focusing on its sensory, motor, vascular, visceral, secretory, and psychic symptoms (*TT*, 21–36). Chapter Three explores the character of the timid individual: a distinction is made between the natural hypersensitivity of the *timide* (*TT*, 54), and the consequences of the crises of timidity. These consequences, Hartenberg argues, begin to take effect once the individual becomes aware of himself as timid — usually in the early stages of puberty (*TT*, 58) — and, in certain unfortunate cases, starts to *cultivate* his timidity. These effects are all negatively coded, and include sadness, misanthropy, and the 'maladie de l'idéal' (after Dugas), egotism and dilettantism, and affected and at times rash behaviour.

It is in Chapter Four, however, that the concept of timidity becomes explicitly enmeshed in a network of cultural beliefs and socially established distinctions pertaining to gender, sexuality, and race. Focusing on the aetiology and evolution of timidity, Hartenberg outlines gender as a key factor determining the effect shyness has on the sufferer: in doing so, he sheds light on the conspicuous lack of female presence in Dugas's study, in which only a handful of references are made to female writers (Ackermann, George Eliot, Bashkirtseff). Hartenberg holds that while the physiological manifestations of timidity are almost identical in men and women, the psychic and social consequences of these manifestations differ widely. At root, these differences reflect the relative levels of passivity and activity each sex is expected and encouraged to present in society. For the nineteenth-century woman, less obliged to 'payer de sa personne' or initiate action in public (*TT*, 128), 'la paralysie émotive de la timidité l'entrave moins et, partant, la préoccupe moins' (*TT*, 128). While attacks of timidity may be momentarily unpleasant for women, Hartenberg suggests, they rarely lead to more complicated psychic consequences since shyness is compatible with a traditional vision of feminine modesty and chasteness. As a result, and paradoxically, female displays of timidity can function as a useful means of sexual attraction (*TT*, 129). Shyness is thus naturalized and normalized for the female, evidence of how, as McDaniel argues, 'shyness norms [...] have often been used to support hierarchies of gender'.[52] In other

52 McDaniel, *Shrinking Violets*, p. 21.

words, the presumption of timidity in women can be used to justify their exclusion from the public sphere. Tellingly, however, Hartenberg does admit that timidity can become a cause of conflict for independent women: 'Plusieurs femmes menant, il est vrai, une existence indépendante, m'ont déclaré avoir, à maintes reprises, pleuré de rage contre leur timidité' (*TT*, 130).

Timidity is not construed as a cause for concern for (dependent) women, then, but rather as a function of their femininity. It is instead for men that shyness becomes problematic, severely reducing their bodily and mental health and, as both cause and effect of this, their social status. Hartenberg's study repeatedly affirms the need for men to succeed socially, promoting a distinctly Darwinian conception of life in which men exist in a state of perpetual struggle, embroiled in 'les conflits quotidiens de la concurrence vitale' (*TT*, 218); 'la lutte pour la vie ou la conquête sexuelle' (*TT*, 130).[53] Heightened sensitivity to a sense of dignity and honour (*TT*, 129), coupled with difficulty in succeeding in professional and personal life, can, Hartenberg suggests, engender a whole spectrum of interconnected pathologies in timid males (*TT*, 51–52; 124; 145–53). These range from the phobia of blushing (erythrophobia) (*TT*, 130; 192–213) to the sexual practices of onanism ('une sorte d'égotisme sexuel', *TT*, 153) or pederasty (an 'inversion[s] sexuelle[s] acquise[s]', *TT*, 154), and severe alcohol and drug abuse (*TT*, 210; 238–39).[54]

In addition to linking timidity with gender and sexuality (as either cause or effect), Hartenberg suggests that timidity is racially determined. He identifies

---

53 On differences between the Lamarckian and Darwinian theories of evolution, and the role of conflict therein, see Nye, *Crime, Madness, and Politics in Modern France*, pp. 119–24 and *The Reception of Charles Darwin in Europe*, ed. by Eve-Marie Engels and Thomas F. Glick (London; New York: Continuum, 2008), II, especially chapter 17, 'The Interminable Decline of Lamarckism in France'. For further discussion of the complex scientific, cultural, and literary reception of Darwin in France, see *The Literary and Cultural Reception of Charles Darwin in Europe*, ed. by Thomas F. Glick and Elinor Shaffer (London: Bloomsbury, 2014), IV, especially Part 7.

54 For discussion of the discourses surrounding sexual health in nineteenth-century France, see Foucault, *La Volonté de savoir* (Paris: Gallimard, 2001); also Nye, *Masculinity and Male Codes of Honor in Modern France*, chapter 10, on the connections between virility, honour, and courage within the gendered discourse on heroism at the *fin de siècle*. Foucault alludes to historical assumptions surrounding timidity and sexual deviance when he writes that nineteenth-century social science 'declared the furtive customs of the timid [...] dangerous for the whole of society' (cited in Nye, *Crime, Madness, and Politics in Modern France*, p. 165). On erythrophobia in the nineteenth century, consult *Histoire de la vie privée*, ed. by Philippe Ariès and Georges Duby (Paris: Seuil, 1985), IV, pp. 450–51; on the blush more widely, see Paul White, 'Reading the Blush', *Configurations*, 24, 3 (2016), 281–301.

people of Slavic and Germanic origin as naturally timid (contradicting the opinion of Max Nordau, he adds, on the subject) (*TT*, 132), along with the Celts (agreeing with Ernest Renan on this point) (*TT*, 133). While the 'peuples latins' (*TT*, 132) of the Mediterranean are much more expansive, the 'Anglo-Saxons' are, surprisingly, the least inclined to timidity for Hartenberg, who explicitly contradicts Stendhal's description of bashfulness as one of the 'vices anglais' (*TT*, 131). Instead: 'Sanguins, vigoureux, doués d'un tonus musculaire élevé — ce qui est un obstacle à l'impressionnabilité nerveuse — ils [les Anglo-Saxons] marchent à travers les hommes avec, dans les regards et dans les gestes, une assurance résolue et une confiance dans l'efficacité de leurs forces' (*TT*, 131). Next to this imposing image of English physical and psychological prowess, Hartenberg paints a more measured picture of the modern French people who, viewed as a collective, are positioned naturally between the two extremes of severe reticence (exemplified by the Slavs) and utter expansiveness (epitomized by the southern Europeans or Anglo-Saxons): 'Il y aurait chez lui [le Français] à peu près équilibre entre la sensation interne et la manifestation externe' (*TT*, 133).

This rather guarded description of the 'natural' French temperament in a book aimed primarily at a French readership is intriguing. It points to the position Hartenberg negotiates in *Les Timides* between a scientific commitment to heredity as the principal cause determining timidity in an individual (*TT*, 134–44), and a belief that medical and educational intervention can be effective in curing or, better still, preventing, pathological forms of it from developing. That is, by positioning French subjects as relatively, but not exceptionally, timid, Hartenberg suggests that certain French subjects may indeed inherit a disposition to timidity, but that it is, generally, mild enough in them to be rectified. This position allows Hartenberg to highlight the real dangers that (male) timidity, if unchecked, poses to both individual and national health, but also the possibilities open to medical and educational professionals to intervene and help fashion a France in which everyone comes to play his (or her) part. As Hartenberg concludes:

> quoi qu'on dise, les voluptés intérieures du dilettantisme et de la création d'art ne saurait suppléer entièrement aux satisfactions que procurent l'activité et l'effort parmi la collectivité humaine. La pensée et le rêve ne remplacent pas l'action et la vie. […] Au degré d'évolution sociale atteint par l'humanité du XXe siècle, c'est dans la vie collective que l'individu normal de notre race puisera ses meilleures distractions et ses satisfactions les plus saines. (*TT*, 263–64)

While not as anxiety-inducing or suspicious as the criminal or prostitute, it is possible to see how the timid individual — anti-social by very definition — could become grouped together with the figures of social deviance which populated the French imagination at the turn of the twentieth century.[55] In the journal co-edited by Hartenberg and his fellow psychiatrist Paul Valentin, the *Revue de psychologie clinique et thérapeutique*,[56] Valentin clarifies the threat posed by those 'natures problématiques'[57] who suffer from ambiguous complaints, like shyness, not (yet) severe enough to warrant confinement in an asylum: 'Les malades soignés dans nos cliniques privés de maladies nerveuses et mentales sont les uns les aliénés en voie de devenir, les autres les psychonévropathes plus ou moins gravement atteints.'[58] Quoting the psychiatrist Richard Von Krafft-Ebing, Valentin continues:

> "Ces hommes ne sont pas encore des fous, mais il y a chez eux quelque chose qui cloche". [...] N'ont-ils pas [ces malades], sous des dehors impérieux, *équivoques* ou séduisants, l'influence la plus délétère sur un grand nombre de ceux qui, de près ou de loin, sont contraints à les subir?[59]

Likewise, Hartenberg's own rhetorical flourishes in the closing pages of *Les Timides* outline a normative vision of society in which seemingly minor behavioural differences — in this case, shyness and solitariness — equate with abnormality and ill-health. And, in an effort to halt the progression and potential spread of morbid timidity, Hartenberg suggests a number of therapeutic treatments which further hint at the sinister turn his utopian dream of human collectivity and uniformity will take later in the twentieth century. Many of the suggestions Hartenberg makes seem legitimate, to the extent that Fairbrother

55 For example, images of prostitution abounded in *fin-de-siècle* French visual art (see work by Degas and Toulouse-Lautrec), while fiction by Zola, amongst others, engaged in representations of criminality; see *Thérèse Raquin* and the Rougon-Macquart cycle (e.g. Jacques Lantier, Roubaud).

56 For a useful study of this short-lived but significant journal, consult J. Postel, 'Une tentative à méditer. Histoire de la première revue française de psychologie médicale 1897–1901', *Psychologie médicale*, 3, 5 (1971), 645–56.

57 Paul Valentin, 'Bulletin', *Revue de psychologie clinique et thérapeutique*, 5, 1 (1901), 1–8 (p. 4).

58 Ibid., p. 2.

59 Ibid., pp. 4–6, my emphasis. The first sentence in this quotation, "Ces hommes ne sont pas encore des fous, mais il y a chez eux quelque chose qui cloche", comes from Von Krafft-Ebing, *Traité clinique de psychiatrie* (Paris: A. Maloine, 1897), p. 40.

sees in them a prescient forerunner of Cognitive Behavioural Therapy.[60] He suggests dramatically improved education, contrasting the poor hygiene, mental overloading, and lack of physical exercise characteristic of French schools with the English model in which 'la vie physique, la liberté, l'initiative, tiennent la première place' (*TT*, 218).[61] At the individual level, his vision of 'auto-thérapie' or self-help stresses the importance of motivational reading, exemplified, through the means of fiction, by Julien Sorel's repeated rereading of Napoleon's *Mémorial de Saint-Hélène* in *Le Rouge et le Noir* (and thus offering the reader two examples of inspirational texts) (*TT*, 223). It also emphasises the importance of early socialization, and strategic props or activities to give the sufferer confidence in public (holding an umbrella, smoking a cigarette, whistling) (*TT*, 223–31). Possible medical treatments include improved hygiene and diet and 'verbal suggestion', as well as hydrotherapy, massage, and electrotherapy, all prescribed or administered by a specialist psychiatric doctor (*TT*, 231–37).

Fairbrother does not mention Hartenberg's recommendation of electrotherapy in her appreciative, but decontextualized, exploration of *Les Timides et la timidité*. By presenting shyness as a discrete phenomenon, she similarly fails to mention Hartenberg's hypothesis that the most serious forms of timidity are linked to the organic defects of congenital degeneration (*TT*, 214–16); that timidity can, as Valentin's comments also suggest, be indicative of a more severe, underlying problem. Degeneration, or *dégénérescence*, was a mid-nineteenth-century psychological theory of inherited (mal)adaptation to unhealthy environments, with roots in Lamarckian evolutionary and heredity theory. As explored by Nye and Pick, degeneration quickly surpassed its original function as a clinical diagnosis to become a compelling means of explaining the many societal ills with which France was seen to be afflicted in the aftermath of the Franco-Prussian war (slow population growth, increasing alcoholism, and the spread of syphilis and tuberculosis).[62] For Hartenberg, the prevention of timidity merges with 'la lutte contre la dégénérescence' (*TT*, 217). To ensure a national population as high in quality as in quantity — thus in which

60 Fairbrother, 'The Treatment of Social Phobia', pp. 1293, 1303.

61 For discussion of the Third Republic debates surrounding the benefits of sport, and comparison with Britain, see Robert Tombs and Isabelle Tombs, *That Sweet Enemy: The French and the British from the Sun King to the Present* (London: Pimlico, 2007), pp. 413–18, and Nye, *Crime, Madness, and Politics in Modern France*, chapter 9.

62 Nye, *Crime, Madness, and Politics in Modern France*; Daniel Pick, *Faces of Degeneration: A European Disorder, c. 1848–c. 1918* (Cambridge and New York: Cambridge University Press, 1989).

chronic timidity is eliminated — parents who have themselves suffered from timidity should do their utmost to create the right environmental conditions for 'la procréation d'enfants normaux, sains, équilibrés et calmes' (*TT*, 217). This, Hartenberg claims, will help stem the tide of degeneration. More disturbingly, he adds:

> À cet égard, on ne peut qu'applaudir aux projets surgis de divers côtés, tendant à réglementer les mariages, ainsi qu'aux campagnes contre l'alcoolisme, la tuberculose, la syphilis, à toutes ces initiatives éclairées et généreuses qui cherchent à soulager l'humanité de ses tares dégénératives. (*TT*, 217–18)

Hartenberg's vision of a nation cleansed of shyness thanks to a eugenical plan of controlled breeding says much about the reach and aspirations of *fin-de-siècle* psychiatry, as well as the reigning belief that France was in major need of both physical and moral regeneration.[63] When compared with Dugas's study, this vision also demonstrates the ambivalence surrounding *fin-de-siècle* theories of shyness. Hartenberg's elision of timidity with alcoholism, tuberculosis, and syphilis — key concerns of the era — shows timidity to be a highly undesirable trait in a society where social and professional ambition was considered increasingly necessary for men. The *timide* is one who struggles to 'get on' in society and thus one whom society struggles to 'get on' with.

For Hartenberg, the emblematic figure of the *timide* is perhaps the erythrophobic 'M. G…, 34 ans', a 'malheureux tombé, par l'effet de sa rougeur, aux derniers degrés de l'échelle sociale' (*TT*, 209–10): a marginalized individual tumbling down the social ladder who threatens, metonymically, to bring the whole nation down with him in the process. Dugas's monograph, devoid of references to degeneration, and maintaining a focus on the 'grands timides' who will go on to be the star subjects of Dugas's later works, presents timidity in a more open sense. Not entrapped in the web of degenerative disorders spun by Hartenberg, timidity is allowed to exist as a potentially enabling trait

63 Degeneration is the subject of several articles by Hartenberg in the *Revue de psychologie clinique et thérapeutique* throughout 1900: he proposes enforced castration, legalized suicide, and euthanasia as legitimate means of fighting against the psychoses and neuroses caused by degeneration. These measures, he suggests, can be applied even when degeneration is at its potential, not yet fully realized, state; Hartenberg, 'Bulletin: Contre la dégénérescence', *Revue de psychologie clinique et thérapeutique*, 4, 5 (1900), 129–33 (p. 132). While Hartenberg does not make such extreme claims in *Les Timides et la timidité*, the comments he does make regarding eugenics need to be seen in this context.

at the creative level, while nonetheless remaining highly debilitating socially. Like Dugas, Hartenberg makes extensive use of literary excerpts to exemplify certain psychic or physiological phenomena associated with shyness, or to provide readers with models for overcoming it (Julien Sorel in *Le Rouge et le Noir*, as we have seen, or Philippe in *Le Culte du moi*). But, explicitly contradicting Dugas, he is adamant that timidity is not in itself a catalyst for literary creation.[64]

Conclusion

Despite the marked differences which emerge from a comparative reading of their work, both Dugas and Hartenberg agree that systematic or chronic timidity is a disorder for which individuals can, and in certain cases *should*, seek help. By focusing on their turn-of-the-century texts, this chapter has shown that the processes through which shyness came to be considered a mental illness were set in motion earlier than is frequently thought.[65] While shyness researchers typically consider the late twentieth century as the moment of shyness's medicalization, perhaps a result of looking primarily at the American context, there is a gradual — but as yet sporadic — move to examine attitudes towards shyness within a broader historical and comparative perspective.[66] By exploring Dugas's *La Timidité* and Hartenberg's *Les Timides et la timidité* in their *fin-de-siècle* contexts, this chapter has sought to understand the epistemological and ideological stakes implicit in the moral and medical attack on timidity at the turn of the century. It has argued that both Dugas and Hartenberg mapped the concept onto their respective philosophical, psychological, and physiological frameworks, assessing the moral weaknesses but also strengths of the

64 As Hartenburg writes: 'Je ne crois pas que ce soit à proprement parler la timidité qui prédispose aux vocations d'art, mais bien plutôt l'hyperesthésie affective, la délicatesse du cœur, la finesse de l'esprit [...]. Or on peut être doué d'un cœur sensible, d'un esprit fin, sans être pour cela timide, sans se retrancher du monde et sans s'interdire exclusivement les joies de la vie pratique' (*TT*, p. 263). Hartenberg makes similar arguments in relation to creativity and mental illness in an earlier discussion of Edmond de Goncourt (Hartenberg, 'Le Tempérament d'Edmond de Goncourt', *Le Lorraine-Artiste*, 14 (1896), 289–93).

65 For example, McDaniel, in her otherwise astute *Shrinking Violets*, suggests that shyness did not attract the attention of psychologists until the 1970s, ignoring *fin-de-siècle* psychopathology entirely.

66 As in, most recently, Joe Moran's *Shrinking Violets: A Field Guide to Shyness* (London: Profile Books, 2016).

sufferer (Dugas), or fashioning timidity — in the male, at least — as an ominous symptom of national degeneration and decline (Hartenberg).

By paying close attention to these monographs and their references, the chapter has also revealed the literary-historical origins of the *fin-de-siècle* debate on timidity, and a paradox lying at its heart: that this undesirable, even deviant, condition may have, at least in part, inspired the very works used to form these psychopathological theories; that shyness can have a productive, creative effect on both the individual and the collective. Hartenberg rejects this possibility, but it is palpable in Dugas's study, connecting his work to that of twenty-first-century writers such as Christopher Lane and Susan Cain who argue for greater appreciation of temperamental and behavioural diversity. And while pointing to new lines of enquiry for shyness researchers in particular, the literary references in these two monographs carry broader implications with regard to nineteenth-century interdisciplinarity, exemplifying the way in which literature shaped, as well as reflected, scientific knowledge in the period.

Bibliography

Anon., 'Chronique', *L'Année psychologique*, 1945, 665

Ariès, Philippe, and Georges Duby (eds), *Histoire de la vie privée*, L'Univers historique, 5 vols (Paris: Seuil, 1985–1987), IV

Berrios, G. E., *The History of Mental Symptoms: Descriptive Psychopathology Since the Nineteenth Century* (Cambridge; New York: Cambridge University Press, 1996)

Binet, Alfred, 'Hartenberg, Les Timides et la timidité [compte rendu]', *L'Année psychologique*, 8 (1901), 510–13

Bourke, Joanna, *Fear: A Cultural History* (London: Virago, 2006)

Buchanan, Heather, and Neil Coulson, *Phobias*, Palgrave Insights in Psychology (Basingstoke: Palgrave Macmillan, 2012)

Cabanès, Jean-Louis, Didier Philippot, and Paolo Tortonese (eds), *Paradigmes de l'âme: littérature et aliénisme au XIXe siècle* (Paris: Presses Sorbonne Nouvelle, 2012)

Cain, Susan, *Quiet: The Power of Introverts in a World That Can't Stop Talking* (London: Viking, 2012)

Chavira, Denise A., Murray B. Stein, and Vanessa L. Malcarne, 'Scrutinizing the Relationship Between Shyness and Social Phobia', *Journal of Anxiety Disorders*, 16 (2002), 585–98

Crozier, W. Ray, *Understanding Shyness: Psychological Perspectives* (Basingstoke: Palgrave, 2001)

——, and P. J. de Jong (eds), *The Psychological Significance of the Blush* (Cambridge and New York: Cambridge University Press, 2012)

Danziger, Kurt, *Naming the Mind: How Psychology Found its Language* (London: Sage, 1997)

Dowbiggin, Ian Robert, *Inheriting Madness: Professionalization and Psychiatric Knowledge in Nineteenth-Century France* (Berkeley: University of California Press, 1991)

Dugas, Ludovic, 'La Timidité', *Revue philosophique de la France et de l'étranger*, 1896

——, 'La Timidité de Waldeck-Rousseau', *Annales de Bretagne*, 34 (1919), 68–76

——, *La Timidité: étude psychologique et morale*, Bibliothèque philosophie contemporaine (Paris: Félix Alcan, 1898)

——, *Les Grands Timides* (Paris: Félix Alcan, 1922)

——, *Les Timides dans la littérature et l'art* (Paris: Félix Alcan, 1937 [1925])

——, 'Un philosophe breton, Théodule Ribot (1839–1916)', *Annales de Bretagne*, 32 (1917), 145–68

Dumasy-Queffélec, Lise, and Hélène Spengler (eds), *Médecine, sciences de la vie et littérature en France et en Europe de la Révolution à nos jours*, 3 vols (Geneva: Droz, 2014)

Engels, Eve-Marie, and Thomas F. Glick (eds), *The Reception of Charles Darwin in Europe*, II (London; New York: Continuum, 2008)

Fairbrother, Nichole, 'The Treatment of Social Phobia — 100 Years Ago', *Behaviour Research and Therapy*, 40 (2002), 1291–304

Foucault, Michel, *Histoire de la folie à l'âge classique* (Paris: Gallimard, 2007)

——, *La Volonté de savoir*, Histoire de la sexualité (Paris: Gallimard, 2001)

Gill, Miranda, 'Self-Control and Uncontrollable Passion in Stendhal's Theory of Love', *French Studies*, 69, 4 (2015), 462–78

Glick, Thomas F., and Elinor Shaffer (eds), *The Literary and Cultural Reception of Charles Darwin in Europe*, IV (London: Bloomsbury, 2014)

Goldstein, Jan Ellen, *Console and Classify: The French Psychiatric Profession in the Nineteenth Century* (Cambridge and New York: Cambridge University Press, 1987)

Guillin, Vincent, 'Théodule Ribot's Ambiguous Positivism: Philosophical and Epistemological Strategies in the Founding of French Scientific Psychology', *Journal of the History of the Behavioral Sciences*, 40 (2004), 165–81

Hartenberg, Paul, 'Bulletin: Contre la dégénérescence', *Revue de psychologie clinique et thérapeutique*, 4 (1900), 129–33

——, 'Bulletin: "La Timidité"', *Revue de psychologie clinique et thérapeutique*, 3 (1899), 33–42

——, *L'Attente* (Paris: P. Ollendorff, 1901)

——, 'Le Tempérament d'Edmond de Goncourt', *Le Lorraine-Artiste*, 14 (1896), 289–93

——, *Les Timides et la timidité* (Paris: Félix Alcan, 1901)

Heiser, Nancy A., Samuel M. Turner, and Deborah C. Beidel, 'Shyness: Relationship to Social Phobia and Other Psychiatric Disorders', *Behaviour Research and Therapy*, 41 (2003), 209–21

Janet, Pierre, *Les Obsessions et la psychasthénie*, 2 vols (Paris: Félix Alcan, 1908), I

Jolibert, Bernard, *L'Éducation d'une émotion: trac, timidité, intimidation dans la littérature*, Collection 'Éducation et Philosophie' (Paris: Harmattan, 1997)

Kagan, Jerome, *Galen's Prophecy: Temperament in Human Nature* (New York: Westview Press, 1994)

Krafft-Ebing, Richard von, *Traité clinique de psychiatrie* (Paris: A. Maloine, 1897)

Lane, Christopher, *Shyness: How Normal Behavior Became a Sickness* (New Haven: Yale University Press, 2007)

La Rochefoucauld, François de, *Maximes et réflexions morales du Duc de La Rochefoucauld* (Paris: Lecointe, 1829)

Lloyd, Stephanie, 'Morals, Medicine and Change: Morality Brokers, Social Phobias, and French Psychiatry', *Culture, Medicine, and Psychiatry*, 32 (2008), 279–97 <https://link.springer.com/article/10.1007/s11013-008-9092-4>

——, 'The Clinical Clash over Social Phobia: The Americanization of French Experiences?', *BioSocieties*, 1 (2006), 229–49

Lyons, William, *The Disappearance of Introspection* (Cambridge, MA: MIT Press, 1986)

Mantegazza, Paolo, *La Physionomie et l'expression des sentiments* (Paris: Félix Alcan, 1885)

McDaniel, Patricia, *Shrinking Violets and Caspar Milquetoasts: Shyness, Power, and Intimacy in the United States, 1950–1995*, The American Social Experience Series, 40 (New York: New York University Press, 2003)

Micale, Mark S., *Hysterical Men: The Hidden History of Male Nervous Illness* (Cambridge, MA: Harvard University Press, 2008)

Mijolla, Alain de, *Freud et la France: 1885–1945* (Paris: Presses universitaires de France, 2010)

Moran, Joe, *Shrinking Violets: A Field Guide to Shyness* (London: Profile Books, 2016)

Nicolas, Serge, and Agnès Charvillat, 'Introducing Psychology as an Academic Discipline in France: Théodule Ribot and the Collège de France (1888–1901)', *Journal of the History of the Behavioral Sciences*, 37 (2001), 143–64 <http://onlinelibrary.wiley.com/doi/10.1002/jhbs.1002/full>

Nordau, Max, *Dégénérescence* (Paris: Félix Alcan, 1894)

Nye, Robert A., *Crime, Madness, and Politics in Modern France: The Medical Concept of National Decline* (Princeton, NJ: Princeton University Press, 1984)

——, *Masculinity and Male Codes of Honor in Modern France* (Berkeley, CA: University of California Press, 1998)

Pick, Daniel, *Faces of Degeneration: A European Disorder, c.1848–c.1918*, Ideas in Context (Cambridge; New York: Cambridge University Press, 1989)

Postel, J., 'Une tentative à méditer. Histoire de la première revue française de psychologie médicale 1897–1901', *Psychologie médicale*, 3 (1971), 645–56

Prévost, M., Roman d'Amat, and Tribout de Morembert (eds), 'Paul Hartenberg', in *Dictionnaire de biographie française* (Paris: Letouzy et Ané, 1986), XVII, 686

Ribot, Théodule, *La Psychologie des sentiments* (Paris: Félix Alcan, 1896)

Schmidt, Louis A., and Jay Schulkin (eds), *Extreme Fear, Shyness, and Social Phobia: Origins, Biological Mechanisms, and Clinical Outcomes*, Series in Affective Science (New York: Oxford University Press, 1999)

Scott, Susie, *Shyness and Society: The Illusion of Competence* (Basingstoke: Palgrave Macmillan, 2007)

Shorter, Edward, *A History of Psychiatry: From the Era of the Asylum to the Age of Prozac* (New York: John Wiley & Sons, 1997)

Shuttleworth, Sally, *The Mind of the Child: Child Development in Literature, Science, and Medicine, 1840–1900* (Oxford: Oxford University Press, 2010)

Sierra, M., and G. E. Berrios, 'Introduction to "A Case of Depersonalization"', *History of Psychiatry*, 7 (1996), 451–54

Smith, Adam, *The Theory of Moral Sentiments* (Cambridge: Cambridge University Press, 2002)

Tarde, Gabriel, *Les Lois de l'imitation: étude sociologique* (Paris: Félix Alcan, 1890)

Tombs, Robert, and Isabelle Tombs, *That Sweet Enemy: The French and the British from the Sun King to the Present*, Pimlico, 786 (London: Pimlico, 2007)

Valentin, Paul, 'Bulletin', *Revue de psychologie clinique et thérapeutique*, 5 (1901), 1–8

Walsh, Richard T. G., Thomas Teo, and Angelina Baydala, *A Critical History and Philosophy of Psychology: Diversity of Context, Thought, and Practice* (Cambridge: Cambridge University Press, 2014)

White, Paul, 'Reading the Blush', *Configurations*, 24, 3 (2016), 281–301

Zimbardo, Philip, and Lynne Henderson, '"Foreword"', in *Shyness: Development, Consolidation and Change* (London: Routledge, 2000), xiii–xv

PART 2

Writing Pathological Experiences

CHAPTER 5

De Karl-des-Monts à Cénéri : lorsque la voix de l'interné entre dans le roman

Mélanie Bhend

Au XIXe siècle, la naissance de l'aliénisme[1] a eu pour effet de modifier radicalement la conception de la folie et le statut du fou. En incluant les folies partielles à sa nosologie, elle a pu déclarer aliéné un individu qui paraissait sain d'esprit et l'enfermer légitimement dans un asile. Placé ainsi à la merci du médecin qui régit l'institution asilaire, cet individu est un aliéné, en dépit de ce qu'il peut dire ou montrer. Ses actes et paroles sont réinterprétés selon une grille psychiatrique et le rejet de son diagnostic apparaît donc au médecin comme la confirmation de son mal. Il ne suffit plus de paraître sensé pour attester la raison. La voix de l'interné se voit ainsi bâillonnée par l'institution asilaire, et un des recours qui lui reste pour s'exprimer réside dans l'écriture. Par ce moyen, l'interné se reconstruit et déclare une intention de communiquer cette perception à l'autre. Cet autre, c'est l'opinion publique qu'il faut convaincre de l'effet dévastateur du diagnostic de l'aliéniste sur l'interné et de l'inefficacité de l'asile à soigner la folie. Mais cette entreprise ne va pas sans obstacles. La première critique de ces internés et sans doute la plus essentielle concerne la contestation de leur diagnostic de folie et le placement en asile qui en a résulté. Or, si, comme l'ont attesté les aliénistes, la folie peut se dissimuler derrière un masque de raison, toute revendication de la part d'une personne potentiellement atteinte d'aliénation mentale paraît suspecte. C'est pourquoi ces individus sont qualifiés dans ce chapitre pour ce qu'ils sont : des internés, soit des individus placés en asile pour aliénation mentale.

Parallèlement au développement scientifique, en littérature, de nouvelles conceptions du 'moi' ont conduit au développement de textes dans lesquels s'exprime la subjectivité de l'auteur.[2] Les mémoires, l'autobiographie, le journal

1 En dépit de son anachronisme et pour des raisons pratiques, ce terme sera employé pour désigner rétrospectivement la science médicale ayant pour objet l'étude de l'aliénation mentale.

2 Sur cette évolution, voir 'La première personne dans l'histoire', dans Sébastien Hubier, *Littératures intimes : les expressions du moi, de l'autobiographie à l'autofiction* (Paris : Armand Colin, 2003), chapitre 1.

 | DOI:10.1163/9789004368019_007

intime ou les correspondances constituent autant de supports sur lesquels l'auteur exploite les possibilités qu'offre l'expression du moi : une construction textuelle du moi à travers la figure du narrateur, l'affirmation de la subjectivité et l'intention de communiquer cette intériorité au lecteur.

Après avoir retracé les conditions par lesquelles la conception de la folie et le statut de l'aliéné ont été problématisés par les changements apportés par l'aliénisme et l'établissement de la loi des aliénés, ce chapitre se penche sur la valeur de la voix de l'interné du point de vue littéraire dans deux textes significatifs des années 1860 : *Un martyre dans une maison de fous* (1863) de Karl-des-Monts[3] et *Un beau-frère* (1869) d'Hector Malot.[4] Le premier est un texte autobiographique,[5] le second un roman qui inclut, à l'intérieur du récit, le journal du protagoniste. Dans les deux cas, le personnage principal a été interné dans un asile pour aliénation mentale et emploie l'écriture comme moyen d'élever sa voix au-delà de son diagnostic. Les deux œuvres visent à offrir au lecteur une description critique de l'asile et des aliénistes, en dénonçant le caractère arbitraire de leur internement ainsi que les pratiques inhumaines et inefficaces de cette science qui prétend soigner la folie. Karl-des-Monts, auteur, narrateur, et personnage d'*Un martyre dans une maison de fou*, livre ainsi sa correspondance privée avec sa maîtresse durant son internement à l'asile de Pau. Dans ces lettres, la folie et l'aliénisme sont représentés dans leur rapport à l'horrible et au grotesque. Céméri d'Eturquerais, pour sa part, est le protagoniste du roman de Malot et narrateur du journal inséré dans le récit

---

3 Karl-des-Monts est le nom de plume d'Ernest de Garay. Bien qu'on ne sache que très peu de choses sur cet auteur, cette correspondance a pu être établie sur un autre ouvrage, *Légendes des Pyrénées*, qui a été publié sous son nom véritable et sous son pseudonyme chez Michel Lévy frères à Paris, en 1857 et 1876 respectivement. *Un martyre dans une maison de fous* a tout d'abord été publié en 1863 aux Éditions Diamant, à Bruxelles. Ce chapitre prendra pour référence la plus récente réédition : *Un martyre dans une maison de fous*, éd. par Jérôme Solal (Paris : Fayard, 2010).

4 Hector Malot (1830–1907) est un journaliste et romancier français connu de son temps pour son engagement dans la défense des droits des enfants et des aliénés, pour lesquels il milite en faveur d'une réforme de la loi de 1838 dès les années 1860. Voir Jean Foucault et Francis Marcoin, *Diversité d'Hector Malot* (Arras : Université d'Artois, 2001). L'édition de référence correspond à la première publication en volume du roman : *Un beau-frère* (Paris : Hetzel, 1869). Toute référence future à *Un beau-frère* et *Un martyre dans une maison de fous* figurera dans le corps du texte du chapitre, abréviés respectivement *B* et *M*.

5 Dans la mesure où il remplit les conditions du 'pacte autobiographique', soit l'identité entre l'auteur, le narrateur et le personnage, en signant ses lettres du même nom que son livre, nous considérons qu'il entre dans cette catégorie. Nous y ferons référence par la suite comme 'témoignage'. Voir Philippe Lejeune, *Le Pacte autobiographique* (Paris : Seuil, 1975).

principal. Il y raconte son expérience au jour le jour dans la ferme Luat, un établissement privé pour le traitement de l'aliénation mentale, donnant à voir les conséquences néfastes de la proximité de la folie sur l'homme sain d'esprit.

À travers l'analyse comparative de ces deux textes, il s'agira dans un premier temps de se pencher sur le thème de la folie afin de dégager les caractéristiques esthétiques et rhétoriques qui rendent ces œuvres représentatives tout d'abord d'une conception particulière de la folie, celle qui la lie à l'horreur et à l'inhumain, mais également d'une posture critique à l'égard de l'aliénisme. Puis, dans un second temps, ces caractéristiques seront étudiées du point de vue de l'expression du moi lorsque la crédibilité du sujet est remise en cause par le diagnostic d'aliénation mentale. Cette analyse peut servir à l'étude de l'autobiographie dans la mesure où elle problématise la relation du texte aux notions de vraisemblance et de fiabilité du narrateur. Ces deux textes présentent chacun des moyens textuels par lesquels le narrateur se reconstruit une identité en opposition à l'aliénation mentale. Ce phénomène permet notamment de renforcer une des thèses de Michel Foucault qui considère l'asile comme un système de répression et d'exclusion de la folie.[6] Dans ce contexte d'enfermement, l'écriture de soi représente une stratégie de résistance au pouvoir médical. Il s'agit donc de voir comment l'agencement de ces textes peut défavoriser ou au contraire soutenir cette opposition, car si l'état mental du narrateur d'*Un martyre dans une maison de fous* reste toujours sujet à caution, Malot, en faisant entrer la voix de l'interné dans le roman, donc en la contextualisant, parvient à surmonter cet obstacle lié à la crédibilité. Ce second pan d'analyse permettra donc de dégager les différents enjeux littéraires de l'expression du moi aliéné.[7]

Contexte : la loi de 1838 et l'aliénisme

L'établissement de la loi des aliénés de 1838 a conduit à la multiplication des asiles en France en vertu de son premier article.[8] D'environ 10 000 internés

6 Michel Foucault, *Histoire de la folie à l'âge classique* (Paris : Gallimard, 1972).

7 La mise en évidence vise à insister sur la valeur problématique de ce terme, dans la mesure où le 'moi' a été déclaré 'aliéné' par une instance extérieure à l'individu et que ce dernier rejette précisément cet attribut.

8 'Chaque département est tenu d'avoir un établissement public, spécialement destiné à recevoir et soigner les aliénés'. *Loi des aliénés*, Titre I (Article I). Cette loi est retranscrite en annexe dans Robert Castel, *L'Ordre psychiatrique : l'âge d'or de l'aliénisme* (Paris : Minuit, 1976), pp. 316–24.

pour à peine plus d'une trentaine de 'maisons royales de santé' en 1834, cette proportion est passée à 37 717 pour 104 asiles d'aliénés dans le pays en 1871.[9] En vertu de cette loi, tout individu pouvait être enfermé dans un asile contre son gré pour autant que certaines conditions fussent remplies : un ordre motivé du préfet pour celui 'dont l'état d'aliénation compromettrait l'ordre public ou la sûreté des personnes'[10] dans le cas de placement d'office ; un dossier d'admission adressé au préfet comprenant une demande formulée par un membre de la famille avalisé par le certificat d'un médecin extérieur à l'établissement et un autre document établi par le médecin de l'asile dans le cas de placement volontaire. Pour un aliéniste comme Étienne Esquirol,[11] ces mesures étaient indispensables dès lors que les aliénistes avaient constaté que, dans certains cas, la folie pouvait n'être que partielle et latente et que le traitement des individus concernés ne pouvait se faire efficacement qu'à travers leur internement :

> Les lois anciennes ne s'étaient occupées que des aliénés furieux ou qui sont dans un état habituel de démence et d'imbécillité ; la loi nouvelle doit s'étendre aux aliénés dont le délire n'est ni général ni habituel, elle doit venir en aide à l'aliéné pour qu'il recouvre sa raison ; pour atteindre ce but la loi ne doit avoir rien à démêler avec l'aliéné lui-même qui ne la comprendrait pas, et qui est hors d'état d'en abuser.[12]

Foucault a montré comment l'aliénisme, loin de 'libérer' la folie, avait au contraire resserré les liens autour de l'aliéné en l'enfermant dans des établissements qui lui avaient été exclusivement dédiés, sous la surveillance étroite et autoritaire du médecin. L'aliéné s'est alors retrouvé dans un espace refermé sur lui-même, observé et jugé.[13] Constamment soumis à l'évaluation de son état mental, l'interné a vu sa liberté réduite à néant. Ses actes étaient soumis à l'examen médical et sa parole discréditée.[14] Pour Foucault, l'asile est donc un

---

9 Claude Quétel, *Histoire de la folie de l'Antiquité à nos jours* (Paris : Tallandier, 2012), pp. 308–12.

10 *Loi des aliénés*, Titre II (Article 18).

11 Étienne Esquirol (1772–1840), disciple de Philippe Pinel (1745–1826), était médecin à la Salpêtrière puis à Charenton. Outre ses contributions dans l'étude de l'aliénation mentale, il a joué un rôle important dans l'établissement de la loi des aliénés de 1838.

12 Étienne Esquirol, *Examen du projet de loi sur les aliénés* (Paris : J.-B. Baillère, 1838), p. 10.

13 Foucault, *Histoire de la folie*, pp. 619–23.

14 Pinel consacre par exemple un chapitre de son traité à l'art de manipuler l'aliéné, révélant la valeur accordée aux paroles de ce dernier. Voir Philippe Pinel, 'Habileté dans l'art de diriger les aliénés, en paraissant se prêter à leurs idées imaginaires', dans *Traité*

appareil d'exclusion, reconduisant la pratique du 'grand renfermement'[15] de l'époque classique.

À l'opposé, Marcel Gauchet et Gladys Swain voient dans l'institution asilaire 'le plus puissant des moyens de guérison',[16] qui fonctionne comme un 'gigantesque dispositif de socialisation'.[17] En effet, le mal de l'aliéné n'affecte pas sa santé physique mais son esprit, soit ce qui fait de lui un être humain. Le rôle de l'aliéniste consiste dès lors à restaurer cette humanité, ce qui implique donc 'une prise en charge totale de son existence'.[18] Cependant, si cette considération s'oppose diamétralement aux thèses de Foucault, Gauchet et Swain s'accordent néanmoins pour reconnaître l'échec de cette institution. Le regroupement des aliénés dans le microcosme de l'asile a en effet conduit à leur effacement à l'intérieur d'une masse uniforme puisque l'individualité de l'aliéné n'était de toute façon pas prise en compte.

Quoiqu'on fasse, la singularité subjective résiste, inaltérable, à la dissolution au sein de l'entité collective, à tel degré que l'effort pour la nier la fait ressortir et l'accuse, et que, tendant à détruire les liens élémentaires de coexistence pour leur substituer une massification sans différences ni distances intérieures, il n'aboutit, à l'inverse, qu'à privatiser et isoler encore davantage les personnes.[19] Or ce refus par le médecin d'admettre cette individualité écarte par là même toute possibilité de traitement, dans la mesure où ce changement (puisqu'il s'agit bien de cela) implique la reconnaissance mutuelle de l'égarement de la raison.

Ce déséquilibre, couplé à la faible proportion de guérisons,[20] a poussé l'opinion publique à émettre des doutes non seulement sur l'efficacité et la valeur thérapeutique de l'asile, mais aussi sur les critères mêmes qui distinguaient l'individu sain d'esprit de l'aliéné, surtout lorsque cette distinction n'était pas apparente. Dès les années 1860, la détermination et le traitement de la folie raisonnante[21] a pris une tournure polémique poussant les médecins à

---

médico-philosophique sur l'aliénation mentale ou la manie (Paris : Richard, Caille et Ravier, 1801), pp. 92–95.

15 Foucault, *Histoire de la folie*, pp. 67–109.

16 Marcel Gauchet et Gladys Swain, *La Pratique de l'esprit humain : l'institution asilaire et la révolution démocratique* (Paris : Gallimard, 1980), p. 95.

17 Ibid., p. 110.

18 Ibid., p. 127.

19 Ibid., p. 161.

20 Quétel signale par exemple qu'entre 1856 et 1860 les statistiques nationales ne faisaient état que de 8, 24% de guérisons, *Histoire de la folie de l'Antiquité à nos jours*, p. 433.

21 Cette appellation est employée pour qualifier le type de folie qui ne fait état d'aucun trouble de l'entendement et fait l'objet du traité éponyme de Moreau de Tours (1804–1884)

devoir se justifier. C'est ainsi notamment que les aliénistes Falret (1824–1902), Delasiauve (1804–1893) et Brierre de Boismont (1797–1881) ont publié en 1866 dans les *Annales médico-psychologiques* un article intitulé 'Discussion sur la folie raisonnante',[22] en réponse à des accusations de séquestration arbitraire qui remettaient en cause les diagnostics des médecins ainsi que l'efficacité de l'aliénisme, tant du point de vue de la loi, jugée insuffisante pour protéger les aliénés d'internements abusifs, que de celui du traitement de la folie. Ces accusations provenaient de séquestrés tels que Karl-des-Monts, Léon Sandon,[23] ou encore Hersilie Rouy,[24] mais aussi de journalistes et écrivains comme Malot, son ami Jules Vallès,[25] ou Yves Guyot.[26]

---

dans *La Folie raisonnante, envisagée sous le point de vue médico-légal* (Paris : Lacour, 1840). Elle est également appelée 'manie sans délire' (Pinel, *Traité médico-philosophique*, pp. 149–55), 'monomanie raisonnante' dans Étienne Esquirol, *Des Maladies mentales, considérées sous les rapports médical, hygiénique et médico-légal*, 3 vols (Paris : Baillière, 1838), II, pp. 49–72 ; ou 'folie lucide' dans le traité éponyme d'Ulysse Trélat, *La Folie lucide : étudiée et considérée au point de vue de la famille et de la société* (Paris : Adrien Delahaye, 1861). La diversité d'appellations ne fait que souligner la complexité de ce type de folie et la difficulté qu'ont les aliénistes à la définir clairement. Pour des raisons pratiques, nous emploierons ici l'expression générique de fou / folie raisonnant/e.

22 Jules Falret, M. Delasiauve et Brierre de Boismont, 'Discussions sur la folie raisonnante', *Annales médico-psychologiques*, 7 (1866), 382–499.

23 Léon Sandon (1823–1872) était un avocat qui a accusé Adolphe Billaut, ministre de l'Empire, d'avoir ordonné son placement à Charenton où il est resté enfermé pour 'monomanie raisonneuse'. 'L'affaire Sandon', dont le plaidoyer a été publié en 1865, est sans doute la plus connue en raison de son succès médiatique qui a entraîné une réponse de Brierre de Boismont en 1873 : 'Examen médico-légal de l'Affaire Sandon, pour servir à l'histoire de la folie raisonnante au XIXe siècle', *Annales médico-psychologiques*, 10 (1873), 73–96.

24 Hersilie Rouy (1814–1881) a été enfermée dans six asiles différents entre 1854 et 1868. À sa sortie, elle a adressé une pétition à la Chambre des députés, demandant réparation pour séquestration arbitraire. Dans son œuvre posthume, *Mémoires d'une aliénée*, publiée en 1883, elle raconte son expérience asilaire ainsi que le combat anti-aliéniste qui s'en est suivi.

25 Jules Vallès (1832–1885) a lui-même fait l'expérience de l'internement en 1851 pendant quelques mois. Il est connu pour son engagement auprès des catégories sociales défavorisées, et sa représentation de l'asile de Saint-Anne reprend les critiques anti-aliénistes. Voir Jules Vallès, 'Sainte-Anne' [1882], in *Le Tableau de Paris* (Paris : Livre Club Diderot, 1969–1970), pp. 751–67. Pour une biographie de Vallès, voir notamment Corinne Saminadayar-Perrin, *Jules Vallès* (Paris : Gallimard, 2013).

26 Outre le roman *Un fou* publié en 1884, Guyot (1843–1928) est également l'auteur de plus d'une trentaine d'articles intitulés 'Les Aliénés par un infirmier' dénonçant le système aliéniste dans *La Lanterne* du 22 octobre au 29 novembre 1879.

Ce chapitre se penche sur les œuvres qui ont figuré parmi les premières dans leur genre. *Un martyre dans une maison de fous*, publié en 1863 est en effet une des premières publications rendant compte des conditions asilaires de la perspective de l'interné. L'auteur, Karl-des-Monts, s'y présente comme un fervent défenseur de la cause ultramontaine, à une époque où la *Question Romaine* créait la polémique.[27] On l'aurait déclaré fou et enfermé à l'asile afin d'étouffer l'influence qu'il exerçait dans le débat politique. À travers les vingt-quatre lettres qui composent le texte, il retranscrit ses impressions et son expérience dans l'asile de Pau d'où il s'est échappé après neuf mois d'internement. En rendant ces lettres intimes accessibles au public, l'objectif, énoncé en préface, est la dénonciation. Il s'agit de 'soumettre au jugement de l'opinion publique les titres du plus curieux procès que les annales contemporaines puissent offrir à l'étonnement et à l'indignation des temps à venir' (*M*, 7).

Outre le thème de la séquestration arbitraire traité dans le roman *Un beau-frère* de Malot, publié tout d'abord dans *Le Journal des débats*[28] puis en volume chez Hetzel en 1869, tire son originalité de sa forme. Selon l'auteur, il s'agit de l'histoire d'un 'homme sain d'esprit, mais que des parents ont un intérêt à faire passer pour fou, [qui] est reconnu fou par des médecins, et enfermé dans un asile d'aliénés où il devient fou'.[29] Le récit est essentiellement assumé par un narrateur extradiégétique et hétérodiégétique,[30] à l'exception de la partie de l'histoire couvrant l'internement du protagoniste. Dans ce passage, le récit incorpore le journal de l'interné, et le narrateur omniscient cède donc momentanément sa place à Cénéri qui assume la fonction de narrateur autodiégétique. Il y rend compte à sa maîtresse de son expérience asilaire, du premier jour de son internement à sa sortie. En employant cette technique du récit enchâssé, Malot redonne à l'interné une voix que l'institution asilaire lui a retirée et la légitime en la contextualisant. Le succès de son roman a encouragé

27 Controverse politique autour du statut de Rome et de l'autorité papale dans le contexte de l'unité italienne en formation. Pie IX était alors soutenu par les ultramontains qui défendaient le pouvoir absolu, spirituel et temporel du pape sur l'État.

28 *Un beau-frère* est paru en feuilleton du 28 août au 18 octobre 1868.

29 Hector Malot, *Roman de mes romans* (Paris : Flammarion, 1896), p. 32.

30 Ces termes renvoient à la formulation de Gérard Genette dans *Figures III* (Paris : Seuil, 1972), pp. 238–59. *Extradiégétique* et *Intradiégétique* renvoient aux différents niveaux narratifs : 'tout événement raconté par un récit est à un niveau diégétique immédiatement supérieur à celui où se situe l'acte narratif producteur de ce récit' (p. 238). Le premier niveau est dit *extradiégétique*, tandis que l'objet de la narration de ce premier niveau est dit *intradiégétique*. Un narrateur est dit *hétérodiégétique* lorsqu'il est 'absent de l'histoire qu'il raconte', par opposition au narrateur *homodiégétique* (p. 252). Un narrateur est dit *autodiégétique* lorsqu'il est le 'héros de son récit' (p. 253) (degré fort de l'*homodiégétique*).

d'autres auteurs à traiter de thèmes similaires dans leurs romans, faisant de la cause des internés, et plus généralement des aliénés, une affaire politique, comme le souligne Aude Fauvel :

> La polémique fut telle qu'elle engagea même le gouvernement à nommer une commission d'enquête et incita Léon Gambetta à déposer le tout premier projet de réforme de la législation sur les asiles. [...] Avec *Un beau-frère* Malot se signala ainsi comme le premier auteur anti-aliéniste de sa génération.[31]

Les critiques formulées à l'encontre de l'aliénisme par les internés ont ainsi été popularisées notamment par leur passage dans le roman qui constitue un support de poids auprès de l'opinion publique pour porter leurs revendications. Mais au-delà de la valeur polémique que le texte de Malot apporte à la cause des aliénés, il est également représentatif d'une conception littéraire de la folie. L'analyse comparative du texte de Karl-des-Monts et du journal de Cénéri permet de dégager les attributs esthétiques de ce thème : son rapport à l'horreur, au grotesque et à l'inhumain, ainsi que le péril qu'il représente.

Folie esthétique et littéraire

Pour Karl-des-Monts, la folie correspond à la perte de l'humanité, les aliénés se rapprochant plus de la bête que de l'homme :

> Dans la préface de son remarquable *Discours sur l'origine et les fondements de l'inégalité parmi les hommes*, Jean-Jacques Rousseau parle d'une statue de Glaucus que le temps, la mer et les orages avaient tellement défigurée qu'elle ressemblait moins à un dieu qu'à une bête féroce. Ainsi en advient-il de ceux que frappe ce terrible fléau de la folie absolue, et, si je souffre tant ici, ma pauvre chère, c'est, hélas ! que cette lugubre ménagerie est toute pleine de ces statues défigurées, de ces dieux tombés qui ne se souviennent guère du ciel. (*M*, 64–65)

La folie qu'observe l'auteur dans l'asile est une folie caractérisée par l'animalité, la difformité, et la déchéance. À cet égard, le dieu tombé du ciel n'est pas sans

31 Aude Fauvel, 'La Voix des fous : Hector Malot et les "romans d'asile"', *Romantisme*, 4, 3 (2008), 51–64 (p. 51).

évoquer Lucifer, rapportant la folie à l'imagerie de l'enfer qui constitue également un thème récurrent. Cette représentation s'inscrit par ailleurs dans une tradition littéraire et artistique qui relie la folie aux thèmes de l'horreur, de la bestialité, et de la difformité :

> Les conceptions les plus sanglantes d'Edgar Poe, les enfantements les plus monstrueux d'Hoffmann, les caprices hybrides de Goya, les fantastiques délires de Louis Boulanger, les diableries de Callot, les sataniques peuplades dont Bruegel a hérissé son enfer [...] Jamais Shakespeare n'a imaginé des comparses plus squalidement dignes de figurer au sabbat des sorcières. (*M*, 43)

Le recours à l'hyperbole accentue le caractère ineffable et extrême de la description. En évoquant ces images, l'auteur réactive une imagerie populaire qui entoure l'asile et les fous d'une aura mystérieuse et effrayante.[32] C'est donc sans surprise que Karl-des-Monts se réfère à ces auteurs qui ont si souvent associé la folie au fantastique et à l'horreur.

Cette représentation catégorique qui refuse toute cohabitation entre la raison et la déraison permet d'une part au narrateur de se distancer des autres internés mais aussi de se prémunir contre la folie elle-même. En effet, s'il refuse toute acception médicale de la folie, l'association à la maladie n'en est pas moins établie dans ce qu'elle peut avoir de contagieux :

> Il y a dans un pareil milieu je ne sais quoi d'étrange, d'indescriptible, qui vous serre le cœur, vous glace le sang et vous poursuit d'une inéluctable terreur rien qu'à la pensée que, d'un moment à l'autre, toutes ces intelligences gangrenées peuvent faire, à tout jamais, sombrer la vôtre dans les insondables et vertigineux abîmes de la démence. (*M*, 117)

La folie étant considérée comme maladie, l'insalubrité attestée de nombreux établissements asilaires ainsi que la théorie des miasmes ont répandu cette crainte de folie épidémique.[33] Pour l'homme raisonnable enfermé parmi les

---

32 Selon Foucault, la 'Grande peur' resurgit dans le courant du XVIIIe siècle, conduisant à la médicalisation de la folie et à la séquestration des aliénés. Voir Foucault, *Histoire de la folie*, pp. 443–76.

33 Les inquiétudes autour de la salubrité et la qualité de l'air dans leur rapport à la santé ont été au centre des préoccupations dès la fin du XVIIIe siècle. Des théories scientifiques mettaient en relation directe l'atmosphère méphitique d'un lieu avec la mort, ce qui a

fous, cette promiscuité comporte donc le risque que lui-même succombe au mal qui l'entoure.[34] De là découle l'idée que l'asile (et par extension l'aliénisme), loin de soigner la folie, l'exacerbe en concentrant tous les fous en un seul lieu, voire la crée lorsqu'il renferme entre ses murs une personne saine d'esprit. Karl-des-Monts revient en effet souvent sur la métaphore de la *fabrique à fous* pour se référer à l'asile. Les véritables responsables de la folie sont en fait ceux qui clament vouloir la soigner. Graduellement, ces 'fabricants de fous' (*M*, 95) font passer l'individu de l'homme sain au fou puis au cadavre, accentuant ainsi le rapport entre la folie et la mort : 'On leur envoie des hommes … En deux tours de main, ils en ont fait des idiots, des fous furieux ou des … cadavres !' (*M*, 43) Le thème de la mort n'est en lui-même pas surprenant dans une représentation insistant sur l'horrible, le difforme, et l'enfer.

En outre, si l'asile est une 'fabrique à fous', les tenants de la norme, soit le directeur, les médecins et les infirmiers, dans la mesure où ils côtoient quotidiennement la folie, sont eux aussi exposés au risque de contagion de la folie. L'auteur l'affirme indirectement dans le choix de ses qualificatifs. On retrouve en effet dans leurs descriptions les mêmes champs lexicaux que pour les fous : la difformité, la bestialité, et le rapport à l'enfer. Le directeur de l'asile est un 'infect hippopotame' (*M*, 20), les médecins des 'équarrisseurs de chair humaine' (*M*, 49–50), inventeurs de 'machines infernales' (*M*, 78).[35] Karl-des-Monts insiste sur ces points notamment dans la lettre XVIII :

> En ce moment terrible où l'intelligence titube et vacille au bord de l'abîme, il faut, pour la sauver, le plus d'égards, le plus de ménagements possible, eux, *les insensés* ! ne trouvent rien de mieux, dans la profondeur de leur stupidité savante, que d'appréhender brutalement au corps la pauvre

conduit à de vastes campagnes de purification des villes tout au long du XIXe. Voir à ce sujet Alain Corbin, *Le Miasme et la jonquille : l'odorat et l'imaginaire social XVIIIe–XIXe siècles* (Paris : Flammarion, 2008).

34 Foucault relève par ailleurs que le caractère épidémique de la folie dans les maisons de force a été un facteur qui a conduit au 'grand partage' à la fin du XVIIIe siècle : 'À force de vivre dans ce monde délirant, au milieu du triomphe de la déraison, comment ne pas rejoindre, par la fatalité des lieux et des choses, ceux-là mêmes qui en sont le vivant symbole', p. 499.

35 L'auteur fait ici référence aux bains thérapeutiques. Il s'agissait de maintenir le corps de l'aliéné dans une baignoire équipée d'un couvercle qui ne laissait dépasser que la tête et qui était remplie d'eau très froide ou très chaude. Dans la lettre 17, Karl-des-Monts raconte comment il a été témoin de son emploi. L'aliéné, plongé dans de l'eau chaude pendant plusieurs heures alors qu'on avait omis de fermer le robinet reliant la baignoire à la chaudière, avait fini par mourir ébouillanté (pp. 77–81).

> créature chez laquelle le rayon divin a pâli, de l'emporter tout effarée, de la précipiter toute frémissante dans une atmosphère gangrenée par une contagieuse agglomération d'idiots, d'épileptiques, de crétins, de forcenés, de gâteux, et de la tenir là, durant des mois entiers, éperdue, atterrée, seule, nuit et jour face à face des plus atroces torturations physiques et morales ! (*M*, 84, je souligne)

C'est un bouleversement que l'on peut observer : les aliénistes, tenants de la norme et experts en matière de folie, sont des 'insensés', stupides, des brutes dont les aliénés sont les victimes. En faisant confondre les caractéristiques de la folie avec celles des aliénistes, Karl-des-Monts discrédite ainsi la légitimité de l'autorité et affirme sa position antagoniste, tout en se plaçant, lui, du côté de la raison.

Dans le journal de Cénéri, les meurtriers constituent une catégorie d'aliénés et pour cela ils sont qualifiés de 'monstres' et de 'bêtes féroces du Jardin des Plantes' (*B*, 274).[36] On retrouve les champs lexicaux de l'animalité et de la brutalité et le 'Jardin des Plantes' était également employé par Karl-des-Monts dans ses qualificatifs (*M*, 46), mais la folie présentée par le personnage de Cénéri se distingue principalement de celle de Karl-des-Monts dans ce qu'elle inclut la folie raisonnante, représentée par deux internés de la ferme Luat : le capitaine Bourdon et Monsieur d'Auvers. En fait, plus que le caractère bestial ou inhumain qui caractérisent les descriptions de Karl-des-Monts, les aliénés chez Malot se distinguent surtout par leur manque de sociabilité. Il s'agit essentiellement d'individus isolés qui n'ont que peu d'interactions entre eux. Ce phénomène est d'autant plus frappant lorsqu'il est question de fous raisonnants, car si ces personnes jouissent de moments lucides, elles manifestent parfois des accès maniaques pendant lesquels elles délirent et perdent tout caractère social. À l'asile, Cénéri entretient souvent des conversations avec le capitaine Bourdon et Monsieur d'Auvers dans leurs moments de lucidité, pendant lesquels ils apparaissent 'parfaitement calme[s] et sensé[s]' (*B*, 269). Cependant, leur sociabilité, donc ce qui les rend humain, cesse dès qu'apparaissent les signes du délire :

36 Le travail effectué au Jardin des Plantes, partie intégrante du Muséum d'histoire naturelle, était de classifier et exposer les plantes et animaux venus du monde entier. Au XIXe siècle, il s'agissait autant d'un lieu de recherche de la science naturaliste que d'un espace public où les visiteurs venaient voir les animaux en cage.

> Mon plus grand tourment […] c'était la conversation de mes camarades, M. d'Auvers, le capitaine Bourdon, qui tout à coup, au milieu d'un entretien, se mettent à déraisonner.
>
> Leurs paroles rapides, qui souvent ne sont pas terminées, leurs phrases qui se suivent au hasard sans aucune liaison, me fatiguaient extrêmement ; et aussi leurs regards inquiets, leurs gestes désordonnés. (*B*, 283)

Le style de ce passage permet d'illustrer les propos du narrateur. Les phrases sont saccadées, les éléments du discours, 'paroles', 'phrases', 'regards' et 'gestes', s'enchaînent dans une accumulation presque essoufflée. De surcroît, à l'instar de ses interlocuteurs, Cénéri semble avoir de la peine à terminer son propos : 'Leurs paroles rapides […] me fatiguaient extrêmement ; et aussi leurs regards …'. Cette correspondance entre la forme et le contenu du texte est indicatrice de l'évolution de Cénéri et du lien qui l'unit au capitaine Bourdon, car ce dernier était également sain d'esprit lorsqu'il est entré à l'asile. C'était en effet suite aux manigances de sa femme et de son amant qu'il s'était retrouvé à la ferme Luat, et c'est le côtoiement prolongé de la folie qui lui aurait finalement fait perdre la raison, 'car vous savez que la folie se propage, par imitation, des fous aux personnes faciles à impressionner. On ne vit pas impunément avec les fous' (*B*, 268). Malot reprend ici le thème de la contagion de la folie et, du point de vue de la construction textuelle, le personnage du capitaine fait figure d'avertissement, de projection proleptique pour le protagoniste, ce dont ce dernier prend peu à peu conscience. Graduellement, Cénéri suit le destin qui a frappé le capitaine, ce qui renforce l'idée que l'asile provoque la folie plus qu'il ne la soigne. Il ne peut donc que constater l'échec de l'aliénisme dans le traitement de l'aliénation mentale, les asiles servant plus une politique d'enfermement et de protection de la société que de traitement :

> Peut-être que le meilleur remède contre la folie est la parole d'un homme sensé ; le meilleur et le seul, car ici je n'en vois mettre aucun en usage ; nous sommes enfermés, voilà tout ; emprisonnement n'est pas traitement. (*B*, 272)

Les moyens thérapeutiques sont en effet peu présents dans le journal, et les rares exceptions concernent essentiellement les moyens de répression et de contrôle, tels que l'emploi de la camisole de force ou les bains :

> Je ne sais pas si ces bains peuvent faire du bien à un malheureux fou ; pour un être raisonnable, c'est quelque chose d'horrible : l'éponge

> imbibée d'eau froide sur la tête, et autour du cou le couvercle de fer qui vous emboîte, il y a de quoi exaspérer un saint. (*B*, 255)

Les doutes sur l'efficacité de l'aliénisme, souligné par l'expression de l'incertitude 'je ne sais pas', sont contrebalancés par le constat radical de ses lacunes : 'c'est quelque chose d'horrible', 'il y a de quoi exaspérer un saint'. Ce contrebalancement montre que Cénéri a recours à la figure du renversement pour remettre en cause l'aliénisme tout en légitimant sa propre réflexion, à l'instar de Karl-des-Monts qui renversait la représentation des tenants de la norme en leur associant les qualificatifs de la folie. Les deux textes sont donc similaires dans les thèmes qu'ils abordent, qu'il s'agisse du caractère inhumain et contagieux de la folie ou de l'inefficacité de l'aliénisme, mais également dans leur rhétorique, notamment à travers la figure du renversement. En revanche, ils diffèrent du point de vue narratif.

En effet, si le journal de Cénéri prend isolément la forme d'un document autobiographique, à l'instar des lettres de Karl-des-Monts, replacé dans son contexte il s'agit d'un récit enchâssé, ce qui l'inscrit donc dans l'univers fictif et romanesque du récit cadre d'*Un beau-frère*. Ce schéma narratif a l'avantage de légitimer la parole de l'interné, dans la mesure où le récit-cadre révèle les tenants et aboutissants de l'internement de Cénéri : il n'a jamais été fou, mais son beau-frère a pu le faire passer pour tel. Les différences principales entre ces deux textes se situent donc dans ce qu'implique l'expression du moi *aliéné*. Pour Karl-des-Monts, l'enjeu se situe essentiellement au niveau de la construction de soi alors que pour Cénéri, il concerne la vraisemblance.

Enjeux littéraires de l'expression du moi *aliéné*

À l'inverse des fous et des aliénistes, Karl-des-Monts se présente comme un homme cultivé et civilisé, 'un homme du monde, un écrivain qu'on [devrait] croire plus ou moins petit-fils de Voltaire' (*M*, 14). Cet écrit d'interné témoigne de l'importance de l'écriture dans la construction de soi et prend d'autant plus de valeur lorsque l'individualité est dissoute au profit d'un diagnostic. C'est ainsi que le déclaré aliéné Karl-des-Monts se reconstruit par l'écriture à travers la figure du martyr. Cette représentation rythme le discours de l'auteur au fil des lettres et permet autant la réaffirmation d'une position que la revalorisation de soi. Réaffirmation dans la cause politique que défend '[l']avocat' (*M*, 9) dans la mesure où le terme de 'martyr' s'emploie pour 'celui ou celle qui souffre pour une religion quelconque, pour ses opinions' (*Littré*). Revalorisation aussi, puisque le martyr est en général élevé au statut de saint. Le narrateur, se considère ainsi leur égal, qu'il s'agisse '[d']Alcippe des Confessions de Saint Augustin' (*M*, 48), ou même du Christ :

> Je passe là des jours et des nuits sans bouger, dans une sorte d'engourdissement léthargique, le corps affaissé, abandonné, plié sur lui-même, comme le corps d'un Christ dans une descente de croix. (*M*, 29)

L'écriture permet donc au narrateur de développer une rhétorique agissant sur plusieurs plans : au niveau de l'identification, à travers son autoreprésentation apologétique ; mais aussi au niveau de l'opposition, face à la folie et à l'autorité en place dans l'asile ; et enfin au niveau de la relation au lecteur. Il déploie en effet ses arguments à travers une imagerie agressive et pathétique qui s'appuie sur de nombreuses hypotyposes et une verve particulièrement vivace, poussant le lecteur à la compassion et à l'indignation. Par exemple, lorsqu'il rapporte son tabassage par des gardiens pour avoir refusé de retourner dans sa cellule :

> Ces cinq brutes se ruèrent sur moi, ivres de fureur et d'exaspération, me saisirent qui par les cheveux, qui par les moustaches, qui par les bras, qui par les jambes, et, une fois terrassé, m'écrasèrent à coups de pied et à coups de poing avec toute la frénésie qu'on apporte à conculquer une bête venimeuse. (*M*, 70–71)

La disproportion de cette rixe est accentuée par l'emploi de l'anaphore 'qui par' et la brutalité des gardiens est soulignée par tout un champ lexical : 'brutes', 'ivres', 'fureur', 'exaspération', 'frénésie'. Il poursuit en invoquant la compassion et l'indignation du lecteur : 'Ce que tu refuseras à croire, ce qui t'indignera, c'est que, lorsqu'ils m'eurent jeté sur la paille, ces sans-cœur me refusèrent un verre d'eau que je les suppliais en grâce de m'aller chercher' (*M*, 71). Cependant, cette autoreprésentation du narrateur pose des problèmes qui peuvent jouer en la défaveur de son objectif de dénonciation. En effet, nous avons déjà mentionné que l'une des particularités du fou raisonnant était son talent dans l'art de la tromperie. Karl-des-Monts insiste néanmoins sur son authenticité dans la préface :

> Certes il m'en a coûté de me résigner à livrer au public ces confidences de cœur à cœur qui ne lui étaient pas destinées, mais, du moment que l'oppression, qui conculque ma pauvre patrie, s'obstinait à ne pas vouloir m'arracher du front ce sanglant stigmate de folie sous lequel elle a brisé

> ma vie, il m'a semblé que je n'avais plus de réhabilitation à attendre que de l'impression de ces lettres telles qu'elles sont tombées de ma plume au milieu des angoisses de mon cachot. (*M*, 7)

Cependant, ici comme dans tout texte à la première personne, il s'agit autant de représentation que de persuasion, et en dernière instance, il revient au lecteur 'd'évaluer la fiabilité du narrateur et la pertinence des valeurs qu'il essaie de transmettre'.[37] Or, dans la mesure où la folie détruit la crédibilité et qu'il a été accepté que la folie puisse se dissimuler derrière un discours construit et raisonnable, le narrateur se retrouve pris au piège de son stigmate, et l'appréciation de son discours, lorsqu'il est question de démentir son diagnostic, suscitera toujours la suspicion du lecteur. De plus, en faisant abstraction du fait que la folie puisse se dissimuler derrière un discours raisonnable, comme l'affirment les aliénistes, Karl-des-Monts néglige un contre-argument essentiel dans son réquisitoire, ce qui peut discréditer la valeur polémique de ses propos. En d'autres termes, si un aliéné peut se faire passer pour un individu sensé et manipuler son entourage, comment croire celui qui affirme être sain d'esprit ? Si, d'un point de vue littéraire, le texte de Karl-des-Monts se distingue par sa qualité stylistique et esthétique, il présente un défaut sur le plan argumentatif. Dans un texte à la première personne, c'est ce critère de persuasion qui entre en compte plus que la vérité empirique qui, elle, demeure toujours indécidable. Sur ce point, le roman de Malot surpasse le témoignage : conscient du manque de crédibilité d'un individu considéré comme aliéné, le romancier lui redonne une voix en la contextualisant dans l'univers fictionnel et légitime ses revendications.

L'enjeu du texte se situe ici au niveau de la vraisemblance et depuis l'avènement du romantisme, 'l'opposition entre vrai empirique et vraisemblance s'estompe ; la vraisemblance rejoint une esthétique du vrai et du réel'.[38] Il ne s'agit plus tant de 'démontrer la vérité d'une proposition mais plutôt [de] convaincre ou [de] susciter l'adhésion'.[39] Dans ce sens, la crédibilité du narrateur interné peut être remise en question du point de vue de la 'vraisemblance

37 Hubier, *Littératures intimes*, p. 16.

38 Andrée Mercier, 'La Vraisemblance : état de la question historique et théorique', *Temps zéro*, 2 (2009), paragr. 8 <http://tempszero.contemporain.info/document393> [consulté le 29 septembre 2015].

39 Ibid., paragr. 15.

pragmatique'[40] puisqu'elle implique précisément la fiabilité du narrateur et la situation énonciative, mais en enchâssant cette voix narrative instable à l'intérieur d'un récit cadre, cet obstacle est surmonté grâce au narrateur omniscient qui se porte garant de la fiabilité du narrateur du récit enchâssé.

Par conséquent, Cénéri a été enfermé parmi les fous parce que des faits bien agencés ont pu le faire passer comme tel. La folie agit comme un stigmate que son porteur ne peut effacer, parce que la folie va de pair avec le mensonge. Contrairement à Karl-des-Monts, Malot reconnaît cette particularité : 'Ah ! oui, les fous disent toujours qu'ils ne sont pas fous, je sais cela' (*B*, 130). Pris au piège, le fou perd sa voix, et le capitaine procure un exemple de ce phénomène :

> Ainsi ces deux passants avaient été un moment attendris [par les discours du capitaine] ; puis l'abbé était venu, et d'un mot il avait refoulé leur émotion ; devant son affirmation, les doutes qu'ils avaient pu avoir sur la folie de cet homme s'étaient changés en certitude. Après tout, quoi de surprenant à cela ? N'est-il pas plus naturel de croire le médecin que le malade ?
>
> « Si vous ne m'aviez pas dit qu'il était fou, je ne m'en serais pas aperçu, » n'est-il pas le mot de plus d'un visiteur ? (*B*, 280–81)

Le constat de Cénéri s'expose dans la force des questions rhétoriques et dans l'intrusion du discours direct qui, sans locuteur spécifique, prend presque la valeur d'un truisme : dans toute cette affaire et comme dans le cas du capitaine, la loi s'avérera inefficace pour protéger Cénéri, et la mort du protagoniste devenu fou à la fin du roman n'est que la confirmation de l'échec de l'asile. Ceci fait écho à la position de Malot, comme il l'explique plus tard dans *Roman de mes romans* :

> Interrogez un préfet, un procureur de la République, consultez surtout un médecin aliéniste, demandez, aux uns et aux autres, s'il est possible qu'une personne raisonnable puisse être enfermée dans une maison d'aliénés, tous vous répondront par la loi de 1838 ; et si vous insistez les fonctionnaires hausseront les épaules, tandis que l'aliéniste vous examinera pour voir si vous n'êtes pas un candidat « à la manie de la persécution ».[41]

Alors certes, dans le débat qui oppose le témoignage 'réel' au récit fictif, n'importe quelle vérité fictionnelle peut être défendue pour peu que l'écrivain

40 Cécile Cavillac, 'Vraisemblance pragmatique et autorité fictionnelle', *Poétique*, 101 (1995), 23–46.

41 Malot, *Roman de mes romans*, p. 32.

agence ses éléments en toute vraisemblance. Pourtant, le roman de Malot est parvenu à défendre la cause des aliénés et à atteindre l'opinion publique, comme en témoigne cet article de *L'Univers illustré* du 10 novembre 1894, qui rapporte un fait pour lequel le docteur Falret s'était vu condamné à une amende pour négligence. Le médecin aurait affirmé que cette pratique était courante dans la profession. L'auteur de l'article conclut en citant le roman de Malot : 'On voit que M. Hector Malot n'exagérait rien quand il publia son célèbre roman intitulé *Un beau-frère*.'[42]

Un martyre dans une maison de fous et *Un beau-frère* avaient donc pour objectif de dénoncer l'autocratie et l'inefficacité de l'aliénisme, et le roman y est parvenu avec plus d'influence que le témoignage. Nous avons pu voir que, sur le plan de la polémique, la crédibilité du narrateur était étroitement liée au concept de vraisemblance qui, dans le cas de rejet de folie, est un facteur essentiel à l'adhésion du lecteur. Toutefois, au-delà de leur force persuasive, ces textes sont représentatifs d'un important changement de perception de la folie et de l'aliéné. Sur le plan esthétique, le thème entre dans la littérature en s'accompagnant d'horreur et de pathétique. L'imagerie de la folie qui provoquait la crainte n'était certes pas tant une innovation, mais, en s'exprimant à travers la voix de l'interné, elle a été dotée d'une dimension perceptive. Le lecteur découvre ainsi l'asile et le narrateur selon la perspective et l'expérience subjective de l'interné. Ainsi, pour Karl-des-Monts, l'écriture occupe une place essentielle, car elle lui permet de se reconstruire vis-à-vis de la folie qu'on lui attribue. En s'élevant au rang de martyr et en se distinguant à la fois des aliénés et des aliénistes, il reprend possession de son individualité et se revalorise. Ceci est d'autant plus important dans un siècle où la folie est devenue objet de détermination externe, de la part de l'aliéniste, d'une part, mais par extension à tout représentant de la raison, de la *normalité* : par opposition à l'aliéné que l'on enferme, 'l'homme libre est devenu le juge premier de la folie'.[43] Le journal de Cénéri, pour sa part, insiste sur l'impact de la proximité de la folie sur la personnalité de l'homme sain d'esprit. À la lecture du journal, le lecteur peut retracer la lente dégradation mentale de Cénéri telle qu'il la ressent lui-même. L'imitation de l'écriture intime favorise cette identification et l'inclusion du journal à l'intérieur du récit accentue son impact en crédibilisant la parole de l'interné. En somme, en faisant entrer la voix de l'interné dans le roman, Malot est parvenu à la fois à lui donner de la visibilité, une crédibilité et une valeur littéraire tant esthétique que critique.

---

42 Maître Guérin, 'Courrier du Palais', *L'Univers illustré*, 10 novembre 1894, p. 715.

43 Foucault, *Histoire de la folie*, p. 555.

Bibliographie

Brierre de Boismont, Alexandre, 'Examen médico-légal de l'Affaire Sandon, pour servir à l'histoire de la folie raisonnante au XIXe siècle', *Annales médico-psychologiques*, 10 (1873), 73–96

Castel, Robert, *L'Ordre psychiatrique : l'âge d'or de l'aliénisme* (Paris : Minuit, 1976)

Cavillac, Cécile, 'Vraisemblance pragmatique et autorité fictionnelle', *Poétique*, 101 (1995), 23–46

Corbin, Alain, *Le Miasme et la jonquille : l'odorat et l'imaginaire social XVIIIe–XIXe siècles* (Paris : Flammarion, 2008)

Esquirol, Étienne, *Des Maladies mentales, considérées sous les rapports médical, hygiénique et médico-légal*, 3 vols (Paris : Baillière, 1838)

——, *Examen du projet de loi sur les aliénés* (Paris : Baillière, 1838)

Falret, Jules, Louis Delasiauve, et Alexandre Brierre de Boismont, 'Discussions sur la folie raisonnante', *Annales médico-psychologiques*, 7 (1866), 382–499

Fauvel, Aude, 'La Voix des fous : Hector Malot et les "romans d'asile"', *Romantisme*, 4, 3 (2008), 5–164

Foucault, Jean, et Francis Marcoin, *Diversité d'Hector Malot* (Arras : Université d'Artois, 2001)

Foucault, Michel, *Histoire de la folie à l'âge classique* (Paris : Gallimard, 1972)

Gauchet, Marcel, et Gladys Swain, *La Pratique de l'esprit humain : l'institution asilaire et la révolution démocratique* (Paris : Gallimard, 1980)

Genette, Gérard, *Figures III* (Paris : Seuil, 1972)

Guérin, 'Courier du Palais', *L'Univers illustré*, 10 novembre 1984

Hubier, Sébastien, *Littératures intimes : les expressions du moi, de l'autobiographie à l'autofiction* (Paris : Armand Colin, 2003)

Karl-des-Monts, *Un martyre dans une maison de fous*, éd. par Jérôme Solal (Paris : Fayard, 2010)

Lejeune, Philippe, *Le Pacte autobiographique* (Paris : Seuil, 1975)

Malot, Hector, *Roman de mes romans* (Paris : Flammarion, 1896)

——, *Un beau-frère* (Paris : Hetzel, 1869)

Mercier, Andrée, 'La Vraisemblance : état de la question historique et théorique', *Temps zéro*, (2009) < http://tempszero.contemporain.info/document393 >

Moreau de Tours, Jacques-Joseph, *La Folie raisonnante, envisagée sous le point de vue médico-légal* (Paris : Lacour, 1840)

Pinel, Philippe, *Traité médico-philosophique sur l'aliénation mentale ou la manie* (Paris : Richard, Caille et Ravier, 1801)

Quétel, Claude, *Histoire de la folie de l'Antiquité à nos jours* (Paris : Tallandier, 2012)

Saminadayar- Perrin, Corinne, *Jules Vallès* (Paris : Gallimard, 2013)

Trélat, Ulysse, *La Folie lucide, étudiée et considérée au point de vue de la famille et de la société* (Paris : Delahaye, 1861)

Vallès, Jules, 'Sainte-Anne' [1882], dans *Le Tableau de Paris* (Paris : Livre Club Diderot, 1969–1970), pp. 75–167

CHAPTER 6

La Maladie comme métaphore chez Baudelaire

Joanna Rajkumar

La Maladie comme métaphore et la poésie comme symptôme

Dans ses œuvres poétiques comme dans *Mon Cœur mis à nu*, Baudelaire interroge les symptômes d'une société guidée par la morale bourgeoise, soumise au grand Monsieur Progrès et à la très puissante Dame Industrie, ces 'despotiques ennemis de toute poésie'.[1] Dans une telle société devenue aveugle à la Beauté et sourde à la vérité poétique, le poète à la 'muse malade' est condamné à vivre en être souffrant.[2] Le thème de la maladie est ainsi développé d'une part, pour désigner les maux du poète, physiques ou moraux, d'autre part, pour évoquer dans un sens métaphorique les maladies de la société, la corruption des esprits et du langage modernes. Le poète ne peut retrouver dans son époque une 'odeur de santé' semblable à celle du passé vigoureux et rythmique, dans lequel le lyrisme avait encore toute sa valeur.

La métaphore du langage malade, comme symptôme d'une société malade, repose sur une conception organiciste, dont le modèle socio-politique et artistique s'effondre dans la seconde moitié du XIXe siècle. Le signe, qui engage le corps — réel, imaginaire, symbolique — fonctionnant sans doute toujours à la fois comme symptôme et utopie, la tendance à utiliser la maladie comme métaphore semble, d'une part, dire quelque chose d'essentiel sur l'imbrication des dimensions physiques et métaphysiques dans notre rapport à la maladie et au concept du mal. D'autre part, elle exprime également quelque chose de constitutif de notre rapport au langage, ordinaire ou littéraire. En tant que 'zone d'ombre de la vie',[3] la maladie bouleverse la pensée et lui résiste. Sur le fond silencieux et inconscient de l'idée abstraite de santé, elle ouvre une brèche, qui est aussi ouverture à l'imagination et à la parole. Comme l'écrit Susan Sontag en préambule de *La Maladie comme métaphore : le sida et ses*

---

1 Charles Baudelaire, 'Théophile Gautier', *Œuvres complètes*, éd. par Charles Pichois and Jean Ziegler, 2 vols (Paris : Gallimard 1975–76), I, 128. Toutes les références, données dorénavant entre parenthèses seulement, renvoient à cette édition.

2 Selon le titre du poème 'La Beauté', dans *Les Fleurs du mal*, *Œuvres complètes*, I, 14–15.

3 Susan Sontag, *La Maladie comme métaphore : le sida et ses métaphores*, trad. par Marie-France Paloméra et Brice Matthieussent (Paris : Seuil, 2005 [1993]), p. 10.

 | DOI:10.1163/9789004368019_008

métaphores (1993), la façon la plus saine d'être malade est d'épurer la maladie de la prolifération métaphorique qui l'accompagne, c'est-à-dire de résister à sa puissance de contamination dans le discours. Appliquée au langage, la métaphore de la maladie désigne précisément des dynamiques implicites de contamination du discours, pensées sur le modèle d'une propagation par contagion.

Si la maladie du sujet, corps et/ou esprit, bouleverse le langage et s'accompagne d'un risque de prolifération métaphorique, cette contamination semble révéler un effet de contamination plus profond et inhérent au langage lui-même, que le sujet soit malade ou non. Le langage, en tant qu'il est à la fois rattaché et coupé du corps, serait en lui-même le lieu de projections et de confusions, mettant en évidence un lien spéculaire entre le normal et le pathologique. Ainsi, l'emploi métaphorique du terme 'maladie', dans une zone floue entre imprécision et abus de langage, mettrait en évidence une tendance pathologique du langage dans son rapport à la métaphore en général, et pas seulement à la métaphore de la maladie. Le risque d'un excès problématique de métaphore ne renverrait pas seulement à un fonctionnement pathologique du langage, mais serait intrinsèque au fonctionnement normal du langage et à la manière dont le réel est pétri d'imaginaire et de symbolique. En effet, d'une part, derrière une certaine prolifération métaphorique, comme celle qui peut se manifester face à l'expérience de la maladie, se Texte cache 'notre mythe séculaire d'autotranscendance'[4] : l'inflation du discours sur la maladie sert à donner une fausse illusion de maîtrise, à laquelle il n'est pas facile de résister. D'autre part, la métaphore répondant à un besoin fondamental de l'homme, l'excès de métaphore est un symptôme qui renvoie à ce besoin, mais le mauvais usage de la métaphore ne doit pas pour autant invalider son usage poétique. *In fine*, il s'agit donc pour le poète de distinguer entre un bon et un mauvais usage des maladies, de même qu'entre un bon et un mauvais usage de la métaphore. L'expérience de la maladie et de ses mystères pousse le poète souffrant à distinguer un usage poétique de la métaphore d'un usage vide, lié à un savoir illusoire et à une logique de pouvoir. Dans les deux cas, le langage n'est qu'un semblant, mais cette limite babélienne est à la fois la malédiction et la bénédiction de l'homme, *a fortiori* du poète. Trop ou pas assez de métaphore, telle serait la question ?

Avec et après les romantiques, la maladie est associée à une marque paradoxale d'élection, elle rejoint ainsi le but de la poésie moderne qui doit, selon

4 Ibid., p. 50.

Friedrich Schlegel, tendre à 'l'intéressant'.[5] À partir de Baudelaire et de ses postérités, cette association du poète et de l'artiste à la maladie redonne aussi paradoxalement une valeur au langage poétique et à l'art. L'ambiguïté et la plasticité du thème de la maladie tient, d'une part, au potentiel fantasmatique et au *pouvoir imagogène* liés à l'idée et à l'expérience qu'elle représente. D'autre part, elle s'explique par sa nature de *diagnostic*, la maladie pouvant être 'épousée aussi bien que combattue',[6] voire les deux. Nous examinerons ce rapport ambigu en évoquant d'abord les notes et les lettres écrites de 1866 à 1868 dans lesquels le poète évoque l'évolution de son mal et ses rapports avec les médecins. Face aux ceux qui masquent par un faux savoir leur impuissance à nommer le mal, Baudelaire fait en tant que patient l'expérience d'une violence irrémédiable du langage associée à l'expression métaphorique 'jet(er) (s)a langue aux chiens'. Parallèlement on assiste à la métamorphose de la figure du chien des *Fleurs du mal* au *Spleen de Paris*. Dans les poèmes en prose, Baudelaire s'intéresse moins à la figure du chat, dont la voix sans mots renvoyait à l'idéal poétique dans *Les Fleurs du mal*, qu'à celle plus prosaïque du chien, déambulant dans la ville comme le poète saltimbanque dans Le *Spleen de Paris*. Nous nous pencherons ensuite plus particulièrement sur le poème en prose 'Mademoiselle Bistouri' dans lequel le narrateur suit chez elle une jeune femme qui le prend pour un médecin et lui raconte son étrange passion pour les chirurgiens. Nous étudierons comment, au fur et à mesure des questions posées à la femme sur l'origine de son mal mystérieux, le poète introduit une subtile distance et utilise la figure du narrateur en médecin malgré lui à la fois comme double et comme repoussoir, suggérant par là-même une ambivalente leçon poétique.

Le poète malade : dire le mal entre expressivité et incommunicabilité

Le poète hystérique et les mots élastiques

On peut remarquer chez Baudelaire une tension entre le désir de nommer le mal, d'en déchiffrer les énigmes et les hiéroglyphes, et celui de le dénommer,

---

5 Friedrich Schlegel, philosophe et écrivain (1772–1829) posant avec son frère August et le 'Cercle d'Iéna' (Tieck, Schelling, Schleiermacher et Novalis) les fondements du premier romantisme allemand, dans *De l'étude de la poésie grecque* [1795], cité par Sontag, p. 44.

6 Catherine Coquio, *L'Art contre l'art : Baudelaire, le 'joujou' moderne et la 'décadence'* (Bandol : Vallongues, 2005), p. 88.

de défaire les faux diagnostics.[7] Le poète souffrant de maux incurables, de la mélancolie à la syphilis, est malgré lui la cible de médecins plus ou moins charlatans et de leurs faux discours d'experts. Dans les remarques sur l'évolution de sa santé de 1866 à 1868, Baudelaire met en avant la tendance du discours médical à masquer par des mots l'impossibilité de guérir et d'expliquer. Mentionnant le fait que le médecin ne prenait pas son mal au sérieux avant qu'il n'ait une crise devant lui, il dénonce le côté à la fois vague et lapidaire du diagnostic d'hystérie, 'lâché' sur lui à la fois comme une sentence, un aveu, et comme on lâche les chiens : 'Le médecin a lâché le mot : hystérie. Cela veut dire : je jette ma langue aux chiens'.[8]

L'application du terme 'hystérique' au poète dandy signale les nouvelles valeurs que prend le terme dans le contexte du XIXe et dans la pensée de Baudelaire. La catégorie de l'hystérie a été étendue aux hommes au XVIIe, lorsqu'elle a été rapprochée de la neurasthénie, sans être limitée à une maladie féminine d'après son étymologie.[9] Charcot (1825–93) la conçoit comme une maladie neurologique, désexualisée et déféminisée, par rapport aux représentations qui y étaient attachées jusque-là, et elle devient au XIXe siècle un paradigme de la maladie mentale. Le poète, considéré comme un 'Boileau hystérique',[10] construit la figure du dandy avec les traits d'une hystérie masculine qui suggère une relation spéculaire entre le poète et la femme. L'hystérie pourrait être une tentative de réponse à l'acédie mélancolique. Par ailleurs, elle partage avec le dandysme une dimension d'ostentation relevant du refus. D'abord analysée comme refus de refouler la sexualité, elle prend aussi une valeur d'expressivité corporelle et s'oppose à l'uniformisation des êtres et des noms.

Si la femme naturelle s'oppose au dandy par sa vulgarité — 'Elle est en rut et elle veut être foutue. Le beau mérite !'[11] — on trouve aussi chez Baudelaire

7 Comme l'écrit Roland Barthes dans la préface des *Essais critiques* (Paris : Seuil, 1964) : 'On entend souvent dire que l'art a pour charge d'exprimer l'inexprimable. C'est le contraire qu'il faut dire : toute tâche de l'art est d'inexprimer l'exprimable', p. 17.

8 Lettre à Madame Aupick du 6 février 1866, dans Charles Baudelaire, *Correspondance*, éd. par Claude Pichois avec la collaboration de Jean Ziegler, 2 vols (Paris : Gallimard, 1973), II, 587–89 (p. 589). Nous reviendrons plus bas sur l'expression 'jeter sa langue aux chiens'. Il s'agit sans doute du médecin de Bruxelles Léon Marcq, à qui le poète récapitule ses symptômes et l'ordre dans lequel ils lui arrivent dans une lettre du 20 janvier 1866, p. 575.

9 Dans un mouvement qui ne faisait d'ailleurs que reprendre une théorie du IIe siècle déjà développée par Sextus Empiricus.

10 D'après l'expression employée par Alcide Dusolier dans sa critique du 6 mai 1863, *Baudelaire. Mémoire de la critique. Un demi-siècle de lectures des Fleurs du mal (1855–1905)*, éd. par André Guyaux (Paris : Presses Universitaires de Paris-Sorbonne, 2007), p. 379.

11 Dans *Mon Cœur mis à nu*, écrit entre 1859 et 1866, publié à titre posthume en 1887 (*OC*, I, 677).

une problématisation des rôles culturels accordés au féminin et au masculin, qui passe par la dissolution des fausses antinomies. Commentant *Madame Bovary*, il décrit l'intérêt littéraire du 'mystère physiologique' qu'est l'hystérie des femmes comme des hommes nerveux : 'L'hystérie ! Pourquoi ce mystère physiologique ne ferait-il pas le fond et le tuf d'une œuvre littéraire, ce mystère que l'Académie de médecine n'a pas encore résolu.'[12] Le terme 'hystérie' peut donc conférer une certaine distinction au poète hypersensible. Mais la confusion entre inspiration poétique et hystérie, développée comme un lieu commun depuis les effusions romantiques, tend à la réduire à une forme d'hypocondrie nerveuse, à une mise en scène visant à attirer l'attention.

Écrivant à Sainte-Beuve que les médecins lui interdisent tout excitant, même la lecture, Baudelaire ironise sur le rapport général au langage que trahit cette rhétorique médicale des noms vides : 'Un autre me dit pour toute consolation que je suis *hystérique*. Admirez-vous comme moi l'usage élastique de ces grands mots bien choisis pour voiler notre ignorance de toutes choses.'[13] L'absence totale d'utilité du diagnostic se retourne contre le patient, qui doit se soumettre à des visites répétées dans les cabinets des médecins, sans parvenir à trouver de contre-diagnostic satisfaisant, ni de remède à ses souffrances :

> Depuis six semaines, je suis plongé dans la pharmacie. Qu'il faille supprimer la bière ; je ne demande pas mieux. Le thé et le café, c'est plus grave, mais passe encore. Le vin ? diable ! c'est cruel. Mais voici un animal encore plus dur, qui dit qu'il ne faut ni lire, ni étudier. Drôle de médecine que celle qui supprime la fonction principale ![14]

Le médecin est ici un 'animal' inhumain qui soumet à des interdictions incertaines le poète, qui n'a, quant à lui, 'soif que d'une liqueur inconnue sur la terre, et que la pharmaceutique céleste elle-même ne pourrait pas [lui] offrir', la poésie.[15]

Le phénomène décrit par Baudelaire a été dessiné par Daumier dans ses caricatures sur les gens de médecine. Pour le poète, le célèbre caricaturiste, dont il connaît bien les œuvres et qu'il évoque à plusieurs reprises dans ses lettres, est un véritable 'génie satirique'.[16] Daumier développe par le dessin la dimension visuelle, grotesque et ironique que Baudelaire situe au cœur de

---

12 Baudelaire, *OC*, II, 83.

13 Lettre du 15 janvier 1866, *Corr*, II, 583–85 (p. 583, Baudelaire souligne).

14 Ibid., 583.

15 Baudelaire, *OC*, I, 185–86.

16 Lettre à Champfleury du 25 mai 1865, *Corr*, II, 502.

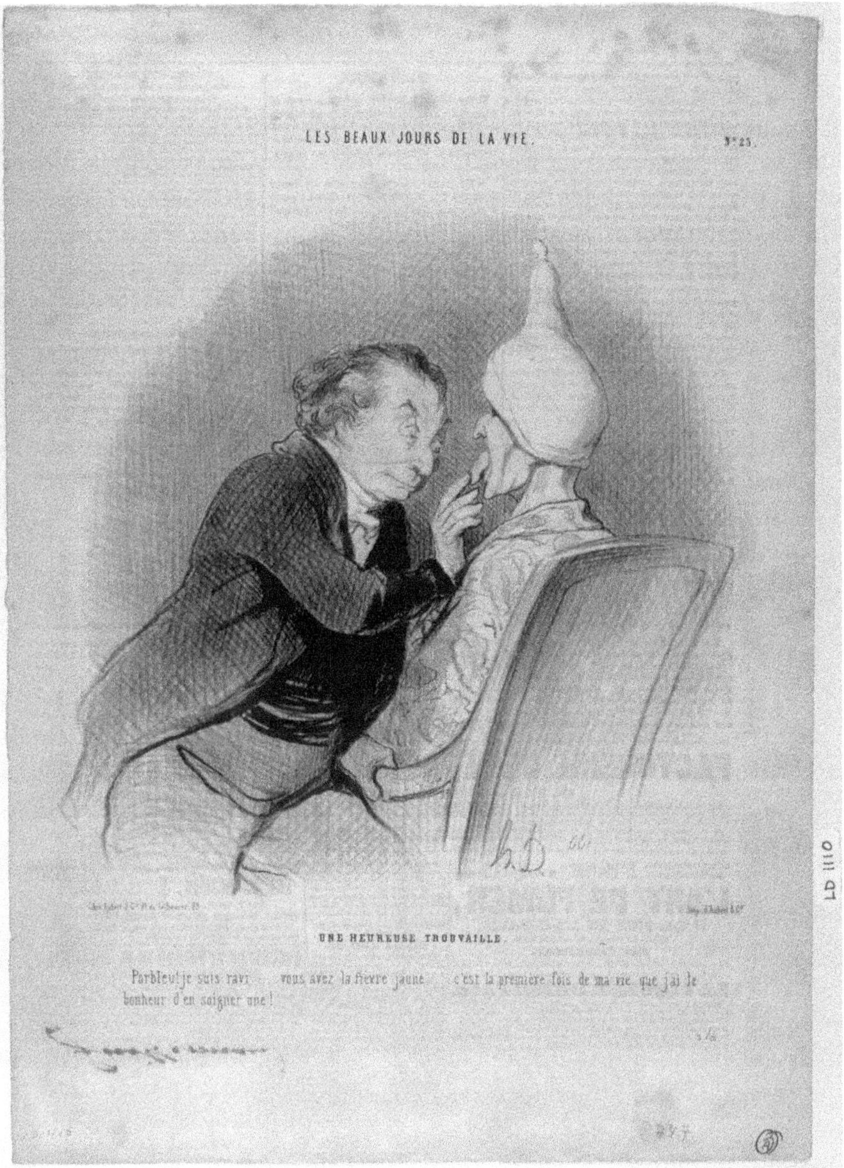

FIGURE 6.1 *Honoré Daumier, 'Une heureuse trouvaille. — Parbleu je suis ravi ... vous avez la fièvre jaune ... c'est la première fois de ma vie que j'ai le bonheur d'en soigner une !', lithographie parue dans Le Charivari du 11 septembre 1844, série 'Les Beaux jours de la vie', n°23.*

sa poétique surnaturaliste. Le rire de la caricature, comme celui de la poésie baudelairienne, permet de montrer toute la violence du réel tout en la transformant en matériau artistique. Dans le dessin 'Une heureuse trouvaille' (Fig. 6.1), on peut voir comment le patient est traité comme un cas et un objet d'étude par un médecin dont l'empathie semble inversement proportionnelle à son intérêt professionnel. La légende jointe au geste du médecin dans le dessin montre comment celui-ci regarde son patient tirant la langue comme une curiosité matérielle de formes et de couleurs ('parbleu', 'fièvre jaune'). Le commentaire, associé au titre de la série et de la gravure, achève de convertir les humeurs corporelles en palette de l'humour, entre rire jaune, humour noir, et ironie.

Nommer / dénommer le mal ou 'jeter sa langue aux chiens'

Ainsi, la seule 'consolation'[17] adressée au poète est ce diagnostic de l'hystérie, donné comme un os à ronger, alors que l'écriture comme fonction principale suppose une économie de la santé autre que celle que conçoit le savoir des médecins :

> À proprement parler, depuis vingt mois j'ai été presque toujours malade [...] Le mal persiste. Et le médecin a prononcé le grand mot : hystérie. En bon français : je jette ma langue aux chiens. Il veut que je me promène beaucoup, beaucoup. C'est absurde. [...] Je cède pour la première fois au désir de me plaindre. Connaissez-vous ce genre d'infirmité ? Avez-vous déjà vu ça ?[18]

Baudelaire, éreinté par les crises qui l'assaillent en Belgique, formule 'en bon français' la violence que masque le 'grand mot', 'hystérie', et son diagnostic apparent. L'expression 'jeter sa langue aux chiens', ajoutée à la précision 'à proprement parler', désigne toute l'agressivité liée à l'expérience de la maladie, l'impuissance face au mal et l'impossibilité de trouver les mots pour décrire ce qui l'assaille étant redoublées par le discours négateur et générique des médecins.

Cette expression a été remplacée en français moderne par l'expression 'donner sa langue au chat', ce qui serait 'une euphémisation, masquant ou adoucissant la brutalité de la castration linguistique dont une telle formule menace le sujet parlant'.[19] Le chien figure ici par excellence ce qui menace les

---

17 *Corr*, II, 583.

18 Lettre à Asselineau du 5 février 1866, *Corr*, II, 586–87 (p. 586).

19 Comme l'écrit Anne E. Berger, 'Donner sa langue au chien', dans *L'Offrande lyrique*, dir. par Jean-Nicolas Illouz (Paris : Hermann, 2009), pp. 175–94 (p. 191), rapportant l'explication

langues humaines, renvoyant au 'spectre d'une démétaphorisation qui touche à l'essence de la fonction langagière et de l'exercice poétique'.[20] La violence radicale de ce qui ne se laisse pas nommer restitue la langue démétaphorisée, comme l'ensemble du corps du sujet, à sa nature de viande, bonne seulement à être mangée, comme dans 'Une charogne' où la chienne inquiète guette le cadavre.[21] L'absence de lien suffisant entre le nom et le corps, comme dans le cas du diagnostic d'hystérie masquant l'inefficacité du savoir, renvoie le sujet à une bestialité proprement inhumaine et horrifiante, l'amputant de son langage alors qu'il est déjà victime de la faillite de son corps.[22] Le poète, qui cède à la plainte à son corps défendant, fait ainsi l'expérience d'une certaine abjection de la langue dans un monde post-lyrique, où ne subsistent que des sursauts et des accidents poétiques. À partir de février 1865, puis de manière aggravée à partir de janvier 1866, Baudelaire est assailli de terribles maux de tête, qui durent jusqu'à plusieurs semaines, sont accompagnés de vertiges, de vomissements et de chutes, qui l'empêchent totalement d'écrire et le forcent à rester allongé. Il parle des 'galops de la névralgie' comme d'un 'supplice'[23] qui continue et qui lui a fait développer 'une peur extrême de tous les maux de tête'.[24] L'impossibilité du déchiffrement de la maladie, par le poète comme par les médecins, donne une acuité redoublée à la question 'Comment guérir ?' : 'Cette maladie, est-elle imaginaire ou réelle ? Est-elle devenue réelle après avoir été imaginaire ?'[25] On peut voir dans la série 'L'imagination' de Daumier une mise en scène du 'mal de tête' avec un cortège de démons diaboliques torturant le malade, que n'aurait pas renié Baudelaire (Fig. 6.2).[26] La représentation

---

donnée par Claude Duneton dans *La Puce à l'oreille, Anthologie des expressions populaires avec leur origine* (Paris : Livre de Poche, 1978), pp. 166–67.

20 Berger, 'Donner sa langue au chien', pp. 191–92.

21 Sur la violence du langage et le retour d'un reste produit par l'inconscient, voir Jean-Jacques Lecercle, *La Violence du langage*, traduit de l'anglais par Michèle Garlati (Paris : PUF, 1996). Sur le rôle de la violence dans l'écriture chez Baudelaire, voir Jérôme Thélôt, *Violence et poésie* (Paris : Gallimard, 1993), et *Au Commencement était la faim* (Fougères : Encre marine, 2005).

22 Claude Duneton voit à l'origine de l'expression 'jeter sa langue aux chiens' la trace laissée dans l'idiome d'une époque où les mutilations humaines n'étaient pas de simples façons de parler.

23 Lettre à Madame Aupick du 22 décembre 1865, *Corr*, II, 551–52 (p. 551).

24 Lettre à Madame Aupick du 5 mars 1866, *Corr*, II, 625–26 (p. 626).

25 Baudealire, *Corr*, II, 342. Dans sa lettre du 12 février 1866, Baudelaire écrit à sa mère : 'Je dois ajouter quelque chose de bien singulier, c'est que *quand je pensais au vertige, le vertige venait*, et ensuite les vomissements. Et la routine du mal recommençait. Si j'avouais cela, on me traiterait de malade imaginaire.' (*Corr*, II, 595, Baudelaire souligne).

26 Les petits diablotins sont de rigueur dans l'imagerie de l'époque, on les retrouve chez Gavarni et ils sont la spécialité d'Ernest Lepoitevin (1806–70). Cette iconographie n'est pas

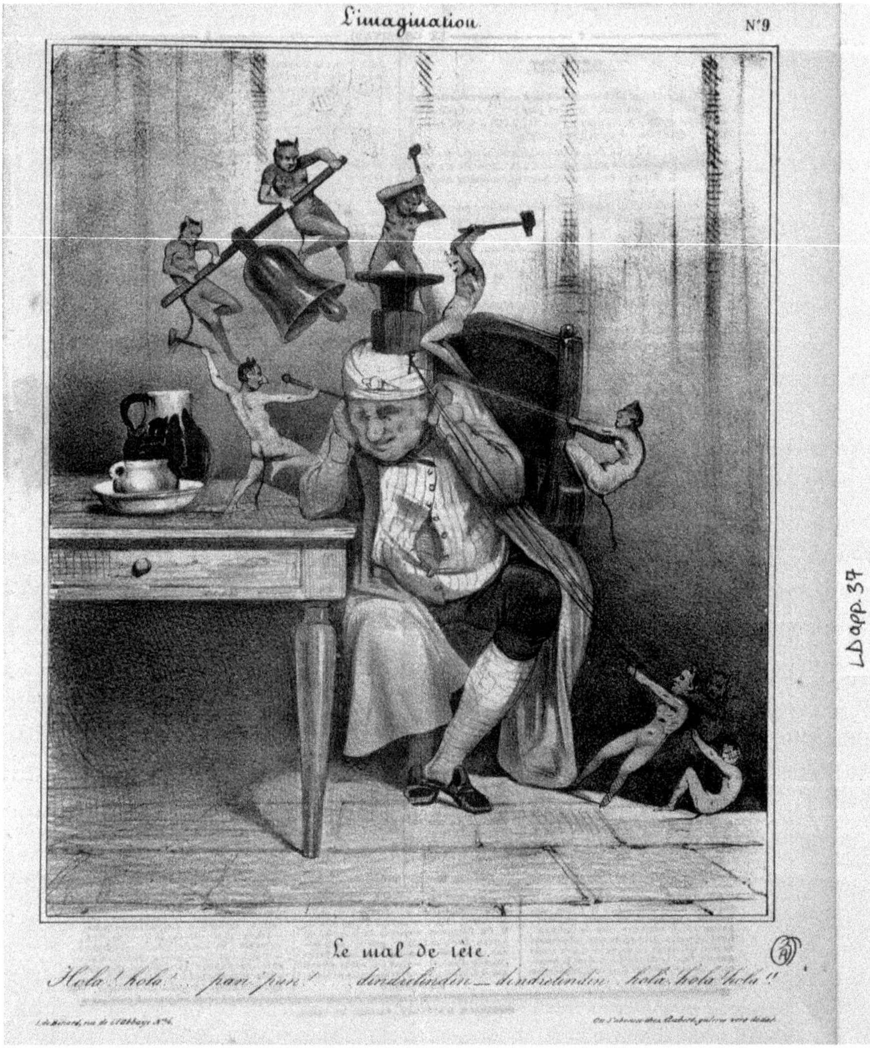

FIGURE 6.2 *Honoré Daumier, 'Le Mal de tête. — Holà ! holà !... pan ! pan !...', lithographie parue dans* Le Charivari *du 23 avril 1833, série 'L'imagination', n°9.*
AVEC L'AIMABLE AUTORISATION DE BENJAMIN A. AND JULIA M. TRUSTMAN COLLECTION OF HONORÉ DAUMIER LITHOGRAPHS, ROBERT D. FARBER UNIVERSITY ARCHIVES AND SPECIAL COLLECTIONS DEPARTMENT, BRANDEIS UNIVERSITY © BRANDEIS UNIVERSITY.

métaphorique de la douleur mêle la profondeur suggestive de l'image avec l'ironie du commentaire, restituant un tintamarre ironique et renversant le mal indicible en comique absolu.

Baudelaire entre chats et chiens

Parallèlement à l'aggravation de cette maladie réelle et/ou imaginaire, Baudelaire s'intéresse dans les poèmes en prose qu'il essaie d'achever à la figure du chien, qui remplace celle du chat dont il écoutait la voix sans mots[27] au timbre profond et poétique dans *Les Fleurs du mal*. Marchant sur les pavés comme un frère des pauvres et des chiens errants, Baudelaire se transforme en un poète de la prose. S'il a affaire à ce qui jette la langue aux chiens dans l'expérience existentielle de la souffrance, dans l'écriture, il cherche à regagner sa langue et sa position de sujet à travers plusieurs figures d'identification privilégiée, notamment les 'bons chiens'. Le cheminement poétique du flâneur baudelairien suit ainsi dans l'ensemble de l'œuvre une ligne d'identification bifide mettant en jeu plusieurs oppositions oscillant entre profane et sacré, normal et pathologique, poésie et prose, chien et chat.[28] D'une part, les beaux chats des *Fleurs du mal* côtoient dans le premier recueil une représentation, marginale et beaucoup moins euphonique, dans laquelle l'animal devenu maigre, et non plus nourri au confort domestique, dans le premier 'Spleen', présente une image allégorique du poète. D'autre part, l'aversion de Baudelaire pour les chiens exprimée dans 'Le Chien et le flacon'[29] se métamorphose

---

sans rappeler les vers du poème liminaire des *Fleurs du mal*, 'Au Lecteur' : 'Serré, fourmillant, comme un million d'helminthes, / Dans nos cerveaux ribote un peuple de Démons' (*OC*, I, 5).

27 'Pour dire les plus longues phrases, / Elle n'a plus besoin de mots', 'Le Chat' (Baudelaire, *OC*, I, 50, v. 15–16).

28 Un article de François Pire s'intéresse à 'Baudelaire entre chien et chat', *La Revue des langues vivantes*, 36, (1977), 612–20, repris dans *'Les Chats' de Baudelaire : une confrontation de méthodes*, dir. par M. Delcroix et W. Geerts (Belgique : Presses Universitaires de Namur, 1981), pp. 67–75. L'article de Berger confirme l'idée d'une nouvelle valeur poétique prise par les chiens dans *Le Spleen de Paris* : 'La défaite du cygne et de l'albatros signe le triomphe du chien. [...] le privilège accordé aux chats [par la critique baudelairienne] tient, d'une part, à la persistance d'une certaine conception de la poésie, d'autre part à la solidarité du pacte lyrique traditionnel avec le pacte anthropothéocratique qui exclut la bête du rapport des hommes à Dieu, c'est-à-dire à leur propre divinité. Les chats ne menacent pas cette entente sacrée de la même manière que les chiens' ('Donner sa langue au chien', pp. 186–88).

29 Il compare le chien au public qui aime flairer les excréments mais refuse les parfums délicats (*OC*, I, 284).

alors en identification fraternelle dans 'Les Bons Chiens', le dernier poème du recueil, même si celui-ci n'étant pas achevé, cela n'en fait le dernier poème de Baudelaire que de fait, et non du choix du poète.[30] Le poète en 'fantôme frileux' est proche du 'vieux saltimbanque', abandonné de tous et réduit à la 'nécessité' :[31]

> Je chante le chien crotté, le chien pauvre, le chien sans domicile, le chien flâneur, le chien saltimbanque, le chien dont l'instinct, comme celui du pauvre, du bohémien et de l'histrion, est merveilleusement aiguillonné par la nécessité, cette si bonne mère, cette vraie patronne des intelligences ![32]

De la langue muette et idéale des chats à l'invocation de 'la muse familière, la citadine, la vivante, pour qu'elle [l']aide à chanter'[33] les chiens solitaires, le poète modifie les accents de son chant au-delà de l'opposition entre prose et poésie.[34] La prose qui naît de la conscience poétique doit trouver une autre musique, pour faire entendre les grincements dysphoriques de la vie moderne. Cette musique, incluant les dissonances et prêtant l'oreille à de nouveaux accords, est au croisement pour Baudelaire d'une exigence poétique de renouveau du vers, et d'une exigence anthropologique, liée aux nouvelles formes de sensibilité et de conscience engendrées par les conditions matérielles des nouvelles agglomérations urbaines. Où va la poésie et 'où vont les chiens'[35] dans ces villes où les habitants des faubourgs sont eux-mêmes considérés comme des rebuts ?

Le Spleen de Paris interroge avec une force brute, tout aussi précise que le maintien des formes dans *Les Fleurs du mal*, le nouveau rôle poétique à donner à tous les fragments et déchets du monde post-romantique, dans une modernité s'inaugurant par le déclin. À la question de la destination des chiens

30 Le poème est écrit en Belgique en 1865 et dédicacé à Joseph Stevens, peintre animalier belge. L'anecdote veut que Baudelaire ait échangé ce poème contre le gilet du peintre, qu'il désirait posséder, voir Berger, 'Donner sa langue au chien', p. 176.

31 Baudelaire, 'Le Vieux Saltimbanque', *Œuvres complètes*, I, 296.

32 Baudelaire, 'Les Bons Chiens', *Œuvres complètes*, I, 361.

33 Ibid., 360.

34 Comme le montre Jean-Marie Gleize dans 'Les Chiens s'approchent, et s'éloignent', *Alea*, Estudos Neolatinos Faculdade de Letras, Unversidade Federal do Rio de Janeiro, 9, 2 (2007), 165–75. Voir aussi *Les Chiens noirs de la prose* (Paris : Seuil, 1999). Le déplacement des chats aux chiens dans le bestiaire du poète marquerait le passage du don lyrique à un goût de la prose, rapprochant Baudelaire de Flaubert : 'Quelle chienne de chose que la prose !', Lettre à Louise Colet, 22 juillet 1852, cité par Berger, p. 190.

35 Baudelaire, *OC*, I, 361. Baudelaire cite une phrase de Nestor Roqueplan recopiée d'un feuilleton, qui renvoie à la prose la plus quotidienne et à l'écriture la plus banale.

parcourant 'les ravines sinueuses des immenses villes', le poète répond aux 'hommes peu attentifs' : 'Ils vont à leurs affaires.'[36] Comme le montrent la tête du cygne tendue vers le ciel et le visage des 'aveugles',[37] le poète ramène le regard des hommes vers le sol et vers les compagnons fraternels qui battent le pavé : 'Comme nous, ils se sont levés de bon matin, et ils cherchent leur vie ou courent à leurs plaisirs.'[38] Le déplacement auquel procède Baudelaire, par et dans son écriture même, transforme 'l'invitation au voyage'[39] et l'ondulation poétique en déambulation sinueuse, sans rime mais toujours sans autre but qu'elle-même. Le poète prosateur s'efforce de correspondre à la nouvelle mission qu'il donne à la poésie, ramasser et recomposer les fragments épars d'une réalité éclatée. Dans un passage de *Du Vin et du hashich*, Baudelaire décrit le poète comme un chiffonnier qui rejoint la figure du saltimbanque en chien errant :

> Voici un homme chargé de ramasser les débris d'une journée de la capitale. Tout ce que la grande cité a rejeté, tout ce quelle a perdu, tout ce quelle a dédaigné, tout ce quelle a brisé, il le catalogue, il le collectionne. Il compulse les archives de la débauche, le capharnaüm des rebuts.[40]

Baudelaire, qui décrit dans la correspondance les conditions de sa misère matérielle et les difficultés à être poète dans la société de son époque, construit entre *Les Fleurs du mal*, *Le Spleen de Paris*, les essais et la correspondance, un parcours du poète en chien ramassant les ordures de la capitale en 'philosophe à quatre pattes'.[41]

L'intérêt de cette identification est de rappeler l'importance de lire *Les Fleurs du mal* avec *Le Spleen de Paris* et vice-versa, Baudelaire ayant lui-même conçu le second recueil comme 'pendant' au premier comme il l'a écrit à Victor Hugo.[42] En affirmant la fraternité du poète et du chien, le texte donne la parole

36 Ibid.

37 Voir Baudelaire, 'Les Aveugles', *Œuvres complètes*, I, 92.

38 Baudelaire, 'Les Bons Chiens', *Œuvres complètes*, I, 361.

39 Baudelaire, version des *Fleurs du mal* (OC, I, 53), version en prose du *Spleen de Paris* (OC, I, 301).

40 Baudelaire, 'Du Vin et du hachisch' : 'Il arrive hochant la tête et butant sur les pavés, comme les jeunes poètes qui passent toutes leurs journées à errer et à chercher des rimes' (OC, I, 381).

41 Baudelaire, 'Les Bons Chiens', *Œuvres complètes*, I, 362.

42 Lettre à Hugo du 17 décembre 1863 : 'Je me propose de vous envoyer prochainement *Les Fleurs du mal* (encore augmentées) avec *Le Spleen de Paris*, destiné à leur servir de pendant. J'ai essayé d'enfermer là-dedans toute l'amertume et toute la mauvaise humeur dont je suis plein', lettre du 8 décembre 1863, *Corr*, II, 338–40 (p. 339).

aux pauvres chiens : 'Prends-moi avec toi, et de nos deux misères nous ferons peut-être une espèce de bonheur.'[43] Donnant sa langue au chat pour se laisser bercer par les rythmes extatiques de sa voix poétique, le poète redonne aussi la parole aux chiens, rendant ainsi hommage à la nécessité comme force du réel et moteur du chant jusque dans la prose. La tension entre 'l'insupportable, l'implacable Vie'[44] et le désir, cruellement formulé au dépens du 'Mauvais Vitrier', de 'voir la vie en beau'[45] s'exprime dans un nouvel équilibre de la langue et du réel, dans un dosage différent du poétique et du prosaïque, que le chien incarne comme symbole des 'formes *nombreuses* de la misère universelle'.[46] Donnant un exemple de la manière dont il souhaite 'exprimer dans une prose lyrique toutes les désolantes suggestions' de la ville, Baudelaire utilise l'image du 'cri strident du *Vitrier*' à 'traduire en une *chanson*'.[47] La tension entre les figures de chats et de chiens dans les textes, et les déplacements de l'écriture de Baudelaire, sont ainsi représentatifs des tensions de la poésie contre et avec elle-même, dans l'autopsie des formes mortes, ou hors d'elle-même, dans les faubourgs de la prose, qui sont autant des vecteurs d'extase que de réel.

'Mademoiselle Bistouri' : le mal, les mots, et la lettre

Le poète en déchiffreur du pathologique

Dans 'Mademoiselle Bistouri', le narrateur croise dans un faubourg une femme ayant une étrange passion pour la chirurgie et voulant absolument le croire médecin. Il accepte de la suivre chez elle et la questionne sur l'origine de ce goût étrange, puis s'en va en invoquant Dieu et en songeant aux 'bizarreries' innombrables que l'on peut voir quand on sait 'se promener et regarder' (*OC*, I, 355). À la fin de cette comédie chirurgicale, 'Mademoiselle *Bistouri*', dont le nom fait écho à 'Madame *Bovary*', est décrite comme un personnage de 'monstr[e] innocen[t]' (*OC*, I, 355). Le poème est souvent interprété comme le face à face d'une femme masochiste et d'un homme à tendances sadiques.[48] Mais le texte

43 Baudelaire, 'Les Bons Chiens', *Œuvres complètes*, I, 361. Le poète n'est pas seulement du côté des faibles et des inadaptés, il est aussi celui qui sait et montre aux autres 'hommes peu attentifs' que ces êtres marginaux et autres monstres innocents sont 'comme nous', *OC*, I, 361.

44 Baudelaire, 'Chambre double', *Œuvres complètes*, I, 282.

45 Baudelaire, 'Le Mauvais Vitrier', *Œuvres complètes*, I, 287.

46 Baudelaire, 'Les Tentations', *Œuvres complètes*, I, 309.

47 Lettre à Arsène Houssaye, *Œuvres complètes*, I, 275–76 (p. 276, Baudelaire souligne).

48 Voir notamment Georges Blin, *Le Sadisme de Baudelaire* (Paris : José Corti, 1948), pp. 36–46, où celui-ci analyse les liens entre l'ironie, l'humour noir, le sarcasme agressif

brouille les catégories, et si le narrateur emprunte certains traits à la figure du poète, il ne s'identifie pas avec lui. La distance, créée au fur et à mesure, entre l'attitude du narrateur et la position de Baudelaire que l'ensemble du poème suggère, met en évidence une complexité du pathologique, ainsi qu'une attention à l'usage réducteur et/ou poétique qui peut en être fait.

Le texte présente implicitement l'héroïne comme une prostituée à la gestuelle aguicheuse. Pourtant, la suite du texte ne donne pas les indications nécessaires pour accréditer cette interprétation : 'J'aime passionnément le mystère, parce que j'ai toujours l'esprit de le débrouiller. Je me laissai donc entraîner par cette compagne, ou plutôt par cette énigme inespérée' (*OC*, I, 353). La scène commence donc par une double méprise : elle le prend pour son fantasme, il l'étiquette comme cas étrange et curiosité à exploiter. Le texte déroule ensuite un dialogue de sourds, en suivant les questions intrusives du narrateur, qui investit le musée mental de Mademoiselle Bistouri pendant qu'elle lui montre les photos de médecins qu'elle collectionne :

> J'aime tant ces messieurs, que bien que je ne sois pas malade, je vais quelquefois les voir, rien que pour les voir. Il y en a qui me disent froidement : « Vous n'êtes pas malade du tout ! » Mais il y en a d'autres qui me comprennent, parce que je leur fais des mines.

La manière dont Mademoiselle Bistouri analyse les réactions des médecins dessine une opposition entre froideur et chaleur. Elle met en évidence une conception unilatérale de la pathologie dont Baudelaire suggère l'insuffisance, voire les effets négatifs. L'alternative 'être malade, ou ne pas l'être et faire des mines' (*OC*, I, 355) trahit une ignorance et un refus des symptômes individuels du patient et de leur expressivité.

La question de psychanalyste, adressée par le narrateur obstiné à Mademoiselle Bistouri, introduit l'idée d'un travail secret de la mémoire : 'Peux-tu te souvenir de l'époque et de l'occasion où est née en toi cette passion si particulière ?' (*OC*, I, 355). Le texte pose donc le problème de l'origine du mal en lien avec la naissance de la compulsion de répétition, en montrant le caractère *inscrit* des fantasmes, la manière dont ils envahissent les opacités du souvenir, ce que Baudelaire appelle, à propos de l'opium, 'tout l'immense et

---

et un sadisme latent ou manifeste, comme dans 'À Celle qui est trop gaie'. Voir également Marie Maclean, *The Baudelairean Experiment* (Londres et New York : Routledge, 1988), p. 154 et pp. 158–60 ; J. A. Hiddleston, *Baudelaire and Le Spleen de Paris* (Oxford : Oxford University Press, 1987), p. 59.

compliqué palimpseste de la mémoire'.[49] Mais la question posée peut aussi être retournée au non moins étrange narrateur, qu'une curiosité excessive pour les énigmes pousse à procéder à un interrogatoire cruel avec la chaleureuse fille qui le reçoit chez elle. Appuyant sur le point de résistance, le faux médecin n'a pas les qualités humaines supérieures de la fausse prostituée qui, elle, ménage ses interlocuteurs : 'Mais tu comprends que je lui ai fait entendre ça par une foule de façons ; je ne lui ai pas dit tout crûment ; j'avais si peur de l'humilier, ce cher enfant !' (*OC*, I, 355). Le chirurgien par défaut use mal du bistouri de la connaissance, sa pulsion 'épistémophilique'[50] ne guérit rien, et l'équilibre construit par Mademoiselle Bistouri, avec ses mécanismes de défense, de croyance, de fiction, lui échappe. Il réduit l'être indéfinissable qu'est 'Mademoiselle Bistouri' à une 'Singulière logique !', résumée par le sobriquet satirique qu'il lui donne et qui déplace son fétiche dans une logique métonymique.

Or la transaction implicite sur les mystères du pathologique fait du narrateur un 'Monsieur Bistouri', ce qui correspond à la formule du fantasme de la femme, et finit par renverser progressivement les rôles. Quand elle décrit son envie qu'un jeune médecin sans le sou lui rende visite, dans son habit de chirurgien taché de sang, le scénario inconscient qui envahit l'esprit du narrateur inverse les places de l'homme et de la femme : 'Elle dit cela d'un air fort candide, comme un homme sensible dirait à une comédienne qu'il aimerait : 'Je veux vous voir vêtue de ce costume que vous portiez dans ce fameux rôle que vous avez créé' (*OC*, I, 355). Cette scène imaginaire fait exactement écho à un passage de 'La Fanfarlo'[51] et s'ajoute à la remarque de Mademoiselle Bistouri sur le physique efféminé d'un des médecins de sa galerie de portraits. La progression du texte suggère ainsi que le masculin et le féminin, le cas limite et le cas dit normal ne sont pas dans une relation d'opposition radicale. L'un peut au contraire révéler les mécanismes de l'autre, et le dépassement des antinomies figées est ce qui permet de comprendre la relation spéculaire plus profonde dans laquelle ils jouent le rôle de 'répondants allégoriques'.[52] La passante oppose sa nature de sphinx de la ville au démon clarificateur du narrateur.

---

49 Baudelaire, 'Un mangeur d'opium, Les Paradis artificiels', *Œuvres complètes*, I, 506.

50 Selon le terme 'épistémophilie' forgé par Steven Murphy pour désigner ce désir de satisfaction herméneutique, *Logiques du dernier Baudelaire* (Paris : Champion, 2003), p. 540.

51 Baudelaire, 'La Fanfarlo', *Œuvres complètes*, I, 576–77. Comme le signale C. Pichois, ce caprice est lui-même un souvenir de *Mademoiselle de Maupin* de Gautier [1835], voir note 1 (p. 577).

52 Selon l'expression utilisée pour 'Une mort héroïque' par Jean Starobinski dans 'Sur quelques répondants allégoriques du poète', *Revue d'Histoire littéraire de la France*, 2 (avril-juin 1967), 402–12 (p. 402).

Les leçons de Mademoiselle Bistouri : 'ne pas être dupe'

Mademoiselle Bistouri donne une nouvelle forme au paradoxe du menteur, qui n'est pas très éloignée du paradoxe du comédien, que l'on trouve dans 'Une mort héroïque' mettant en scène le bouffon Fancioulle. Quand elle pense mentir en disant aux médecins qu'elle est malade, elle dit vrai, et ses mines sont bien les symptômes d'une distorsion, même s'ils ne renvoient pas à une maladie physiologique. Le symbolisme du bistouri, qui revêt de multiples connotations, renvoie à cette idée d'un instrument unique de la médecine, dans une conception biologique et réductrice de la guérison. La valeur phallique du bistouri, comme fétiche de cette femme qui fantasme les hommes 'aim[ant] couper, tailler, rogner !' (*OC*, I, 353), établit une correspondance entre sexualité et chirurgie.[53] Le passage de 'Fusées' souvent rapproché de 'Mademoiselle Bistouri' décrit en effet l'amour comme 'une torture' ou 'une opération chirurgicale', l'un étant 'l'opérateur ou le bourreau', l'autre 'le sujet, la victime'. Comparant les gémissements, les cris, et autres signes de l'amour, à l'effet de 'la question appliquée par de soigneux tortionnaires' (*OC*, I, 651), Baudelaire renvoie toute volupté au mal et à la Chute irrémédiable de l'homme, qui ne peut faire l'amour 'qu'avec des organes excrémentiels'.[54] Ailleurs dans ses notes, le poète définit la question, au sens de 'torture', comme 'l'application d'un moyen matériel à un but spirituel'.[55] Dans le poème, la torture de la 'question' prend une forme linguistique et morale, mais renvoie bien à ce même croisement entre libido, libido *sciendi* et libido *dominandi*. La métaphore du bistouri exprime aussi une 'domination masculine',[56] qui repose sur un discours de pouvoir et des arguments d'autorité, méconnaissant la valeur de ce qui leur échappe, en l'occurrence un savoir poétique du pathologique incarné ici par le personnage féminin. Dans la seconde moitié du XIXe siècle, l'aveuglement bourgeois à la poésie entraîne une féminisation de la figure de l'écrivain. La morale bourgeoise, toute accaparée par ses rêves de pouvoir, ses désirs de normes et de confort, consiste à ne tendre qu'au même, à ne reproduire que le même, même quand elle tente d'aller vers l'autre. En choisissant le 'mystère physiologique'[57] comme nerf central de l'écriture et pouls du texte de 'Mademoiselle Bistouri', Baudelaire fait

---

53 Le terme 'bistouriser' a eu le sens érotique que l'on devine, voir Marie-Françoise Le Pennec, *Petit Glossaire du langage érotique aux XVIIe et XVIIIe siècles* (Nyons : Borderie, 1979), p. 505.

54 Baudelaire, *Mon Cœur mis à nu*, *Œuvres complètes*, I, 688.

55 Ibid., 683.

56 Selon le titre du célèbre ouvrage de Pierre Bourdieu, *La Domination masculine* (Paris : Seuil, 'Liber', 1998).

57 Baudelaire, 'Madame Bovary', *Œuvres complètes*, II, 583.

ici écho à la citation apocryphe de Flaubert déclarant 'Madame Bovary, c'est moi',[58] en suggérant que le poète s'identifie en partie au narrateur et en partie à l'héroïne.

Dans le poème en effet, Mademoiselle Bistouri fait preuve d'une lucidité qui montre qu'elle n'est pas qu'un pur objet de discours, mais qu'elle est un sujet moral, capable de distinguer l'âme et le corps,[59] l'esthétique et l'éthique, comme le poète. À propos des médecins qu'elle connaît, elle ironise sur les critiques faites de l'un à l'autre, et ne se montre 'pas dupe'[60] de leur belle apparence.[61] Identifiant l'inadéquation entre les apparences et les essences, déjà développée par Baudelaire dans 'Une charogne', 'Mademoiselle Bistouri' montre l'impossibilité herméneutique de réduire l'identité à une cohérence. À travers les erreurs de déchiffrement des deux personnages, Baudelaire construit un propos esthétique et politique qui introduit la catégorie du 'monstre innocent'[62] et une dimension inconsciente, se manifestant de manière privilégiée par le rire et la sexualité. La santé de Mademoiselle Bistouri reposant sur son imagination représente ainsi un savoir poétique de l'ivresse et de l'oubli, pour supporter 'l'horrible fardeau du Temps'[63] et les autres maîtres dont l'homme est l'esclave. Baudelaire suggère que cette logique chimérique est bien supérieure au savoir rationaliste du narrateur, dont la médication produit un jugement et non une guérison.

À l'opposé, dans 'Assommons les pauvres' qui suit de peu 'Mademoiselle Bistouri', après avoir lu des ouvrages socialistes utopistes assimilés à un dictionnaire de 'formules de bonnes femmes', le narrateur assiste à la

58 À propos du roman de Flaubert, il rappelle l'incompréhension du curé Burnisien déclarant à Madame Bovary désemparée : « Puisque vous êtes malade, madame, et puisque M. Bovary est médecin, pourquoi n'allez-vous pas trouver votre mari ? » (OC, II, 85). Cette remarque fait écho à la blague de carabin que fait le narrateur au début du texte quand il se défend d'être médecin et répond à la femme lui promettant qu'il sera bien content d'elle : « Sans doute, j'irai vous voir, mais plus tard, *après le médecin*, que diable ! » (OC, I, 353, Baudelaire souligne).

59 Dans *Mon Cœur mis à nu*, Baudelaire, dans une opposition typique du XIXe, explique la naturalité de la femme, à laquelle est déniée, comme à l'animal, toute sensibilité complexe par le fait qu'elle 'ne sait pas séparer l'âme du corps' (OC, I, 694).

60 L'expression est employée à plusieurs reprises à propos de Delacroix et de sa méfiance face aux idées politiques et techniques de progrès des temps modernes (OC, II, 321, 757, 759).

61 'Tiens, voilà K. celui qui dénonçait au gouvernement les insurgés qu'il soignait à son hôpital. C'était le temps des émeutes. Comment est-ce possible qu'un si bel homme ait si peu de *cœur* ?' (OC, I, 354, nous soulignons).

62 'La vie fourmille de monstres innocents' (OC, I, 355).

63 Dans 'Enivrez-vous' : 'Il faut être toujours ivre. Tout est là : c'est l'unique question' (OC, I, 337).

germination de '[l']idée d'une idée' (*OC*, I, 358) : il finit par rosser un mendiant en écoutant la voix de son démon intérieur.[64] Cette poétique de l'agression, guidée par le 'Démon d'action' et de 'combat', aboutit à un formidable renversement de situation qui s'oppose à celui de 'Mlle Bistouri' et produit un 'miracle' de rencontre entre la théorie et la pratique. Le clochard, martyrisé et attendri comme un 'beefteack' (*OC*, I, 358) par les coups de son agresseur, aussi 'obstin[é]' que le narrateur de 'Mademoiselle Bistouri', se rebelle contre la violence de l'arbitraire et *donne* doublement *une leçon* au philosophe en promenade. Face à la rébellion de la victime, le narrateur se félicite de la validité de sa théorie et partage sa bourse avec celui qu'il reconnaît finalement comme son 'égal' : 'Celui-là seul est l'égal d'un autre qui le prouve, et celui-là seul est digne de la liberté, qui sait la conquérir' [...] Par mon énergique médication, je lui avais donc rendu l'orgueil et la vie' (*OC*, I, 358–59). Mais là aussi, Baudelaire met à distance le narrateur, qui finit par s'auto-féliciter dans un discours paternaliste, en demandant au clochard '[d']obéir à [s]es conseils' et de propager sa bonne méthode de partage. Puisqu'il est impossible de sortir du monde,[65] et que les utopies politiques perdent leur sens si elles nient l'aliénation de l'homme par l'homme, en la réduisant à un mécanisme rationnel que l'on pourrait défaire, il faut inventer des moyens de mettre les théories à l'épreuve de leur efficacité pratique. Si le réveil d'une 'carcasse' (*OC*, I, 359) détraquée, trouvant des forces insoupçonnées face au règne de l'arbitraire, vaut mieux que tous les discours politiques, Baudelaire dénonce, jusque dans cette scène de poésie à coups de poing, la menace qui peut toujours resurgir de réduire la force vitale et ses ressources poétiques à une 'langue insuffisante'.[66]

Poétique du malentendu

À travers le dialogue qui n'a pas lieu entre Mademoiselle Bistouri et le narrateur, Baudelaire exprime tout le décalage entre l'apparence et l'essence, pose le problème de l'origine du mal et de ses fins, entre critique des réductions physiologistes et questionnement des extensions métaphysiques. Le narrateur

64 Ce poème en prose 'Assommons les pauvres' semble transposer dans les personnages du narrateur et du clochard le scénario du fainéant et du fouetteur que Baudelaire décrit dans 'Fusées' (*OC*, I, 655).

65 Comme le souhaite explosivement l'âme du narrateur dans '*Anywhere out of the world*', qui prend place entre 'Mademoiselle Bistouri' et 'Assommons les pauvres !', *Le Spleen de Paris* (*OC*, I, 356–57).

66 Baudelaire, 'Notes nouvelles sur Poe' (*OC*, II, 320). Parlant de la situation de Poe et de son 'admirable protestation' dans une Amérique positiviste et matérialiste, il montre comment il ne fut 'jamais dupe' des discours masquant 'la grande vérité oubliée — la perversité primordiale de l'homme,' et se félicite de ces bribes d'antique sagesse revenant à l'Europe d'outre-Atlantique, contrairement à ce que l'on pourrait attendre (p. 322).

qui veut '*voir l'âme*' du monstre innocent et féminin fait preuve d'une 'manie enfantine', qui renvoie à la 'tendance métaphysique' à casser le joujou.[67] Comme le poète en a fait douloureusement l'expérience pour lui-même, le langage ne permet pas de se comprendre et on ne peut pas dire comment il est relié à la réalité, pas plus que les motifs et les causes, présidant ou non à la genèse des formes et à la naissance des analogies, ne peuvent être élucidés à la manière d'un jouet qu'on ouvrirait. Le texte met en place les éléments fondamentaux d'une poétique du malentendu que l'on retrouve dans *Mon Cœur mis à nu* à propos du Monde et de l'amour, qui en est l'exemple privilégié :

> Dans l'amour comme dans presque toutes les affaires humaines, l'entente cordiale est le résultat d'un malentendu. Ce malentendu, c'est le plaisir. L'homme crie : « Oh ! mon ange ! » La femme roucoule : « Maman ! maman ! » Et ces deux imbéciles sont persuadés qu'ils pensent de concert. — Le gouffre infranchissable, qui fait l'incommunicabilité, reste infranchi.[68]

La conscience du 'Malentendu universel', et la différenciation entre l'éthique et l'esthétique qu'elle suppose, peut seule servir de repère pour un bon usage des métaphores.[69] Le gouffre de l'incommunicabilité ne se franchit pas, mais une certaine liberté peut se gagner en renversant les masques du langage : contre l'usage élastique des grand mots qui masquent le vide et tiennent les hommes en leur pouvoir, Baudelaire prône le transport poétique de la métaphore, qui, au contraire, montre le vide au cœur du réel.

Le poète montre, pour la maladie comme pour le désir, que l'imaginaire renvoie à des effets de langage échappant à la conscience du sujet. Mais que le mal du *patient*, au sens étymologique, soit réel ou imaginaire, sa souffrance est bien réelle quelle qu'en soit la cause. Aussi, ce que permet de révéler la question de l'hystérie, c'est que face à l'imbrication des dimensions physiques et métaphysiques, la maladie du médecin consiste à réduire le sujet à ses symptômes pour rester dans un discours de savoir et de pouvoir, c'est-à-dire d'une

---

67 Voir 'Morale du joujou' : 'La plupart des marmots veulent surtout *voir l'âme*, les uns au bout de quelque temps d'exercice, les autres *tout de suite*. [...] Je ne me sens pas le courage de blâmer cette manie enfantine : c'est une première tendance métaphysique. [...] L'enfant, comme le peuple des Tuileries, fait un suprême effort ; enfin il l'entrouvre, il est le plus fort. Mais *où est l'âme* ? C'est ici que commencent l'hébétement et la tristesse' (*OC*, I, 587).

68 Baudelaire, *Mon Cœur mis à nu*, *Œuvres complètes*, I, 696.

69 Baudelaire, *Mon Cœur mis à nu*, 'Fusées', *Œuvres complètes*, I, 704.

part, à méconnaître l'incommunicabilité fondamentale et l'absence de sens qui dépassent les hommes dans la maladie comme dans l'amour, et d'autre part à manquer de cœur, comme le beau médecin évoqué par Mademoiselle Bistouri qui dénonçait ses patients insurgés. L'hystérie du poète comme la maladie du médecin fonctionnent comme des cas limite qui révèlent une dimension essentielle du langage, à savoir le 'Malentendu universel' comme source de souffrance et ruse du plaisir, mécanisme d'aliénation mais aussi rouage de l'amour (*OC*, I, 704).

Conclusion : vertus de la métaphore et conversion du cœur, ou comment bien user du bistouri de la métaphore ?

Face au défaut du langage et au risque d'une violence radicale de démétaphorisation de la langue que lui font éprouver l'expérience de la maladie, on peut observer comment, dans ses poèmes en prose, Baudelaire renverse le mécanisme grâce aux puissances recréatrices de la métaphore, en s'appuyant en retour sur une animalité et une marginalité vectrice d'humanisation. Appartenant au cortège des figures privilégiées d'identification dans le recueil, le chien est ainsi associé à un sujet lyrique pris dans une complexe dynamique d'identification projective.[70] Projetant l'intensité et l'énigme de son mal dans le spectacle d'autres êtres souffrants — petites vieilles, pauvres, veuves, ou vieux saltimbanque — le poète exploite toutes les potentialités d'invention que cette vision lui fournit, dans le but est de *convertir* la solitaire douleur indicible et la violence innommable en création poétique.

Mais au-delà de cette projection et de ses vertus compensatoires et alchimiques, le subtil renversement des rôles à l'œuvre dans 'Mademoiselle Bistouri' suggère une double leçon. Le texte met clairement en scène la loi fondamentale que Baudelaire a formulée dans *Mon Cœur mis à nu*, selon laquelle 'le monde ne marche que par le Malentendu' (*OC*, I, 704). Mais il ne suffit pas de s'appuyer sur cette conscience ironique pour en tirer une morale *cynique*. Tout en mettant en œuvre la lucidité poétique supérieure qu'est la conscience du Mal et du Malentendu, Baudelaire suggère que le narrateur, tout occupé à son déchiffrement des pathologies de l'autre, risque de passer à côté de la leçon

70 Sur cette notion et son jeu complexe avec d'autres notions freudiennes et lacaniennes dans *Le Spleen de Paris*, voir Leo Bersani, *Baudelaire et Freud*, trad. de l'anglais par Dominique Jean (Paris : Seuil, 1981), sur le clivage et la dimension psychotique de la relation au monde, voir notamment pp. 128–31, puis sur l'identification aliénante mais rédimante et 'l'hypocondrie faite allégorie', voir pp. 137–38.

d'humanité que lui offre exemplairement ce 'monstre innocent', comme les médecins font preuve d'inhumanité en traitant leur patient comme un cas. Si l'entente ne peut être que le fruit du 'Malentendu universel', c'est parce qu'il a une fonction et renvoie à un mécanisme de défense à la fois nécessaire et inévitable : 'si, par malheur, on se comprenait, on ne pourrait jamais s'accorder' (*OC*, I, 704). Le poète, œuvrant entre accords et désaccords, harmonie et dissonance, ne doit pas pour autant réduire à sa seule pulsion allégorique les êtres souffrants au miroir desquels il contemple l'énigme indéchiffrable du sujet qui s'écrit. À la fin du poème, la cruauté du narrateur est rachetée par sa pitié finale, son appel à une conversion de son cœur par le Créateur tout puissant, qui seul connaît le secret de la genèse des formes et sait comment les 'monstres' — maux des sujets ou mots du poète, êtres ou signes — se font et ne se font pas. Dans un clivage et une oscillation typiquement baudelairiennes, le poème, comme d'autres textes du *Spleen de Paris*, fait signe vers le nécessaire dépassement de la puissance projective par un mécanisme d'identification et d'empathie plus profond, seul porteur d'une puissance *implicite* de dépassement, dans un rapport à l'autre qui, au-delà du pathologique, est de toute manière plus ou moins un *malentendu*, dialogue de sourds dans lequel chacun est d'abord et surtout en conversation avec ses propres images.

La poésie, à la fois humaine et inhumaine comme la médecine, pose par excellence la question évoquée en introduction : trop ou pas assez de métaphore, et pour quels usages ? À la fin de 'Mademoiselle Bistouri', le poète suggère que pour bien user du bistouri de la métaphore, pour que ses puissances agissent comme des vertus, 'comme la guérison au bout d[e la]lame' (*OC*, I, 356) du langage, celles-ci doivent être portées par une conversion du cœur.

Bibliographie

Barthes, Roland, *Essais critiques* (Paris : Seuil, 1964)

Baudelaire, Charles, *Correspondance*, édition de Claude Pichois avec la collaboration de Jean Ziegler, 2 vols (Paris : Gallimard, 1973)

——, *Correspondance*, édition de Claude Pichois et Jérôme Thélot (Paris : Gallimard, 2000)

——, *Œuvres complètes*, édition établie par Claude Pichois et Jean Ziegler, 2 vols (Paris : Gallimard, 1975–76)

Berger, Anne E., 'Donner sa langue au chien', dans *L'Offrande lyrique*, dir. par Jean-Nicolas Illouz (Paris : Hermann, 2009), pp. 175–94

Bersani, Leo, *Baudelaire et Freud*, trad. de l'anglais par Dominique Jean (Paris : Seuil, 1981)

Blin, Georges, *Le Sadisme de Baudelaire* (Paris : José Corti, 1948)

Bourdieu, Pierre, *La Domination masculine* (Paris : Seuil, 'Liber', 1998)

Coquio, Catherine, *L'Art contre l'art : Baudelaire, le 'joujou' moderne et la 'décadence'* (Bandol : Vallongues, 2005)

Delcroix, M., et W. Geerts (éds), *'Les Chats' de Baudelaire : une confrontation de méthodes* (Paris-Namur : Presses Universitaires de Namur, 1981)

Duneton, Claude, *La Puce à l'oreille. Anthologie des expressions populaires avec leur origine* (Paris : Livre de Poche, 1978)

Gleize, Jean-Marie, *Les Chiens noirs de la prose* (Paris : Seuil, 1999)

——, 'Les Chiens s'approchent, et s'éloignent', *Alea*, 9, 2 (2007), 165–75

Guyaux, André (éd.), *Baudelaire. Mémoire de la critique. Un demi-siècle de lectures des Fleurs du mal (1855–1905)* (Paris : Presses Universitaires de Paris-Sorbonne, 2007)

Honoré Daumier, les gens de médecine, catalogue raisonné de Jean Adhémar (Paris : André Sauret, 1960)

Hiddleston, J. A., *Baudelaire and Le Spleen de Paris* (Oxford : Oxford University Press, 1987)

Lecercle, Jean-Jacques, *La Violence du langage*, traduit de l'anglais par Michèle Garlati (Paris, PUF, coll. 'Pratiques théoriques', 1996)

Le Pennec, Marie-Françoise, *Petit Glossaire du langage érotique aux XVIIe et XVIIIe siècles* (Nyons : Borderie, 1979)

Maclean, Marie, *The Baudelairean Experiment* (London & New York : Routledge, 1988)

Murphy, Steven, *Logiques du dernier Baudelaire* (Paris : Champion, 'Romantisme et modernité', 2003)

Sontag, Susan, *La Maladie comme métaphore : le sida et ses métaphores* [1993], traduit de l'anglais par Marie-France Paloméra et Brice Matthieussent (Paris : Seuil, 2005)

Starobinski, Jean, 'Sur quelques répondants allégoriques du poète', *Revue d'Histoire littéraire de la France*, 2 (avril-juin 1967), 402–12

Thélot, Jérôme, *Violence et poésie* (Paris : Gallimard, 1993)

——, *Au Commencement était la faim* (Fougères : Encre marine, 2005)

CHAPTER 7

Emaciation as a Subversive Strategy in *Renée Mauperin* and an Early Case of 'Hysterical Anorexia'

Susannah Wilson

The wasting female heroine of the nineteenth century is a familiar image to readers of European literature. From Madame Bovary's crisis and the chlorotic women in Baudelaire's 'L'Idéal' (1857), to the consumptive 'Mimi' in *La Bohème* (1896); from Lefebvre's painting *La Blanche Ophélie* (1890) to the English Pre-Raphaelites, the paradoxical fascination with enfeebled and yet captivating women has been repeated in the critical attention paid to the subject. Most research to date in French studies has focused either on the literary representation of emergent diseases such as anorexia nervosa or on the historical analysis of female case studies in male-authored nineteenth-century psychiatric treatises.[1] Increasingly, however, medical humanities scholars have brought to bear the tools of textual and rhetorical analysis on scientific writings and patients' utterances in order to expose ideological biases and to probe the depths of self-expression.[2] The appeal of naturalist fiction is often attributed

1 Patricia A. McEachern, *Deprivation and Power: The Emergence of Anorexia Nervosa in Nineteenth-Century French Literature* (London: Greenwood Press, 1998); Asti Hustvedt, *Medical Muses: Hysteria in Nineteenth-Century Paris* (London: Bloomsbury, 2011); and Lisa Appignanesi, *Mad, Bad and Sad: A History of Women and the Mind Doctors from 1800 to the Present* (London: Virago, 2008) are all fascinating and well-researched examples. There are also pan-cultural histories of anorexia, such as Joan Jacobs Brumberg, *Fasting Girls: The History of Anorexia Nervosa* (New York: Vintage, 2000) and Rudolph M. Bell, *Holy Anorexia* (London: University of Chigago Press, 1985).

2 See for example Michael Finn, 'Physiological Fictions and the Fin-de-Siècle Female Brain', *Nineteenth-Century French Studies*, 39 (2011), 315–31 and Miranda Gill, *Eccentricity and the Cultural Imagination in Nineteenth-Century Paris* (Oxford: Oxford University Press, 2008). The importance of the patient's voice has for some time now been validated in scholarly discussion, whether this emanates from historical archive material or literary texts. For a recent discussion, see 'Tales from the Asylum. Patient Narratives and the (De)construction of Psychiatry', ed. by Alexandra Bacopoulos-Viau and Aude Fauvel, *Medical History*, Special Issue, 60, 1 (January 2016). In this chapter I use the noun 'anorectic' and the adjective 'anorexic'.

 | DOI:10.1163/9789004368019_009

to the ability of authors to be shrewd observers of life; likewise, historians of medicine have asserted the value of using literary texts as supporting evidence of how people endured illness and perceived medical practice.[3] Nineteenth-century literature shared with the psychological sciences a preoccupation with the most extreme of human behaviours, and the value of bringing together the two fields has been reinforced in recent years.

This chapter continues in this critical trend through a comparison of the theme of wasting women in two texts from the later nineteenth century, taking as its focus one literary example, *Renée Mauperin* (1864) by the Goncourt brothers, and a case of 'anorexie hystérique' reported by Dr Georges Gasne and photographed in the *Nouvelle Iconographie de la Salpêtrière* in 1900.[4] The Gasne case study analyses a letter written by the patient, transcribed within the text, in which she narrates the experience of illness. I argue that, as one might expect, a certain idealization of the wasting female body can be identified in the voices of (implied or assumed) male narrators and commentators, but that physical frailty also paradoxically functions as a source of intense power. This force goes beyond the stereotypical view of the weak, wasting female heroine as a transcendent and pure form of beauty. Instead, the power of these young women emerges as an extreme act of aggression. The refusal to grow into women is seized upon by girls — whether in fictional representations or ostensibly factual reports — as a means of defying the expectations of the bourgeois family and patriarchal institutions.

These two texts describe similar constellations of symptoms, which are presented as a subversive act and a rejection of adult feminine 'normality'.[5] However, the attribution of cause is markedly different. The texts also offer complementary commentaries on the cultural meaning of the female body wasting away. The recording or observation of such wasting diseases is made all the more interesting by the context in which they were produced: a contradictory era in which the rights of women had been severely curtailed by the

---

3 See for example Roy Porter and George Rousseau, *Gout: The Patrician Malady* (New Haven: Yale University Press, 1998).

4 Edmond and Jules de Goncourt, *Renée Mauperin* [1864] (Paris: Flammarion, 1990); Georges Gasne, 'Un cas d'anorexie hystérique', *La Nouvelle Iconographie de la Salpêtrière*, XIII (1900), 51–56. Page numbers to these editions will be given in parentheses after citations.

5 The theme of anorectics seeking to avoid growing up or to be androgynous is explored in Hilde Bruch, *The Golden Cage: The Enigma of Anorexia Nervosa* (London: Harvard University Press, 2001). Yannick Ripa has offered a compelling assessment, based on extensive archival research, of feminine 'normality' in psychiatric discourse as being the view of woman as a good bourgeois wife and mother, uninterested in the cultural or political sphere. See *La Ronde des folles: femme, folie et enfermement au XIXe siècle* (Paris: Aubier, 1986).

institution of the Napoleonic Civil Code at the beginning of the nineteenth century, but one also traditionally associated with great medical progress and the making of modern France. Whilst a dynamic and optimistic feminist movement, particularly towards the end of the century, fought inequality, many women isolated in their distress found that their voices were not heard.[6] As Jan Goldstein has shown, alienist (psychiatric) medicine grew to prominence through the process of professionalization alongside the rapid rise of the bourgeoisie as the ruling class.[7] Despite the generally limited status of women, it has been noted by historians and critics that the second half of the nineteenth century was a period when society changed dramatically for French girls. In particular, the typical age of marriage for girls was delayed by several years, extending adolescence and increasing educational and social freedoms that conflicted with the subsequent expectation that these young women become compliant and obedient wives and mothers.[8]

Although the women examined in this chapter are depicted as starving to death, they cannot be called 'anorectics' in the modern sense: indeed, such a suggestion falls into the dubious category of 'retrospective diagnosis' — a popular pursuit in the nineteenth century.[9] A disorder characterized by the act of wilful self-starvation, mainly affecting young women, was first named by Dr Charles Lasègue at La Pitié hospital, Paris in 1873 as 'anorexie hystérique'; the same condition was labelled 'anorexia nervosa' by the eminent Victorian physician, Sir William Gull, a few months later in England in 1874.[10]

6 See Diana Holmes and Carrie Tarr (eds), *A Belle Époque? Women in French Society and Culture, 1890–1914* (Oxford: Berghahn, 2005) and Claire Goldberg Moses, *French Feminism in the Nineteenth Century* (Albany: State University of New York Press, 1984).

7 Jan Goldstein, *Console and Classify: The French Psychiatric Profession in the Nineteenth Century* (Cambridge: Cambridge University Press, 1987).

8 See Beth W. Gale, 'Renée Mauperin as "Vierge Moderne": Documenting Adolescence', *Romance Quarterly*, 53, 1 (2006), 43–48. On the marriage controversy, see Gabrielle Houbre, *La Discipline de l'amour: l'éducation sentimentale des filles et des garçons à l'âge du romantisme* (Paris: Plon, 1997), pp. 155–56 and the introduction to Yvonne Knibiehler et al. (eds), *De la pucelle à la minette: les jeunes filles de l'âge classique à nos jours* (Paris: Temps actuels, 1983), pp. 9–12.

9 See Michael Finn, 'Retrospective Medicine, Hypnosis, Hysteria and French Literature, 1875–1895', in *Framing and Imagining Disease in Cultural History*, ed. by G. S. Rousseau et al. (Basingstoke: Palgrave Macmillan, 2003), pp. 173–89.

10 There is some debate over which of these men named the disease first. Marcé also described the phenomenon of self-starvation in young women in 1860, but it was not named anorexia until the following decade. See Joseph A. Silverman, 'Lasègue's Editorial Riposte to Gull's Contributions on Anorexia Nervosa', *Psychological Medicine*, 22 (1992), 307–08; Louis-Victor Marcé, 'Note sur une forme de délire hypochondriaque consécutive

The nineteenth-century naming of the disease is historically considered to be distinct from the modern diagnosis of anorexia nervosa, which many commentators view as being intrinsically linked to twentieth- and twenty-first-century culture. The psychiatrist Hilde Bruch pioneered work on eating disorders in the post-war era, and her sensitive and impassioned work reaches far beyond her own field. Bruch argues the case for recognizing anorexia nervosa today as a modern disease due to the great increase in its prevalence from the 1960s onwards and the excessive cultural preoccupation with thinness in women that appears to (literally) consume sufferers.[11]

The obsession with weight loss is an aspect of self-starvation that is less obvious in nineteenth-century literary and medical cases of anorexia. In *Renée Mauperin*, the lack of nourishment occurs at an implied level, whereas in Gasne's case study it is explicitly attributed to food-refusal. Previous discussions of the novel have identified this paradox in the Goncourts' novel in particular: illness is the defining feature of the heroine, but it also makes the character opaque due to the limited amount of information given to the reader, for novelistic purposes.[12] Naturalist authors were also responding to and drawing upon nascent clinical discourses of disease and degeneration, which informed later medical thinking on 'anorexie hystérique'.[13] Although there are not always overt references to the refusal of food, the idea of appetite in both texts functions as a metaphor for power over others, and the subversion of sex-role expectations. In addition, these two examples represent the voice of the starving woman, whether through real clinical cases or imagined scenarios. In these two texts pain is communicated, through language as well as physical symptoms, in ways that go far beyond the stereotypical portrayal of the transcendent, enfeebled woman. In this sense, they challenge the dominant view that physical pain has no voice by blurring the boundary between bodily and mental distress.[14]

---

aux dyspepsies et charactérisée principalement par le refus d'aliments', *Annales Médico-psychologiques*, 6 (1860), 15–28.

11 Bruch, *The Golden Cage*, xi. See also Susie Orbach, *Hunger Strike: The Anorectic's Struggle as a Metaphor for our Age* (London: Karnac, 2005).

12 See Éléonore Roy-Reverzy, 'Le Romanesque de la maladie: *Renée Mauperin*', Cahiers Edmond et Jules de Goncourt, 1, 9 (2002), 61–76 (p. 64).

13 See Barbara Giraud, 'A Reflection of the Medical Discourse in the Goncourt Brothers' *Renée Mauperin* (1864)', in *Reflections: New Directions in Modern Languages and Cultures*, ed. by Sarah Buxton et al. (Newcastle upon Tyne: Cambridge Scholars Publishing, 2008), pp. 29–39.

14 Discussing physical pain, Elaine Scarry has offered the compelling argument that 'pain has no voice', because of the difficulty in language of speaking such an unspeakable

These portraits can also be placed in the culturally significant context of the figure of the 'jeune fille' in late nineteenth-century France. Literary depictions offer astute observations of a set of ideologies that underpin medical discourse; indeed, they help us to understand the conflicted nature of the typical 'jeune fille' of this era, particularly those who seized upon the passive-aggressive strategy of self-starvation as a direct means of arresting a sexual and emotional development that they did not desire.[15]

Renée Mauperin

In their preface to the second edition, the Goncourt brothers claim that *Renée Mauperin* is a faithful depiction of the typical 'jeune bourgeoise' of their era:

> Les auteurs, en effet, ont préférablement à tout, cherché à peindre, avec le moins d'imagination possible, *la jeune fille moderne* telle que l'éducation artistique et garçonnière des trente dernières années l'ont faite.[16]

Basing their depiction on observations of conflicted young women, the Goncourt brothers show their eponymous heroine to be an independent, spirited, and intelligent young woman who expresses a profound dissatisfaction with the disappointing life choices available to her.[17]

The novel approaches the theme of matchmaking through a failed version of the sentimental marriage plot; however, beneath this it offers a dark investigation of the hypocrisies and injustices of the French bourgeoisie. Renée sabotages her parents' attempts to pair her off with a series of suitors, and her

---

experience. She suggests that when pain finds or is given a voice, that 'it begins to tell a story', and her comments resonate with what we find in the texts studied here. See Scarry, *The Body in Pain: The Making and Unmaking of the World* (Oxford: Oxford University Press, 1985). I am grateful to Hannah Thompson for the idea of linking Scarry's ideas to nineteenth-century French literature in her article, 'Savage Poetry: Torture and Cruelty in Mirbeau and Barbey d'Aurevilly', *French Studies*, 64, 4 (2010), 410–22 (pp. 410–11).

15 See V. Duzer, 'Le Fruit défendu', *Romantisme*, 165, 3 (2014), 3–12. This article, about secret reading by young girls, presents some interesting primary material showing how many nineteenth-century authors foregrounded the dissimulation of emotion and repression of desire among young girls.

16 See the Goncourts' short preface to the second edition of *Renée Mauperin* (reproduced on p. 281 of the 1990 Flammarion edition).

17 On the inspiration for the novel, see Jules et Edmond de Goncourt, *Journal: mémoires de la vie littéraire, I* (Paris: Laffont, 1953), entry from 22 September 1856, p. 274.

refusal to rise to their expectations takes the form of an excessive emotional investment in her father. In the second half of the novel, this refusal manifests itself in a vaguely defined illness, eventually leading to her emaciation and death. The general movement of the narrative traces a significant shift from the protagonist's position as a rebellious, masculine, healthy, and yet powerless, young woman, to a sick, feminine, compliant, and yet tremendously powerful force in the text. Renée's negative strength in her sickness resides in her ability to extend her misery and pain over a number of other key characters' destinies.[18]

Renée's death is implicitly announced at the opening of the novel when a suitor, Reverchon, asks: 'Vous n'aimez pas le monde, mademoiselle?' (51). Renée's rejection here of 'le monde', carrying the dual and ambiguous connotations of 'society' but also 'the world', contains the suggestion that she will depart from it. The pair are swimming in the river Seine, and Renée says that she envies Reverchon's freedom, 'Vous pouvez aller partout, vous ... vous êtes bien heureux' (52), and complains that she is discouraged from reading and other cultural pursuits. Yet what emerges as the dominant theme in this opening section is Renée's freedom of spirit, expressed through her daring and defiant behaviour. She revels in the fact that spontaneous bathing in the river is 'pas convenable' (54). This freedom of spirit, however, is not matched by true liberty. In the water, her pose is described as 'suspendue et fuyante' (53), simultaneously fixed and yet fugitive. This narratorial intervention seems to announce the immobile, wasting figure of Renée that will dominate the final chapters of the book. It also directly reflects the theme of fixed adolescence: a fleeting state that, in this case, never reaches its natural conclusion.

Remarkably, at this stage Renée's appetite — unusually healthy for a woman – is highlighted. When invited to join Reverchon for dinner after their swim, and immediately after her commentary on the inappropriate nature of the activity, Renée triumphantly announces: 'Ah! je vous préviens, je mange' (54). Hearty appetite is paralleled with female rebellion. As the conversation continues, Renée leaps from a comment on eating to a dismissal of the idea of marriage (she wonders why men would ever choose to marry), which again creates a logical link between appetite and masculinity. This co-opting of an idealized masculine image connects the healthy Renée with the later sick character, for both positions entail a rejection of corporeal, feminine normality. The emaciated form, as we shall later see, is androgynous, defusing the body's

18 Renée indirectly causes her brother's death, by inciting a rival to challenge Henri to a duel which he loses. As a result his fiancée is left alone, and her mother sinks into despair as a result of the failed marriage plan.

potentially sexual power. This theme is announced at this earlier point in the novel through references to Renée's tomboyish actions: for example, cutting a lock of her friend Denoisel's hair, she hurls it into the fire, then takes her father's cigarette and proceeds to smoke it, declaring 'Pouah! que c'est mauvais!' (77). Renée's calculated and deliberately provocative behaviour backfires, and she lacks the strength to be convincingly masculine.

Renée's excessive identification with her father is a recurrent motif in the novel, and it is her status as the favoured child, who behaves like the son Monsieur Mauperin wished he had, that creates the unsolvable tension in her character between freedom and the need to conform. Renée describes herself as completely wrapped up in the person of her father, selecting the adjectives 'remplie, possédée' (119) to describe her feelings. A conversation between Denoisel and Henri reveals Renée to be the painfully contradicted result of her education, unable to find an accommodating adult role for her independence in a world that has not changed. It is this impossible position that presented as causing her maladaptive traits: Henri says that it is 'la façon dont elle a été élevée [...] qui enfin la rend si difficile à marier' (79). Renée has been educationally prepared for a masculine adulthood, and the prospect of a stereotypically feminine one is impossible for her to accept.[19] This split in Renée's nature, between passivity and rebellion/aggression, is evoked in an early reference to her as 'une mélancolique tintamarresque' (81). The noun 'tintamarre', a terrible din or hullabaloo, carries connotations that sit strangely with the notion of a withdrawn, melancholic woman. It is this paradox at the centre of her being that will be Renée's undoing; her refusal to accept her destiny will not just be characterized by sadness and passivity ('mélancolie') but also by aggression and punishment of others. Renée is a subversive force in both her melancholic/passive and aggressive/active states.

Renée passes through a series of failed attempts to meet a suitable match. A turning point occurs in the novel when Renée first becomes ill. Her malaise is initially described as heart palpitations suffered after confronting her brother Henri about his calculated liaison with his fiancée's (and Renée's best friend's) mother. The medical discourse of somatic heart disease has traditionally been emphasized in prior discussions of the novel.[20] However, it is important to

19 For further discussion of the theme of Renée's stereotypically masculine upbringing and the subsequent medicalisation of difference presented in the novel, see Barbara Giraud, *L'héroïne goncourtienne: entre hystérie et dissidence* (Oxford: Peter Lang, 2009), pp. 122–23.

20 See Giraud, 'A Reflection of the Medical Discourse in the Goncourt Brothers *Renée Mauperin* (1864)', for a detailed analysis of the Goncourts' recourse to the medical discourse of heart disease.

note that Renée's chief 'mal' is portrayed as having a psychological root cause, its clearest symptom being an intractable sadness: 'Le mal cédait à un régime doux […] mais elle demeurait triste, d'une tristesse que le temps ne guérissait pas' (170). Although not yet indicative of self-starvation, this 'régime doux' contrasts with Renée's usual healthy appetite. We are also told that Henri knows why Renée has fallen ill, and that she rejects his guilty efforts to make amends: 'Il sentait toujours en elle une froideur, une répugnance, une espèce de résolution sourde qui lui faisait vaguement peur' (170). Renée has adopted a position of passive and yet stubborn resistance in protest against her brother's hypocrisy and, in suffering, she causes him to feel the pain he has coolly ignored. Renée's demise is gradual, beginning when she abandons her previously insubordinate façade and adopts the apparently compliant position of the shrinking, sick woman with no remaining trace of her rebellious and audacious former self. However, the switch to this position of passive resignation is matched by an increase in Renée's power.

No overt reference is made to Renée's refusal to eat, and her illness is periodically described as having a physiological cause. The organic aspect to her illness is, however, ill-defined and unspecified.[21] Renée's newly emaciated form symbolizes dissatisfaction, or a metaphorical form of hunger that will never be satiated. The doctor assesses her 'heart disease' in terms that describe a condition closer to hysteria: her weakness is to have been 'impressionable', tearful, fiery, lively, and passionate (223). Renée's troubling, shrinking body functions as an inverted metaphor of the power she has to change her family situation: where previously her defiant behaviour was ineffective, her self-destructive actions wreak permanent havoc on her entourage. The most evocative image in these later chapters comes when her parents, in desperation, decide to attempt treatment with a cupping-glass. Both parents literally unwrap Renée from her cotton wool protection. No detail is spared in the evocation of the deathly thinness of her form: 'elle avait déjà des angles tout prêts pour le cercueil […] Les omoplates saillaient. L'épine dorsale faisait toucher à l'œil chacun de ses nœuds' (235). In her illness Renée has found the ability to take control of her family, to 'touch' them visually, and to decide her own destiny. In answer to her own prayer, she dies and puts an end to her parents' hopes, leaving them in an overwhelming state of grief. Marilyn Lawrence would later call this behaviour the 'control paradox', and she argued it was central to the experience of anorexia nervosa: the self-starving woman imposes excessive control over her

21 See Roy-Reverzy, 'Le Romanesque de la maladie', for an extended analysis of the novelistic function of the character's vaguely defined illness (pp. 64–65).

food intake, but simultaneously experiences a loss of control over the process ravaging her body.[22]

The Goncourt brothers call their book 'une étude' rather than 'un roman', and the text studies the ways in which adolescence — the symbolic function of which is to be a preparatory state on the way to achieving fulfilment in marriage and motherhood — can become the site of extreme resistance to bourgeois norms. Sophie Pelletier argues that the strength of the bourgeois 'doxa' that women become virtuous wives and mothers was such that it is surprising the naturalist novel should foreground failed adolescence as frequently as it does:

> Il est par conséquent étonnant de rencontrer dans le roman naturaliste (aux prétentions de *mimesis* notoires) tant de jeunes héroïnes qui ne deviendront jamais des femmes accomplies et demeureront figées dans un état pourtant par définition transitoire.[23]

Arguably, in their focus on adolescent girls, authors such as the Goncourt brothers presented first-hand observations of the dilemmas that caused and sustained anorexic behaviour. In this respect, they highlighted and offered a critique of the type of double bind faced by young women who were given a liberal upbringing but nevertheless brought into the world of the traditional bourgeoisie.

Béatrice Gill

In a short article published in 1900, entitled 'Un cas d'anorexie hystérique', Dr Georges Gasne describes the patient 'Béatrice Gill ...', who was treated at the Salpêtrière in the years preceding 1898. Photographic illustrations included in the case study reveal the severity of Beatrice's illness. She is photographed naked and emaciated, close to death, with her face obscured. The study, although short, includes a transcription of a letter written by the patient

22 Marilyn Lawrence, 'Anorexia Nervosa — The Control Paradox', *Women's Studies International Quarterly*, 2 (1979), 93–101 (p. 93).

23 Sophie Pelletier, 'De la jeune fille à la jeune femme, un passage impossible? L'exemple de Chérie', *Romantisme*, 165, 3 (2014), 31–42. In addition to *Renée Mauperin*, Pelletier cites examples from Zola's *Rougon Macquart* novels of young women who fail in the adolescent transition to womanhood: Pauline Quenu (*La Joie de vivre*), Miette (*La Fortune des Rougon*), and Angélique (*Le Rêve*).

describing her experience of illness and the strategies she employed to sustain it before being admitted for treatment. What stands out here, when compared to similar clinical texts, is the attempt on the part of the reporting doctor to both listen to and to give voice to the patient in the process of her treatment. In terms of the themes addressed, close parallels can be drawn between this case of self-starvation and the nebulous wasting disease hauntingly evoked in *Renée Mauperin*. In particular, the family environment is presented as a pathogenic space in which disease thrives.

Sir William Gull's 1873 paper on anorexia asserts that the doctor must take an authoritarian attitude to the patient, and he vigorously endorses forced feeding: 'Food should be administered at intervals varying inversely with the exhaustion and emaciation. The inclination of the patient must be in no way consulted.'[24] Lasègue, for his part, does concede that disordered appetite is 'le mieux analysé par les malades et le moins facilement étudié par les médecins', but he provides little room for the patient's self-analysis in his paper.[25] However, Gasne's case report of his anorexic patient does seem to take seriously her self-analysis, and indeed his conclusions are drawn from the interpretation of Béatrice's description of her troubled family relationships.

The theme of feeding is introduced as a recurrent problem from the beginning of the patient's short life. Interestingly, although Béatrice mentions that she is threatened with forced feeding as a means of blackmailing her into eating, unlike his predecessor Gasne does not advocate this as a first-line treatment. The doctor insists that the best treatment for anorexia is isolation, where he claims most sufferers recover quickly:

> ces malades guérissent comme par enchantement, lorsqu'elles sont séparées de leur milieu [...] elles sont hors de chez elles, cela suffit, à l'instant même elles recouvrent l'appétit, elles digèrent et elles sont sauvées de la mort. (56)

Gasne presents himself as the patient's saviour who brings about the magical cure, 'comme par enchantement' (56), but also as her adversary. In a vignette included at the end, used to illustrate the frustration of treating patients in their own family milieu, Gasne says: 'J'ai essayé [...] je n'ai pas gagné un gramme' (56). The use of the adversarial verb 'gagner' reveals the conflictual

24 William Withey Gull, 'Anorexia Nervosa', in *A Collection of the Published Writings of William Withey Gull* (London: The New Sydenham Society, 1874), pp. 305–14 (p. 310).

25 Charles Lasègue, 'De l'anorexie hystérique', *Archives générales de médecine*, 6, 21 (April 1873), 385–403 (p. 386).

nature of the clinical encounter, and Gasne frequently appears to be in conflict with himself over this patient.

Where Lasègue notes that he has never seen a case of anorexia lead to death, and Gull triumphantly presents 'before' and 'after' portraits of his successfully treated anorectics, Gasne is more circumspect. He is unequivocal in his assessment of how deadly this disease could be: 'on meurt d'anorexie hystérique' (51). As with Renée, Béatrice's illness is from the outset established as being psychological in origin: 'la preuve en est dans l'effet immédiat d'un traitement purement psychique' (51). This psychological treatment consists in isolating the patient in a neutral place, away from the nefarious influence of her family. The apparent success of the treatment provides a counterpoint to the fictional depiction of the progress of Renée's disease, which occurs in the home and at the heart of the family.

The problematic nature of feeding in the family is foregrounded as a theme throughout Gasne's analysis. We are told that Béatrice was initially bottle-fed, but then Gasne adds a curious detail: at four months Béatrice, being 'mal nourrie', needed to be 'mise au sein' (52). This reference is presumably to her being placed with a wet-nurse, after which she began to grow properly.[26] The next reference is to an 18–month-old Béatrice, now back with her birth family, as being 'toujours chétive'; we also learn that 'elle végéta jusqu'à 4 ans' (52). Failing to thrive, Béatrice was sent back to the countryside and to her foster-family where she continued to grow healthily until she returned to Paris to attend school. Here, her health suffered once more and she experienced her first hysterical episode in 1898. The suggestion throughout Gasne's case history is that her family environment was inadequate and stifling to her growth, even from birth. The question as to why her mother did not nurse her child — artificial feeding being almost certainly fatal even in the late nineteenth century — is not asked, but Béatrice's early years are marked by the fragmentation of emotional attachments and by multiple disruptions in the caregiving environment; this seems to have been intolerable to an already fragile individual.[27] The irony is, however, that these disruptions are presented as having

26 Wet-nursing, involving long periods of separation from the infant's birth family, was very common among people of all classes. For a more detailed discussion of this practice and its relevance to psychiatric case studies see Hustvedt, *Medical Muses*, pp. 225–26.

27 Evidence from England and Ireland shows that 'dry nursing' (i.e. artificially feeding babies) was usually fatal. One extreme example is that the Dublin Foundling Hospital was closed down because 99.6% of 'dry-nursed' babies died. See Valerie A. Fildes, *Breasts, Bottles and Babies: A History of Infant Feeding* (Edinburgh: Edinburgh University Press, 1986), p. 275.

saved her, for the same need to remove her from the sickening effect of her family is emphasized in her later treatment.

As with Renée Mauperin, Béatrice's lively and engaging character is foregrounded. The medical commentary is inflected with a tone of ambivalence: on the one hand, it is as though the reporting doctor is genuinely fond of this beguiling child, as he selects the adjectives 'gai', 'émotif', 'douce' and 'sensible' to describe his charge. He seems to feel a combination of captivation and horror. When dressed, Béatrice adheres to the expectations of the male, bourgeois, medical gaze: Gasne notes both her 'gracilité' and the 'jeunesse de son allure' (53). On the other hand, commenting on her naked body, Gasne is attentive to Béatrice's hideous, skeletal features and uncannily full breasts. Gasne describes the presence of these breasts as 'remarkable', and alludes to them several times in the study, as though trying to solve the puzzle of their stubborn presence:

> N'était la conservation (remarquable du reste en la circonstance) de la glande mammaire chez cette jeune fille, on pourrait vraiment dire qu'il ne lui reste que la peau et les os (53–54)

Gasne emphasizes Béatrice's budding sexuality, but her skeletal form also troubles him; in particular, the effect this has on her facial appearance. In total contrast to the previous depiction, her face is said to be 'complètement décharnée', giving her 'un aspect de vieillard' (51).

Gasne makes three further references to these troubling breasts, which also seem to bother Béatrice. Gasne writes, 'les seins tranchent par leur volume sur la maigreur générale' (53); they seem not to fit this emaciated body. These breasts present an enigma for both doctor and patient, and are an illustration of the paradox of the body being hyper-controlled and yet recalcitrant: the body is determined to grow, but Béatrice is resolute in her attempt to stunt it. We are told that the patient has never menstruated, but that her breasts act as a constant physical reminder of the latent forces of puberty, causing her pain and discomfort: 'ses seins sont toujours un peu douloureux et la malade a toujours peur qu'ils soient heurtés' (53). The ever-present force of change is stressed by the use of the adverb 'toujours', and Béatrice's fear of being knocked reinforces the suggestion that she experiences her body as being in conflict with her determinedly childlike sense of self.

In the photographic image, Béatrice subverts many of the expectations of her sex, without completely disconnecting from it. One of the most striking aspects of the image is that Béatrice's face is obscured; the patient is literally defaced. Gasne insists that this was a necessity without explaining why: 'La face, que nous avons dû supprimer ici' (51), or whether this blanking out had been carried out at the request of the patient, her family, or because of the intimate and yet troubling quality of the image. The erasure of the patient's face has the effect of dehumanizing her image, adding to her words a potentially fictional and unreal quality.[28] The mild sexualization and indeed idealization of the anorexic body, also common in literary portrayals,[29] is counterbalanced by a sense of revulsion expressed towards her skeletal form, her weight loss being described as 'épouvantable', and her thinness at the most extreme: 'son poids était de 55 livres [...] on ne peut imaginer squelette mieux décharné' (53). Béatrice's ability to disrupt norms (of gender and of weight) is remarkable, and it is her sole means of escaping the unsatisfactory environment of her family.

In a fascinating moment of self-revelation, a letter to her doctor (cited in full in the case study) reveals most strongly the subversive nature of Béatrice's illness. Although the patient has previously been described as gentle and likeable, we are explicitly warned about her manipulative character; our reading of her words as sincere is pre-empted and shaped by this warning. Gasne writes: 'le médecin doit énergiquement refuser sa confiance aux promesses qu'on lui fait. Ces promesses ne seront pas tenues' (56). These verbal manipulations, whether lies or fantasies, repeat the calculating behaviour that we are told anorectics typically exhibit: Béatrice is enthralling, sweet, and engaging but she is also utterly untrustworthy.[30]

Her complicated nature is brought to the fore via the theme of appetite, a subject on which both Gasne and Béatrice offer commentary. Béatrice's appetite fluctuates in relation to the proximity of her family. The first reference, one we have already noted, is her less than enthusiastic appetite for the milk offered by her mother; Béatrice was only able to grow when nursed by another woman. Later, after her first hysterical crisis, she was sent to stay with other family members in the countryside at Epernon. Here, we find the first reference to her food refusal: 'elle mangeait peu et digérait mal' (52). Returned to her family in Paris, she became acutely anorexic. In both places, Béatrice

---

28 For a longer discussion of photographic images of anorexic patients, see Susannah Wilson, 'The Iconography of Anorexia Nervosa in the Long Nineteenth Century', in *Picturing Women's Health*, ed. by Kate Scarth et al. (London: Pickering and Chatto), pp. 77–104.

29 McEachern (1998) explores this theme in relation to Balzac's *Pierrette* and *Le Lys dans la vallée*, Maupassant's *Fort comme la mort* and two other novels by the Goncourt brothers, *Sœur Philomène* and *Madame Gervaisais*.

30 Indeed, hysteria expert Charles Lasègue claimed that all hysterics were liars in 'Les hystériques, leur perversité, leurs mensonges', a paper that was read to the Société medico-psychologique on March 28 1881 and re-edited in Lasègue, *Écrits psychiatriques*, ed. by J. Corraze (Toulouse: Privat, 1971), pp. 165–71.

employs 'toutes sortes de stratagèmes pour ne pas manger' (53), as if in reflection of the verbal strategies she employs to hoodwink her reader. By contrast, at the point of being admitted to hospital the mere fact of being separated from her family immediately lifts her spirit:

> Le lendemain on trouve une jeune fille gaie qui tout de suite nous apprend qu'elle a un appétit féroce et qu'elle a pris tout le lait que nous avons mis à sa disposition; [...] la guérison fit des progrès extraordinaires. (53)

Soon after being admitted, her appetite and digestion returned to normal and Gasne reports that she only retained a particular distaste for wine.

Béatrice also explores the theme of appetite in her letter to Gasne, and it is principally through this idea that she evokes her absolute suppression of bodily needs. There is clear evidence here of the paradox of controlling the body and yet the disease controlling her. This is demonstrated by Béatrice's repeated use of the construction 'un changement / un revirement s'est opéré en moi', which reveals a major shift in her behaviour. Béatrice's actions are presented as controlled, as if 'operating' like an automaton. And yet, at the same time, Béatrice, when she is not eating, seems to have achieved complete control, saying: 'je ne mangeais presque pas eh bien, je ne sentais pas le besoin de manger, l'estomac ne me demandait jamais rien, je ne me fatiguais pas' (55). The use of the verb 'demander' creates an image of a disembodied and personified stomach with a will of its own: so fragmented is her sense of self and so effective her self-deception that she does not experience her mind and body as unified and feelings of hunger are prevented from reaching the brain.

A further aspect of the 'control paradox' evident in Béatrice's own writing about her case is the commentary on the strategies to which she resorts in order to avoid eating. The difficulty of her feeding is once again emphasized as being most marked in the context of her family, in which she uses food refusal as a means of resisting their demands. In asserting absolute control over her food intake and therefore her body weight, as with Renée's illness in its latter stages, Béatrice overturns traditional structures of authority and renders her family powerless. Feeding is presented as a matter of force: whether her uncle's threat of sending her to hospital where she would be force fed (55), or her uncle's bullying behaviour, 'mon oncle me forçait à manger une chose que je ne voulais pas manger' (55), Béatrice is not allowed to choose for herself. And yet, paradoxically, she does choose. She describes the use of subterfuge to avoid eating whilst maintaining a compliant front: she spits food into her handkerchief (she reiterates this twice) and sneaks away to the cellar, pretending to drink her milk but in fact disposing of it. Béatrice stubbornly resists her family's attempts to control her, using whatever means she has at her disposal, 'je faisais tout ce que je pouvais' (55). At the same time, Béatrice is at the mercy of her disease and is controlled by it.

This contradiction, the feeling of being pulled in two directions at once, is expressed as both a daring achievement, as if in celebration of Béatrice's defiance, and as a sinful tendency from which she seeks to detach her authentic self. She suggests that she has 'l'aplomb' to spit out her meat, and uses the verb 's'esquiver' to describe successfully outmanoeuvring her aunt. Yet, in a simultaneously subversive and compliant turn, she also describes these actions as sins, 'vices', and as shameful, 'honteux'. She presents these sinful manipulations as being external to her and controlling her, stating: 'tous ces vilains vices qui étaient odieux seront chassées de cette cervelle qui était buttée, anéantie complètement, bornée' (55). The use of the idea of banishment, 'chasser', and the positioning of the brain as the object of the constrictive verbs that follow (butée, anéantie, bornée) characterizes her mental processes as beset by conflict. This reflects Gasne's own assertion, previously noted, that he has entered into a struggle with the symptoms of this intractable disease.

Literary depictions of self-starvation observe and portray in detail the personal, social, and ideological conflicts experienced by adolescent girls, who have since the late nineteenth century become increasingly vulnerable to anorexia nervosa. Alongside the detailed clinical picture offered in the medical literature, they explain, to some extent, the puzzle of this disorder. Medical accounts alone do not sufficiently unpack the meaning of this destructive and yet perversely empowering behaviour. In seeking to account for the effect of the stifling expectations placed upon young girls, literary narratives anticipate later twentieth-century clinical explanations of anorexia that focus more closely on the meaning of the disease in its sociological context. In this respect, they provide a more satisfying reading of anorexic behaviour by explaining its possible cultural meaning without fixating on the eradication of symptoms. Nineteenth-century clinical accounts offer little direct appreciation of the psychological significance of food refusal. But, in foregrounding interesting, individual case studies, they leave a valuable record of the ideological assumptions brought to the clinical encounter and they also provide a unique outlet for the patient's self-expression, which would not otherwise survive. Taken together, these two documents provide a rich account of some of the meanings attached to emaciation, whether obviously self-inflicted or incidental. They can in turn be interpreted as an important record of the refusal of young women to accept the narrowly defined adult role imposed upon them.

Bibliography

Appignanesi, Lisa, *Mad, Bad and Sad: A History of Women and the Mind Doctors from 1800 to the Present* (London: Virago, 2008)

Bacopoulos-Viau, Alexandra and Aude Fauvel (eds), 'Tales from the Asylum. Patient Narratives and the (De)construction of Psychiatry', *Medical History*, 60, 1 (January 2016)

Bell, Rudolphe M., *Holy Anorexia* (London: University of Chigago Press, 1985)

Bruch, Hilde, *The Golden Cage: The Enigma of Anorexia Nervosa* (London: Harvard University Press, 2001)

Brumberg, Joan Jacobs, *Fasting Girls: The History of Anorexia Nervosa* (New York: Vintage, 2000)

Duzer, Virginie, 'Le Fruit défendu', *Romantisme*, 165, 3 (2014), 3–12

Fildes, Valerie A., *Breasts, Bottles and Babies: A History of Infant Feeding* (Edinburgh: Edinburgh University Press, 1986)

Finn, Michael, 'Physiological Fictions and the Fin-de-Siècle Female Brain', *Nineteenth-Century French Studies*, 39 (2011), 315–31

——, 'Retrospective Medicine, Hypnosis, Hysteria and French Literature, 1875–1895', in *Framing and Imagining Disease in Cultural History*, ed. by G. S. Rousseau et al. (Basingstoke: Palgrave Macmillan, 2005), pp. 173–89

Gale, Beth W., 'Renée Mauperin as "Vierge Moderne": Documenting Adolescence', *Romance Quarterly*, 53, 1 (2006), 43–48

Gasne, Georges, 'Un cas d'anorexie hystérique', *La Nouvelle Iconographie de la Salpêtrière*, XIII (1900), 51–56

Gill, Miranda, *Eccentricity and the Cultural Imagination in Nineteenth-Century Paris* (Oxford: Oxford University Press, 2008)

Giraud, Barbara, 'A Reflection of the Medical Discourse in the Goncourt Brothers' *Renée Mauperin* (1864)', in *Reflections: New Directions in Modern Languages and Cultures*, ed. by Sarah Buxton, Laura Campbell, Tracey Dawe, and Elise Hugueny-Leger (Newcastle upon Tyne: Cambridge Scholars Publishing, 2008), pp. 29–39

——, *L'héroïne goncourtienne: entre hystérie et dissidence* (Oxford: Peter Lang, 2009)

Goldstein, Jan, *Console and Classify: The French Psychiatric Profession in the Nineteenth Century* (Cambridge: Cambridge University Press, 1987)

Goncourt, Edmond and Jules de, *Renée Mauperin* (Paris: Flammarion, 1990 [1864])

——, *Journal: mémoires de la vie littéraire, I* (Paris: Laffont, 1953)

Gull, William Withey, 'Anorexia Nervosa', in *A Collection of the Published Writings of William Withey Gull* (London: The New Sydenham Society, 1874), pp. 305–14

Holmes, Diana and Carrie Tarr (eds), *A Belle Époque? Women in French Society and Culture, 1890–1914* (Oxford: Berghahn, 2005)

Houbre, Gabrielle, *La Discipline de l'amour: l'éducation sentimentale des filles et des garçons à l'âge du romantisme* (Paris: Plon, 1997)

Hustvedt, Asti, *Medical Muses: Hysteria in Nineteenth-Century Paris* (London: Bloomsbury, 2011)

Knibiehler, Yvonne, Marcel Bernos, Élisabeth Ravoux-Rallo, and Éliane Richard (eds), *De la pucelle à la minette: les jeunes filles de l'âge classique à nos jours* (Paris: Temps actuels, 1983)

Lasègue, Charles, 'De l'anorexie hystérique', *Archives générales de médecine*, 6, 21 (April, 1873), 385–403

Lasègue, Charles, 'Les Hystériques, leur perversité, leurs mensonges', in *Écrits psychiatriques*, ed. by J. Corraze (Toulouse: Privat, 1971 [1881]), pp. 165–71

Lawrence, Marilyn, 'Anorexia Nervosa — The Control Paradox', *Women's Studies International Quarterly*, 2 (1979), 93–101

Marcé, Louis-Victor, 'Note sur une forme de délire hypochondriaque consécutive aux dyspepsies et caractérisée principalement par le refus d'aliments', *Annales Médico-psychologiques*, 6 (1860), 15–28

McEachern, Patricia, *Deprivation and Power: The Emergence of Anorexia Nervosa in Nineteenth-Century French Literature* (London: Greenwood Press, 1998)

Moses, Claire Goldberg, *French Feminism in the Nineteenth Century* (Albany: State University of New York Press, 1984)

Orbach, Susie, *Hunger Strike: The Anorectic's Struggle as a Metaphor for our Age* (London: Karnac, 2005)

Pelletier, Sophie, 'De la jeune fille à la jeune femme, un passage impossible ? L'exemple de Chérie', *Romantisme*, 165, 3 (2014), 31–42

Porter, Roy and George Rousseau, *Gout: The Patrician Malady* (New Haven: Yale University Press, 1998)

Ripa, Yannick, *La Ronde des folles: femme, folie et enfermement au XIXe siècle* (Paris: Aubier, 1986)

Roy-Reverzy, Éléonore, 'Le Romanesque de la maladie: *Renée Mauperin*', *Cahiers Edmond et Jules de Goncourt*, 1, 9 (2002), 61–76

Scarry, Elaine, *The Body in Pain: The Making and Unmaking of the World* (Oxford: Oxford University Press, 1985)

Silverman, Joseph A., 'Lasègue's Editorial Riposte to Gull's Contributions on Anorexia Nervosa', *Psychological Medicine*, 22 (1992), 307–08

Thompson, Hannah, 'Savage Poetry: Torture and Cruelty in Mirbeau and Barbey d'Aurevilly', French Studies, 64, 4 (2010), 410–22

Wilson, Susannah, 'The Iconography of Anorexia Nervosa in the Long Nineteenth Century', *Picturing Women's Health*, ed. by Francesca Scott, Kate Scarth, and Ji-Won Chung (London: Pickering and Chatto, 2014), pp. 77–104

CHAPTER 8

'Dictante Dolore': Writing Pain in Alphonse Daudet's *La Doulou*

Steven Wilson

Although many writers were contaminated by syphilis in nineteenth-century France, few used the disease to transcribe into words the physical and psychological torments it put them through. Drawing on Elaine Scarry and Joanna Bourke's contemporary theories of pain expression, this chapter will take as its focal point Alphonse Daudet's first-person written account of syphilis in order to examine the relationship between pain and the expressive capacity of language.[1] Daudet's personal reflections, which seek to convey a sense of the embodied experience of actual sufferers of syphilis in nineteenth-century France, will be read in the light of Maupassant's suggestion that the pain of syphilis defies articulation in human language. Maupassant and Daudet's accounts thus represent two conflicting attempts to find the words to capture the bodily agony and mental torture engendered by the disease that Alain Corbin has argued was most closely associated with 'le morbide' in the nineteenth century.[2] While, as we shall see, Maupassant claims that words cannot express the raw realities of syphilis-induced pain, Daudet's notebook on life with syphilis, *La Doulou*, suggests that the experience of suffering from a painful disease need not render the patient speechless. By unravelling the multifaceted representations of pain through an examination of the key metaphorical paradigms in *La Doulou*, our analysis will propose that it is the use of figurative language that permits the sufferer to communicate his lived experience of syphilis and, in the process, offer a richly-textured account of the painful effects of syphilis to complement the many medical narratives of the disease in nineteenth-century France. However, we will also question whether Daudet's attempts to draw pain into explanatory realms, where it is embellished by the

1 Elaine Scarry, *The Body in Pain: The Making and Unmaking of the World* (Oxford and New York: Oxford University Press, 1985) and Joanna Bourke, *The Story of Pain: From Prayer to Painkillers* (Oxford: Oxford University Press, 2014).

2 Alain Corbin, in 'L'Hérédosyphilis ou l'impossible rédemption. Contribution à l'histoire de l'hérédité morbide', *Romanticisme*, 31 (1981), 131–49, argues that: 'Il va de soi que la maladie vénérienne symbolise et résume le morbide' (p. 140).

 | DOI:10.1163/9789004368019_010

use of metaphorical and figurative language, may, in fact, have the effect of diminishing the visceral qualities of his account of the realities of life with the tertiary stages of 'la grosse vérole'. In this way, we will reflect on what *La Doulou* tells us about the complex relationship between pain and writing whereby, on the one hand, pain acts as an incitement to writing, and on the other, it presents a significant creative challenge to writers who seek to express, communicate, and capture it.

'Literary Syphilitics'

Associated with sexual temptations, deadly pleasures, decadence, and socio-scientific anxieties concerning contamination and contagion, syphilis is a distinguishing feature of the fictional landscape of nineteenth-century France and provides an entry point into literary reflections on life's mortiferous pleasures.[3] The STD of its day, it provoked fear and yet, at the same time, a morbid attraction, as we see in the erotically alluring woman of Baudelaire's 'À une Passante', where the poet notes: 'Dans son œil, ciel livide où germe l'ouragan, / La douceur qui fascine et le plaisir qui tue'.[4] Paris's international reputation as the nineteenth-century capital of vice and depravity captivated many writers of the time, including Baudelaire, who not only succumbed to the city's carnal, sensual, and sexual temptations, but saw in them some of the constituent elements of modernity, including decomposition, decay, rot, and putrefaction. As des Esseintes, the morbid hero of Huysmans's *À Rebours*, puts it in his characterization of the socio-cultural climate of the time, 'Tout n'est que syphilis'.[5] However, syphilis was also endowed with an idealized image:

---

3 As Claude Quétel writes in 'La Syphilis: Présentation', in *Peurs et terreurs face à la contagion*, ed. by Jean-Pierre Bardet et al. (Paris: Fayard, 1988), pp. 285–95, 'la plus culturelle de toutes [les maladies sociales], celle qui a le plus terrorisé la société du XIXe siècle et de le première moitié du XXe, qui a le plus imprégné les discours non seulement de la médicine à une époque où celle-ci avait encore un discours, mais aussi de l'hygiène du travail, de la morale et de la littérature, c'est la syphilis' (p. 285).

4 Charles Baudelaire, 'À une Passante', in *Œuvres complètes*, ed. by Yves-Gérard Le Dantec and Claude Pichois (Paris: Gallimard, Bibliothèque de la Pléiade, 1966), 88, ll. 7–8.

5 Joris-Karl Huysmans, *À Rebours* (Paris: Gallimard, 1977), p. 193. As Susan Sontag notes in *Illness as Metaphor and AIDS and its Metaphors* (London and New York: Penguin, 1991), 'throughout the nineteenth century, disease metaphors became more virulent, preposterous, demagogic', to the extent that disease became synonymous with anything that was deemed 'unnatural' or unhealthy. In this context, it is hardly surprising that the (often decadent) fin-de-siècle spirit places such emphasis on the aesthetics of disease, for 'disease', in Sontag's

associated with literary creation, it was thought that the disease may have stimulated the creativity of the imagination; hence the hackneyed notion of the *génie syphilitique*, as reflected in Baudelaire's maxim in *Mon Cœur mis à nu*: 'Le jour où le jeune écrivain corrige sa première épreuve, il est fier comme un écolier qui vient de gagner sa première vérole'.[6] Of course, the nineteenth-century author's interest in syphilis was also motivated by more personal concerns. Baudelaire, along with Flaubert, Jules de Goncourt, Guy de Maupassant, Alphonse Daudet, and others, was a member of that infamous nineteenth-century French club deemed the 'literary syphilitics' by Julian Barnes.[7] Given the sheer prevalence of syphilis in France during the nineteenth century, the number of writers infected by the disease is, in some ways, hardly remarkable. As Flaubert's sardonic entry in the *Dictionnaire des idées reçues* puts it, 'Syphilis: plus ou moins, tout le monde en est affecté'.[8] Moreover, Flaubert's letter to his friend Bouilhet, written from Constantinople in 1850, reflects a desire at the time to use an infection with syphilis to project an image of sexual bravura:

> Il faut que tu saches, mon cher monsieur, que j'ai gobé à Beyrouth [...] VII chancres, lesquelles ont fini par se réunir en deux, puis en un. [...] Je soupçonne une Maronite de m'avoir fait ce cadeau, mais c'est peut-être une petite Turque. Est-ce la Turque ou la Chrétienne, qui des deux? problème? pensée!!! [...] Rien n'est bon pour la santé comme les voyages.[9]

Inspired by some of the emphases on illness and disease brought forward by current reflections on texts described in the medical humanities as 'illness narratives', through which we seek to understand better the ways in which sufferers give shape and meaning to the trauma of pathological disease — that is, to understand the human (as opposed to simply the scientific or medical) dimension to illness — the focus of this chapter is on the 'embodied' experience of syphilis in nineteenth-century France. In a context where the self

commentary on the tendency towards metaphorical extremes in the nineteenth century, is anything that 'opposes life' (p. 75).

6 Charles Baudelaire, *Mon Cœur mis à nu*, in *Œuvres complètes*, p. 1288.

7 Julian Barnes, 'Introduction' to Alphonse Daudet, *In the Land of Pain*, ed. and trans. by Julian Barnes (London: Jonathan Cape, 2002), v–xv (vii).

8 Gustave Flaubert, *Dictionnaires des idées reçues*, in *Œuvres complètes*, 18 vols (Paris: Conard, 1910), I, 415–45 (p. 443).

9 Gustave Flaubert, Lettre à Louis Bouilhet, 14 novembre 1850, in *Correspondance*, I (Paris: Gallimard, Bibliothèque de la Pléiade, 1973–2007), 707.

depends on the body for expression, and the body mediates our relationship with the external world, illness has always been one of the prevailing subjects of life-writing.[10] As Rita Charon observes:

> Illness intensifies the routine drives to recognise the self. It is when one is ill that one has to decide how valuable life is, which relationships are most meaningful, and what terrors or comforts the end of life holds. When people become sick or disabled, they question their existence in new ways.[11]

For medical humanist Anne Hunsaker Hawkins, the value of the illness narrative — or what she terms 'pathography', 'a form of autobiography or biography that describes personal experiences of illness, treatment, and sometimes death' — is that it 'returns the voice of the patient to the world of medicine, a world where that voice is too rarely heard, and it does so in such a way as to assert the phenomenological, the subjective, and the experiential side of illness'.[12] Physician and medical anthropologist Arthur Kleinman has further commented that illness narratives create a 'symbolic bridge that connects body, self and society' in a network which meshes 'physiological processes, meanings and relationships so that our social world is linked recursively to our inner experience'.[13] Read in this context, Daudet's first-person account of syphilis will be used to probe the following questions: how did the literary syphilitic of the nineteenth century capture the spectre of *mors syphilitica*? How did he find the words to express not only bodily agony but also the mental torture engendered by syphilis? And how, given the prevalent assumption that pain is the classic enemy of descriptive powers, did he prevent language and creativity from being suppressed in his account?[14]

10 As Simone de Beauvoir puts it in *Le Deuxième sexe*, 2 vols (Paris: Gallimard, 1976), acknowledging her debt to analyses of embodiment offered by Heidegger, Sartre, and Merleau-Ponty: 'Le corps n'est pas une chose, il est une situation: c'est notre prise sur le monde et l'esquisse de nos projets', I, p. 73.

11 Rita Charon, *Narrative Medicine: Honoring the Stories of Illness* (Oxford: Oxford University Press, 2006), p. 87.

12 Anne Hunsaker Hawkins, *Reconstructing Illness: Studies in Pathography*, 2nd ed. (West Lafayette, IN: Purdue University Press, 1999), pp. 1, 12.

13 Arthur Kleinman, *The Illness Narratives: Suffering, Healing and the Human Condition* (New York: Basic Books, 1988), xiii.

14 Explaining why modern culture has 'willingly, almost gratefully, handed over to medicine the job of explaining pain', David Morris, in *The Culture of Pain* (Berkeley and Los Angeles:

The Pain of Words

Some initial insights into the power and capacity of words to articulate illness, which will serve as an important contrast to Daudet's approach to describing his experience, are provided in the correspondence of arguably the most famous member of the nineteenth-century literary syphilitics' club, Guy de Maupassant. In a letter to his friend (and municipal librarian of Rouen) Robert Pinchon, dated 2 March 1877, Maupassant tells of his reaction to his doctor's declaration that he had contracted syphilis:

> Tu ne devineras jamais la merveilleuse découverte que mon médecin vient de faire en moi [...]. La vérole [...]. J'ai la vérole! enfin! la vraie! pas la misérable chaude-pisse, pas l'ecclésiastique christalline (sic) [...] — non, la grande vérole, celle dont est mort François 1er. La vérole majestueuse et simple, l'élégante syphilis [...]. J'ai la vérole [...] et j'en suis fier, morbleu! [...]. Alléluia, j'ai la vérole, par conséquent je n'ai plus peur de l'attraper et je baise les putains des rues, les rouleuses des bornes, et après les avoir baisées, je leur dis: 'J'ai la vérole'. Et elles ont peur de moi et je ris...[15]

Maupassant uses his initial diagnosis to boast, as Flaubert did, of his sexual vigour, but later that year, he begins to complain about serious hair loss and severe migraines, indicating that syphilis had reached its secondary stage. From this point on, we notice an important change in tone in his correspondence alluding to or explicitly mentioning his syphilis. Maupassant evokes ocular troubles as a particular handicap in 1880 in a letter to his literary mentor in which he writes: 'Je n'y vois presque plus de l'œil droit — Mon médecin est un peu inquiet et croit à une congestion de je ne sais quelle partie de l'organe. Enfin c'est à peine si je puis vous écrire en fermant cet œil...'.[16] The Swiss ophthalmologist Edmund Landolt observes a further deterioration in Maupassant's sight in 1888 when he detects that his pupils no longer react to the light and, in

University of California Press, 1991), reminds us that 'pain not only hurts but more often than not frustrates, baffles, and resists us', pp. 18–19.

15 Letter of 2 March 1877 to Robert Pinchon, cited in Jean Goens, *De la syphilis au sida: cinq siècles des mémoires littéraires de Vénus* (Bruxelles: Presses Interuniversitaires Européennes, 1995), p. 109.

16 See Maupassant's letter of 18 February 1880 to Gustave Flaubert, in Gustave Flaubert–Guy de Maupassant, *Correspondance*, ed. by Yvan Leclerc (Paris: Flammarion, 1993), p. 231.

1891, Maupassant describes his situation in particularly despairing terms in a letter to a doctor, addressed simply to 'mon cher ami':

> Mes douleurs de tête sont si fortes que je la serre entre mes deux mains et il me semble que c'est une tête de mort.
>
> Certains chiens qui hurlent expriment très bien mon état. C'est une plainte lamentable qui ne s'adresse à rien, qui ne va nulle part, qui ne dit rien et qui jette dans les nuits, le cri d'angoisse enchaînée que je voudrais pouvoir pousser… Si je pouvais gémir comme eux, je m'en irais quelquefois, souvent, dans une grande plaine ou au fond d'un bois et je hurlerais ainsi, durant des heures entières, dans les ténèbres. Le cerveau usé et vivant encore, je ne peux pas écrire. Je n'y vois plus. C'est le désastre de ma vie…[17]

The progressive deterioration in Maupassant's condition and his diminishing ability to convey the frightening experience of syphilis within the structures of human language — as we see in the reference to 'certains chiens qui hurlent' which 'expriment très bien [s]on état' in the quotation above — are echoed in the observations made by David Le Breton in his *Anthropologie de la douleur* where he argues:

> La douleur est un échec radical du langage. […] Elle […] laisse [l'individu] impuissant à nommer cette intimité torturante. Incommunicable, elle n'est pas un continent dont les explorateurs pourraient dessiner la géographie tangible. Sous sa lame, le morcellement de l'unité de l'existence provoque la fragmentation du langage. Elle suscite le cri, la plainte, le gémissement, les pleurs ou le silence, c'est-à-dire autant de défaillances de la parole et de la pensée; elle brise la voix et la rend méconnaissable.[18]

The contention that pain shatters language and, by extension, suppresses the literary imagination, has become something of an *idée reçue*: as Henri Mitterand observes, 'la représentation de la douleur, et la réflexion sur la douleur, tant morale que physique, occupent dans la littérature romanesque une place mineure par rapport à la place dominante qui est réservée à la

---

17 Maupassant, Lettre à un médecin, décembre 1891, in *Correspondance*, ed. by Jacques Suffel (Evreux: Le Cercle du Bibliophile, 1973), letter 694.

18 David Le Breton, *Anthropologie de la douleur* (Paris: Métailié, 1995), p. 39.

scénographie du désir et du plaisir, sous toutes leurs formes'.[19] Referring to the expressibility of pain in her 1926 essay, 'On Being Ill', Virginia Woolf famously argues that people have a deep reservoir of language to describe love, but only a shallow one for articulating suffering: 'among the drawbacks of illness as a matter for literature there is the poverty of the language. [...] Let a sufferer try to describe a pain in his head to a doctor and language at once runs dry. There is nothing ready made for him.'[20] In *The Body in Pain*, Scarry contends that pain is a sensation that is outside of language, is essentially private, and therefore cannot be articulated within textual structures:

> If one were to move through all the emotional, perceptual, and somatic states that take an object — hatred for, seeing of, being hungry for — the list would become a very long one and, though it would alternate between states we are thankful for and those we dislike, it would be throughout its entirety a consistent affirmation of the human being's capacity to move out beyond the boundaries of his or her own body into the external, shareable world. This list and its implicit affirmation would, however, be suddenly interrupted when, moving through the human interior, one at last reached physical pain, for physical pain — unlike any other state of consciousness — has no referential content. It is not *of* or *for* anything. It is precisely because it takes no object that it, more than any other phenomenon, resists objectification in language.[21]

Those in pain, Scarry claims, are unable to translate their experience into words, for pain cannot be accommodated by the structures of language in the face of a paucity of directly expressive words for painful sensations. This raises a number of issues, not only concerning the meaning of pain, but also its articulation: if pain 'resists objectification in language', and the absence of a direct language of pain causes the sufferer to feel isolated from the external world, then it would appear that pain cannot be shared, and that the person in pain feels cut off from any sense of community. As Jacques Poirier and

19 Henri Mitterand, 'Jouir/souffrir: le sensible et la fiction', in *Pleasure and Pain in Nineteenth-Century French Literature and Culture*, ed. by David Evans and Kate Griffiths (Amsterdam: Rodopi, 2008), pp. 31–52 (p. 35).

20 Virginia Woolf, 'On Being Ill', in *The Essays of Virginia Woolf*, ed. by Andrew McNeillie, 4 vols (London: Hogarth Press, 1994), IV, 317–29 (p. 318).

21 Scarry, *The Body in Pain*, p. 5 (emphasis in original).

Françoise Salaün put it: 'parce qu'[elle] est avant tout intime, la douleur est une expérience dont ni la nature ni l'intensité ne se communique aisément'.[22]

Communicating Pain

Scarry's theory of pain expression and the associated questions raised by Maupassant's account provide a framework for an analysis of Alphonse Daudet's first-person account of syphilis. Daudet acquired syphilis at the age of seventeen, not from one of the many prostitutes of nineteenth-century Paris, but from a woman employed to read aloud at the Imperial Court. The first manifestations of the disease in the author were examined by Dr Philippe Ricord, the founder of syphilography who first classified the three stages of syphilis.[23] Daudet was immediately treated with mercury and the disease lay dormant for a long time. He got married, had three children and established himself as one of France's foremost literary figures. However, given that syphilis progresses with time in scope and severity, Daudet's troubles were not over: he experienced a number of what he termed 'warning signs' (aches, shooting pains, burning sensations in the eyes) and, over the years, his syphilis progressed to its tertiary stage, extending into the disabling neurological syndrome of progressive locomotor ataxia, also known as *tabes dorsalis* — an atrophy of the dorsal columns of the spinal cord — which caused twelve final years of suffering and debility, before he died in 1897 at the age of 57. In his notebook on life with syphilis, *La Doulou* (the Provençal word for pain that he used as a child), Daudet declares that the expression of pain — or, at least, any sense of accurate, coherent enunciation of pain — is beyond words. Telling the story of a night of excruciating pain, when only howls of anguish could express his agony, he writes: 'Ce que j'ai souffert hier soir — le talon et les côtes! La torture… pas de mots pour rendre ça, il faut des cris'.[24] Daudet's reversion to pre-language cries and inarticulate groans recalls some of Maupassant's observations on the unsharability of pain and appears to support Scarry's assertion

22 Jacques Poirier and Françoise Salaün, *Médecin ou malade? La Médecine en France aux XIXe et XXe siècles* (Paris: Masson, 2001), p. 108.

23 For more on Dr Philippe Ricord, see, for example, Deborah Hayden, *Pox: Genius, Madness, and the Mysteries of Syphilis* (New York: Basic Books, 2003), pp. 29–32; 51–52.

24 Alphonse Daudet, *La Doulou* (Paris: Mercure de France, 2007), p. 38. Subsequent references are from this edition and are given in parentheses only.

that pain engenders 'an immediate reversion to a state anterior to language, to the sounds and cries a human being makes before language is learned'.[25]

Critics of Daudet's posthumously-published journal which records the anguish of the tertiary stage of syphilis tend, unsurprisingly, to consider *La Doulou* for what it reveals about the inadequacy of language to express physical suffering. Michael Worton, for instance, focuses on the heavily fragmented nature of the text — the gaps, the fissures, the lack of proper syntax, the absence of punctuation — and argues that the deficiency of narrative coherence in it reflects the contingency of a life of suffering.[26] Worton suggests, however, that the writer of *La Doulou* is someone who is 'confronting the inadequacy of language in situations of suffering', and that the text may be read as a response to a need to fracture or transcend the solitude produced by illness, an 'attempt to do something with the suffering, to make it matter':

> What is important and valuable about *La Doulou* is that Daudet does not deny pain, that he forces himself to speak it here — haltingly, fragmentedly, painfully. And he is saying his pain in writing, because writing and reading enable a relationship that is honest but, usefully, not direct and immediate. [...] Daudet undoubtedly believes that suffering can open up an ethical dimension within the sufferer, in the sense that an individual's pain — which has no point in itself — can nonetheless take on a charge of meaning if it becomes the occasion for the empathetic, even suffering response of a reader.[27]

The focus of the present analysis is less on the reader's response to Daudet's attempts to communicate his experience of pain than on the metaphorical, rhetorical, and structural mechanisms the author deploys in his quest to convey an experience that is resistant to expression. As such, it draws on the recent scholarship of Joanna Bourke, which has advocated a fundamental shift from the 'ontological fallacy' of considering pain as an entity to regarding it instead as an interpretation of experience: 'pain describes the *way* we experience something not *what* is experienced. It is a manner of feeling [...] not an intrinsic quality of raw sensation.'[28] In this respect, Bourke supports an approach to pain narratives that focuses on the person-in-pain if the sensation

25 Scarry, *The Body in Pain*, p. 4.

26 Michael Worton, 'Of Sapho and Syphilis: Alphonse Daudet on and in Illness', *L'Esprit Créateur*, 37 (1997), 38–49.

27 Ibid., pp. 45–46.

28 Bourke, *The Story of Pain*, pp. 5, 7 (emphasis in original).

of pain and its effect on lived experience are to be appreciated. Recognizing that 'if we are to understand how people in the past suffered, we need to pay attention to the languages they seized hold of in order to overcome some of the obstacles to pain-speech', Bourke places particular emphasis on an analysis of figurative language and 'rhetorical figures of speech that employ association, comparison or resemblance', all of which allow for the transfer of concepts into a context in which they are not usually found and thereby offer a potentially instructive means of conveying experiences that are most resistant to expression.[29] Grouping these linguistic concepts under the shorthand term of 'metaphor', Bourke suggests: 'Crucially, by using metaphors to bring interior sensations into a knowable, external world, sufferers attempt to impose (and communicate) some kind of order onto their experiences'.[30] There are three such organizational metaphors that Daudet uses in *La Doulou*, each of which presents a possible opportunity for the author to circumvent barriers to the communication of syphilis-induced pain.

The most common metaphor in Daudet's first-person account of syphilis objectifies pain as a belligerent, self-governing entity. As his symptoms begin to suggest bodily dysfunction, Daudet pays a rather unpleasant visit to his urologist, the renowned Dr Félix Guyon, and describes his condition in terms of a hostile subversion: 'Il me sonde: contraction de la vessie, prostate un peu nerveuse, rien en somme. Et ce *rien*, c'était *tout* qui commençait: l'Invasion' (28; emphasis in original). The experience of syphilis is conceptualized here as a foe assaulting a passive body, with Daudet's resigned sense of despair — of defeat, almost — encapsulated in the *majuscule* of 'Invasion'. The mighty enemy is presented as an antagonist, its potency encrypted in a language which suggests that the bodily defences of the vulnerable assailant are unable to withstand the attack that is underway. These are '[les] premiers temps du mal qui me tâte partout, [qui] choisit son terrain' (29). This analogy underlines the reified nature of a pain which is considered dominant and uncontrollable. The discourse of invasion is replicated in connected metaphors, one of which — infiltration — is commonly used in modern narratives documenting viral infections whereby, in the use of 'metaphors of aggression', viruses are seen to 'attack', 'devour', and 'destroy' the body by 'intruding' into a host cell.[31] In Daudet's case, pain is presented as an enemy which invades and progressively occupies his entire body: 'Douleur qui se glisse partout, dans ma vision, mes

29 Ibid., pp. 53–54.

30 Ibid., p. 55.

31 Priscilla Wald, *Contagious: Cultures, Carriers, and the Outbreak Narrative* (Durham, NC: Duke University Press, 2008), p. 170.

sensations, mes jugements; c'est une infiltration' (47). As Bourke argues, 'embodied events (including painful ones) routinely test the limits of conventional language'.[32] Yet Daudet's seemingly idiosyncratic communication of his experience of being in pain by recourse to discourses of invasion and infiltration may be seen as constituting an early version of the now ubiquitous militarized rhetoric that Susan Sontag has suggested first developed in the late nineteenth century with the identification of bacteria as agents of disease, but which, over time, came to designate diseases in general, casting them as 'evil predators', 'demonic enemies' and 'alien others'.[33]

Daudet's articulation of pain as external exogenous entity, separate from the body of the patient but threatening its defences, gives rise to a second prominent group of metaphors in *La Doulou*, namely pain as analogous to something that ruptures, shatters, and rips apart the body. Daudet recounts '[des] coups lancinants' in his legs (27), 'grands sillons de flammes découpant et illuminant [s]a carcasse' (28), '[la] brûlure des yeux' (28), 'la douleur en petit oiseau-*pück* sautillant ici, là, poursuivi par la piqûre' (53), 'fulgurations dans le pied, muscles broyés par un camion, coups de lance dans le petit doigt' (53). This rich collection of metaphors not only articulates the intensity of pain, but once more conceptualizes pain as an entity that breeches bodily integrity and transgresses the materiality of the body's external defences. As Daudet retreats into himself, becoming ever more introspective and defensive, seeking as best he can to fend off external aggression, the body then becomes a *site* where terror is wrought. We see this in his references to specific bodily locations and his use of prepositions in a brief exposition of what he calls 'formes de la douleur':

> Quelquefois, sous le pied, une coupure, fine, fine, un cheveu. Ou bien des coups de canif sous l'ongle de l'orteil. Le supplice des brodequins de bois aux chevilles. Des dents de rats très aiguës grignotant les doigts de pied. (44–45)

These allusions to a body-in-pain which is violated by an aggressive, reified other find their parallel in the battle metaphors so common in modern autopathography. In turn, these are rooted, Hawkins suggests, in the antagonistic paradigms that conceptualize the human struggle in Christian culture — good versus evil, light versus darkness, the flesh versus the spirit, and life versus death:

32 Bourke, *The Story of Pain*, p. 59.

33 See Sontag, *Illness as Metaphor*, pp. 65–67.

> Christianity's habit of dualism becomes an explicit military metaphor in the familiar passage from Ephesians urging the believer to "put on the whole armour of God" and with the breastplate of righteousness, the shield of faith, the helmet of salvation, and the sword of the spirit, to fight against the "rulers of the darkness of this world" (6: 11–17). [...] The pervasiveness of military metaphor in our contemporary understanding of illness and its therapies is thus not at all surprising; indeed it seems almost predetermined.[34]

Read in this way, we can see that the patient's fight against pain as an external, reified agent seeking to breech the body's defence systems is often motivated by a desperate hope for an ultimate victory.

While there is no evidence for religious faith on Daudet's part, the subsuming of pain into the richly evocative tenets of Christian suffering is rendered explicit in one final, and remarkable, metaphor he turns to in his account of life with syphilis. Describing a night of particular agony, Daudet provides a theological interpretation for the pain he suffers:

> *Il Crociato*. Oui, c'était cela, cette nuit. Le supplice de la Croix, torsion des mains, des pieds, des genoux, les nerfs tendus, tiraillés à éclater. Et la corde rude sanglant le torse, et les coups de lance dans les côtes. Pour apaiser ma soif sur mes lèvres brûlées dont la peau s'enlevait, desséchée, encroûtée de fièvre, une cuillerée de bromure iodé, à goût de sel amer: c'était l'éponge trempée de vinaigre et de fiel.
>
> Et j'imaginais une conversation de Jésus avec les deux Larrons sur la Douleur. (49)

As Bourke has discussed, pain has, for centuries, been ideologically interpreted using the figurative languages of religion, with suffering being justified in terms of its divine function, whether it be instruction, expiation, test, or even grace.[35] However, in Christian doctrine, pain is most often entangled with the notion of transgression. Etymologically, the word 'pain' derives from the Greek 'poine' meaning suffering and the Latin 'poena' connoting punishment. In French, the phrase 'avoir mal', used to designate physical pain, evokes moral fragility. While the notion of 'douleur', which might be translated as 'anguish' given that it does not separate physical from mental pain, does not carry the same associations with moral transgression or divine punishment, its use in the Passion

34 Hawkins, *Reconstructing Illness*, p. 63.

35 See Bourke, *The Story of Pain*, chapter 4, 'Religion', pp. 88–130.

narratives of the Bible suggests a sense of suffering and subsequent purification which gives access to God. As Le Breton puts it, 'l'acceptation de la douleur est une forme possible de dévotion qui rapproche de Dieu, purifie l'âme'.[36] Pain — 'la douleur' — may therefore also be conceptualized as a form of penance for, and expiation from, sin.

In Judeo-Christian cultures, the so-called sins of the flesh have often been perceived as a catalyst of pain, with venereal and sexually-transmitted diseases in particular, from gonorrhoea to syphilis to modern-day AIDS, inviting theological speculation on the perishable 'sinful' body.[37] Daudet's portrayal of himself on the Cross, nerves stretched and pulled to breaking point, skin pulling from his lips, bodily integrity falling apart, may suggest that he imagines that he is being punished for wrongdoing with his courtly lover. The additional reference to the coarse rope whipping blood from the torso and the spear prodding at the ribs — acts which are outside the act of crucifixion itself but also find clear parallels in the biblical Passion narrative — reinforces his sense of divine castigation, as does the fact that, in 1889, he reported to Edmond de Goncourt a dream in which he was caught up in the Last Judgement, defending himself against a sentence of 3500 years in hell for 'the crime of sensuality'.[38] Whatever Daudet's personal religious beliefs, or lack thereof, what is clear from an analysis of the crucifixion metaphor in *La Doulou* is that the writer is drawn to situating his syphilitic body within a religious and cultural framework that allows him to interpret and communicate his pain. Daudet's pain is therefore much more than a sensation he *feels*; rather, its articulation in writing corroborates Morris's suggestion that:

> pain is not just [...] unreflectively endured as a series of biochemical impulses. [...] We experience our pain as it is interpreted, enfolded within formal or informal systems of thought that endow it with a time-bound meaning — whether theological, economic, scientific, or psychological.

36 Le Breton, *Anthropologie de la douleur*, p. 90.

37 See Peter Allen, *The Wages of Sin: Sex and Disease, Past and Present* (Chicago: University of Chicago Press, 2000). This book includes a quotation, in translation, from the seventeenth-century French physician, Monsieur Flamand, pontificating that syphilis was to be seen as 'the just rewards of unbridled lust' (p. 42).

38 Cited in Sebastian Dieguez and Julien Bogousslavsky, 'The One-Man Band of Pain: Alphonse Daudet and his Painful Experience of Tabes Dorsalis', in *Neurological Disorders in Famous Artists*, ed. by Julien Bogousslavsky and François Boller (Basel: Karger, 2005), pp. 17–45 (p. 21). Daudet also reportedly told Anatole France just before his death that he had been 'justly punished for having loved life too much' (cited in Dieguez and Bogousslavsky, p. 28).

> We make sense of pain in much the same way that we make sense of the world.[39]

The Aesthetics of Pain

While pain resists direct articulation in human language, as Woolf and Scarry have proposed, Daudet's writings demonstrate that it need not have no communicable meaning at all. As Lucy Bending has argued, '[pain] is given meaning — has meaning imposed on it — when the sufferer, or someone acting benevolently or malevolently on behalf of the sufferer, draws suffering into association with something else'.[40] Pain is then, she suggests, 'compelled to move outwards from the direct description of pain itself into a metaphorical and explanatory realm in which pain is fitted into another and distinct framework of reference'.[41] Daudet's articulation of pain within the ideological tenets of religious discourse thus offers an interpretative framework that allows him, unlike Maupassant, to capture and communicate his experience of syphilis. For Hawkins, such a scenario presents certain key advantages in any bid to share an experience of illness:

> If pathography is an imaginative reformulation of experience that reconnects the isolated individual sufferer with his or her world, the connecting "formula" needs to be both culture-specific and transcultural, for the patient's world includes both a particular society at a certain moment in history and the larger and more timeless human community that underlies it.[42]

That said, the conventional nature of the metaphorical paradigms used in Daudet's text raises an important question about the extent to which figurative interpretations of pain blunt the rawness and, by extension, the authenticity of accounts of subjective experience.[43] When Daudet, or indeed any patient-author, takes pain out into metaphorical and explanatory realms, does he not

---

39 Morris, *The Culture of Pain*, p. 45.

40 Lucy Bending, *The Representation of Bodily Pain in Late Nineteenth-Century English Culture* (Oxford: Clarendon Press, 2000), p. 86.

41 Ibid., p. 85.

42 Hawkins, *Reconstructing Illness*, p. 27.

43 George Lakoff, in 'The Meanings of Literal', *Metaphor and Symbolic Activity*, 1 (1986), 291–96, famously argues that only literal language can claim truth.

run the risk of ritualizing and therefore trivializing the experience, not least when he resorts to archetypal language and allegory? As Le Breton writes with reference to the ubiquitous stabbing and biting metaphors used to describe pain:

> celui qui annonce ces images approximatives n'a jamais reçu de coups de couteau et n'a jamais été mordu par un chien. Il reprend à son usage des métaphores devenues lieux communs et qui finissent par organiser une expérience autrement informulable.[44]

By giving pain expression and presence in metaphor, Daudet succeeds in drawing it into the realm of the explanatory; at the same time, however, it is precisely because the quest to communicate an experience of illness depends upon commonly-understood analogies that *La Doulou* becomes metaphorically heavy and references to pain are harnessed to language which is somewhat formulaic and, as a result, limiting. The effect is that the metaphorical paradigms used to capture, communicate, and share pain in *La Doulou* often hebetate its subjective qualities. Even if Daudet's ordeal is interpreted as an example of what Bourke terms 'retrojection', whereby the religious metaphor of the crucifixion is 'mapped back into the body' and 'literally felt and absorbed by the body [...], not only providing meaning for painful events but also fundamentally affecting the way people actually *perceive* those events in their bodies', it remains the case that his identification with Christ on the Cross draws attention to a heightened use of language, as illustrated in his prefacing of the account with the mythical inscription '*Il Crociato*', The Crusader.[45] Furthermore, Daudet reveals at one point an awareness of the importance of reliving and rewriting pain: 'à quoi ça sert, les mots, pour tout ce qu'il y a de vraiment senti en douleur [...]? Ils arrivent quand c'est fini, apaisé. Ils parlent de souvenir, impuissants ou menteurs' (38). This disclosure that words can only articulate the raw realities of pain in retrospect testifies to the levels of stylistic reflection that inform *La Doulou* and casts a shadow over the authenticity and veracity of Daudet's written account of pain.

The presence of an epigraph — the highly-symbolic inscription '*dictante dolore*' — in *La Doulou* exposes a certain reception anxiety on the part of the

---

44 Le Breton, *Anthropologie de la douleur*, p. 40.

45 Bourke, *The Story of Pain*, p. 92 (emphasis in original). Daudet's enigmatic reference to '*Il Crociato*' also recalls Meyerbeer's 1824 opera, *Il Crociato in Egitto* (The Crusader in Egypt), which tells the story of a Christian prisoner who escapes a death sentence and is reunited with his lover.

author and further suggests that pain is not, in fact, the *object* of enquiry in Daudet's writing, but the *incitement* to an act of writing. This is underlined in one of the most vivid and highly-stylised metaphors used in the text:

> Depuis que je sais que c'est pour toujours — un toujours pas très long, mon Dieu! — je m'installe et je prends de temps en temps ces notes avec la pointe d'un clou et quelques gouttes de mon sang sur les murailles du *carcere duro*. (48; emphasis in original)

Here, Daudet conceptualizes the materiality of the cell wall as his notebook, and spilled blood as ink, the symbolic blood trope corroborating the suggestion that bodily rupture is the impetus for the production of the written account rather than the object of its attention. This highlights once again that what we are dealing with in *La Doulou* is the articulation of pain by a professional writer as well as a suffering subject, for what Daudet's account demonstrates, ultimately, is that writing about pain necessarily incentivizes a reflection on the function, nature, and power — or otherwise — of language. As Mitterand writes:

> *La Doulou* de Daudet [est] le "carnet", tenu entre 1887 et 1895, des souffrances physiques qui assiègent [l'auteur], ainsi que des analyses qu'il en fait, qui parviennent non à vaincre la douleur mais seulement à imposer à celle-ci une coexistence durable avec la double volonté de lucidité et d'art.[46]

The 'double volonté' that drives the writing of Daudet's account of pain — which we might also think of as a desire to understand the nature of the pain he is suffering and to interrogate the effects that pain has on writing — reminds us that he is concerned to approach the task of keeping a notebook on syphilis not simply as a patient but also as a literary *personnage*.

The crafted metaphorical language in *La Doulou* and the high degree of literary self-consciousness that pervades the text situate Daudet within a demonstrable literary heritage of writers who have tried to give expression to pain, not least through recourse to the crucifixion metaphor. While Daudet's use of culturally-ubiquitous metaphors of pain draws attention to some of the inherent limitations in *La Doulou*, the writer's self-identification with Christ invites us to re-evaluate this understudied text as much more than an attempt

46 Henri Mitterand, 'Jouir/souffrir: le sensible et la fiction', p. 36.

to communicate the pain that results from syphilis. As Claire Moran has argued, the nineteenth-century literary and artistic *imaginaire* in France gave rise to 'a reinvention of the representation of crucifixion'.[47] With reference to Nerval's poem 'Le Christ aux Oliviers' (1844) and Huysmans's decadent portrayal of the decomposition of Jesus's body in *Là-bas* (1891), Moran notes that the crucifixion motif in mid to late nineteenth-century France held a curious appeal for writers concerned with probing not just pain but, more particularly, the limits of self-expression. Following on, as it does, from Ernest Renan's 'humanized' depiction of Christ as an ordinary suffering man in *Vie de Jésus* (1863), and anticipating some of the expressionist and surrealist works of the late nineteenth and early twentieth centuries, including by Alfred Jarry, Max Ernst, and Edvard Munch, *La Doulou* takes its place in a rich cultural environment that questions the ways in which pain simultaneously disrupts language and prompts a range of creative strategies to overcome this challenge. In this way, it makes an important contribution to broader European fin-de-siècle literary and artistic traditions concerned with finding the structures to give expression to what it means to be in pain. To return to Mitterand's phrase, the 'double volonté' that motivates *La Doulou* originates not only from an aspiration to record the experience of pain, but, more particularly, to experiment with stylistic literary devices that shape the ways in which that pain is communicated. It is precisely this 'double volonté' that sets Daudet apart from his otherwise more prominent *confrères* in the nineteenth-century literary syphilitics' club.

Bibliography

Allen, Peter, *The Wages of Sin: Sex and Disease, Past and Present* (Chicago: University of Chicago Press, 2000)

Bardet, Jean-Pierre, et al. (eds), *Peurs et terreurs face à la contagion* (Paris: Fayard, 1988)

Barnes, Julian, 'Introduction' to Alphonse Daudet, *In the Land of Pain*, ed. and trans. by Julian Barnes (London: Jonathan Cape, 2002), v–xv

Baudelaire, Charles, *Œuvres complètes*, ed. by Yves-Gérard Le Dantec and Claude Pichois (Paris: Gallimard, Bibliothèque de la Pléiade, 1966)

Beauvoir, Simone de, *Le Deuxième sexe* (Paris: Gallimard, 1976)

---

47 Claire Moran, 'Creative Crucifixions: The Artist as Christ in Nineteenth-Century France and Belgium', in *Pleasure and Pain in Nineteenth-Century French Literature and Culture*, pp. 253–71 (p. 253).

Bending, Lucy, *The Representation of Bodily Pain in Late Nineteenth-Century English Culture* (Oxford: Clarendon Press, 2000)

Bourke, Joanna, *The Story of Pain: From Prayer to Painkillers* (Oxford: Oxford University Press, 2014)

Charon, Rita, *Narrative Medicine: Honoring the Stories of Illness* (Oxford: Oxford University Press, 2006)

Corbin, Alain, 'L'Hérédosyphilis ou l'impossible rédemption. Contribution à l'histoire de l'hérédité morbide', *Romantisme*, 31 (1981), 131–49

Daudet, Alphonse, *La Doulou* (Paris: Mercure de France, 2007)

Dieguez, Sebastian, and Julien Bogousslavsky, 'The One-Man Band of Pain: Alphonse Daudet and his Painful Experience of Tabes Dorsalis', in *Neurological Disorders in Famous Artists*, ed. by Julien Bogousslavsky and François Boller (Basel: Karger, 2005), pp. 17–45

Evans, David, and Kate Griffiths (eds), *Pleasure and Pain in Nineteenth-Century French Literature and Culture* (Amsterdam: Rodopi, 2008)

Flaubert, Gustave, and Guy de Maupassant, *Correspondance*, ed. by Yvan Leclerc (Paris: Flammarion, 1993)

Flaubert, Gustave, *Correspondance*, 5 vols (Paris: Gallimard, Bibliothèque de la Pléiade, 1973–2007)

——, *Dictionnaires des idées reçues*, in *Œuvres complètes*, 18 vols (Paris: Conard, 1910), I, 415–45

Goens, Jean, *De la syphilis au sida: cinq siècles des mémoires littéraires de Vénus* (Bruxelles: Presses Interuniversitaires Européennes, 1995)

Hayden, Deborah, *Pox: Genius, Madness, and the Mysteries of Syphilis* (New York: Basic Books, 2003)

Hunsaker Hawkins, Anne, *Reconstructing Illness: Studies in Pathography*, 2nd ed. (West Lafayette, IN: Purdue University Press, 1999)

Huysmans, Joris-Karl, *À Rebours* (Paris: Gallimard, 1977)

Kleinman, Arthur, *The Illness Narratives: Suffering, Healing and the Human Condition* (New York: Basic Books, 1988)

Lakoff, George, 'The Meanings of Literal', *Metaphor and Symbolic Activity*, 1 (1986), 291–96

Le Breton, David, *Anthropologie de la douleur* (Paris: Métailié, 1995)

Maupassant, Guy de, *Correspondance*, ed. by Jacques Suffel (Évreux: Le Cercle du Bibliophile, 1973)

Morris, Davis M., *The Culture of Pain* (Berkeley and Los Angeles: University of California Press, 1991)

Poirier, Jacques, and Françoise Salaün, *Médecin ou malade? La Médecine en France aux XIXe et XXe siècles* (Paris: Masson, 2001)

Scarry, Elaine, *The Body in Pain: The Making and Unmaking of the World* (Oxford and New York: Oxford University Press, 1985)

Sontag, Susan, *Illness as Metaphor and AIDS and its Metaphors* (London and New York: Penguin, 1991)

Wald, Priscilla, *Contagious: Cultures, Carriers, and the Outbreak Narrative* (Durham, NC: Duke University Press, 2008)

Woolf, Virginia, 'On Being Ill', in *The Essays of Virginia Woolf*, ed. by Andrew McNeillie, 4 vols (London: Hogarth Press, 1994), IV, 317–29

Worton, Michael, 'Of Sapho and Syphilis: Alphonse Daudet on and in Illness', *L'Esprit Créateur*, 37 (1997), 38–49

PART 3

Reading Body, Mind, and Environment

CHAPTER 9

Against 'Neuronormativity': 'Volcanic' Temperament in Mirbeau's *L'Abbé Jules*

Elizabeth Emery

The word *colère* is repeated forty-one times in Octave Mirbeau's 1888 novel, *L'Abbé Jules*, not including derivatives such as *s'encoléra*.[1] It is, in fact, the determining characteristic of the eponymous protagonist, Jules Dervelle, a delinquent-turned-priest who is unable to control the violent eruptions of fury that he regularly vents, much to the consternation of his family: 'Il avait des colères si terribles que tout le monde tremblait devant lui, et que lui-même, la crise passée, restait, pendant des heures, malade, le cerveau brisé, et tout pâle, semblable à un épileptique terrassé par son mal' (53). These rages are, as Mirbeau makes it clear, internal and uncontrollable, welling up from within Jules and leaving him shattered as would an epileptic fit. Like his sadism, they are constants of his personality, inherited vestiges, as Jules himself admits, of his mother's mysticism (217) and his drunken, womanizing father's cruelty (54). As a child, he was, like his father, difficult and nasty: 'sournois, tracassier, cruel, il ne se plaisait que dans les méchants tours' (54). He beat his schoolmates, ratted them out, and revolted against his teachers. Yet he was also extremely intelligent, active, and hard-working (if primarily for his own interests); he led others in anti-social activities such as petty crime, tavern brawls, and womanizing (53–54).

Given the novel's explicit references to bodies, behaviour, environment, and heredity, it is tempting to read *L'Abbé Jules* in a Naturalist light, identifying the ultimate sinning ancestor not as a woman (Zola's Tante Dide of *Les Rougon-Macquart*), but as Jules's violent horse-breeding father, or interpreting Jules Dervelle as the brother of Zola's 'bad' priests Frère Archangias and l'abbé Faujas (or as a perverted model of the saintly but hysterical Serge Mouret).[2] Pierre Michel has shown that a number of contemporaries, such as Alphonse Daudet,

1 Octave Mirbeau, *L'Abbé Jules* (Angers: Éditions du Boucher, 2003). All page references will be to this edition and will appear in the text. The novel was first published in March 1888 after serialization in *Le Gil Blas*.

2 On the links between Zola's and Mirbeau's priest characters see Yannick Lemarié, 'Ovide Faujas et Jules Dervelle: deux curés en enfer', *Les Cahiers Octave Mirbeau*, 6 (1999), 100–21.

 | DOI:10.1163/9789004368019_011

did just this, reading *L'Abbé Jules* as a Naturalist text, much to Mirbeau's chagrin. In fact, Michel has also shown that Mirbeau had sought neither to study biological or environmental determinism nor to emulate Zola or Goncourt. Instead, influenced by an 1887 reading of Dostoyevsky's *Idiot*, in *L'Abbé Jules* Mirbeau wished to explore 'la vie psychique dans toute sa complexité, ses fluctuations, ses contradictions, ses ténèbres [...] Suggérer au lieu de tout dire'.[3] Furthermore, while the character of Jules Dervelle owes a great deal to a popular French literary tradition in which environment and sexual impulses exacerbate the psychic torment of 'bad priest' characters (Claude Frollo in Victor Hugo's *Notre-Dame de Paris*, Frère Archangias in *La Faute de l'abbé Mouret*, and l'abbé Faujas in Zola's *La Conquête de Plassans*, to name just three), Mirbeau was also much less interested in analysing a 'type' than in building recognition for the psychological 'fluctuations' inherent in each individual.[4] But because he did not wish to 'tout dire', he did not adopt a third-person omniscient narrator who might make this goal clear. Instead he created an awkward first-person narrative structure and what Michel has called a 'chronologie boiteuse'.[5]

L'Abbé Jules is told largely in the voice of Albert Dervelle, Jules's nephew, who recalls his childhood impressions of his uncle in two short chapters (twelve pages each) before flashing back in a 100-page third chapter to evoke the uncle's life story, allegedly based on 'research' that the adult narrator has undertaken retroactively. This seeming digression is critical to building sympathy for Jules and characters like him, unable to balance reason and

3 While it is tempting to read *L'Abbé Jules* as a kind of rewriting of *La Faute de l'abbé Mouret*, particularly in 1888, at a moment when Mirbeau's admiration for Zola had made way for criticism of his commercial success and bourgeois complacency, Mirbeau himself rejected such readings. Michel summarizes the goals Mirbeau expressed in a letter dated 20 June 1887 to Paul Hervieu. 'Préface', in *L'Abbé Jules* (Paris: Éditions du Boucher, 2003), 3–18 (pp. 5–9). In *Octave Mirbeau et le roman* (Angers: Société Octave Mirbeau, 2005), Michel analyses at length Mirbeau's refusal of the realist novel and its conventions because of what he considers hypocritical claims to depict 'reality'.

4 The 'bad priest' genre has a long history in French literature. See, for example, Ray P. Bowen, 'An Analysis of the Priest Genre in the Modern French Novel', PMLA, 37, 4 (1922), 722–34. Despite his desire to distance himself from the overtly scientific premises expressed in Zola's 1880 *Le Roman expérimental*, early Naturalist novels such as the Goncourts' 1861 *Sœur Philomène* or Zola's 1867 *Thérèse Raquin* contained similarly complex studies of 'la vie psychique'. For more about the often fraught yet complex relationship between Mirbeau and Zola see Yannick Lemarié, 'Zola, Émile', an entry in the online *Dictionnaire Octave Mirbeau*. [http://mirbeau.asso.fr/dicomirbeau/index.php?option=com_glossary&id=550].

5 Pierre Michel, *Octave Mirbeau*, p. 86.

impulse, personal creativity and social constraints. Chapter Three, the account of Albert's 'research' into his uncle's past, quickly slips into a *style indirect libre* in which the reader is privy to Jules's thoughts even though Albert is still narrating. Seeing Jules in action, understanding his frustrations, regrets, and furies helps readers come to the realization that Jules is a bad priest not by choice or because of environment, but because of his physiological constitution: he lives in a state of near-constant inner turmoil in which his instincts vie with reason. *L'Abbé Jules*, in short, echoes the raging scientific debates of the 1880s, which pitted spiritualists and metaphysicians against doctors and experimental scientists as they attempted to understand and explain the physical and psychological mechanisms responsible for human behaviour.[6]

Scholars such as Jean-Louis Cabanès have already studied Mirbeau's first novels as a virulent critique of inflexible social norms imposed and upheld by institutions such as the law and the church.[7] The present chapter continues in this vein, focusing more precisely on the ways in which Mirbeau, who was intimately familiar with medical discourse, deploys a poetics of physiological difference — a language of fluids, pressure, and balance borrowed from the medical treatises of his day — to build sympathy for members of society ostracized for their perceived moral failures.[8] Mirbeau's treatment of Jules's 'choleric temperament' particularly calls into question *fin-de-siècle* medical discourses that classified behaviours by the dominant fluids said to be circulating in the body. Albert's attempts to understand his uncle reveal 'fluctuations'

---

6 Marc Jeannerod provides an excellent overview of the international 'development of neurophysiological thought', the subtitle of *The Brain Machine* (Cambridge, MA: Harvard University Press, 1985) while John I. Brooks focuses more specifically on the French philosophical and scientific context in *The Eclectic Legacy: Academic Philosophy and the Human Sciences in Nineteenth-Century France* (Newark, DE: University of Delaware Press, 1998).

7 Jean-Louis Cabanès, 'Le Discours sur les normes dans les premiers romans de Mirbeau', *Octave Mirbeau. Actes du colloque international d'Angers du 19 au 22 septembre 1991*, ed. by Pierre Michel and Georges Cesbron (Presses universitaires d'Angers, 1992), pp. 153–63.

8 Mirbeau's father was a doctor (an *officier de santé*) and newspaper articles, essays, and fictional passages dedicated to medical symptoms and techniques (like the technical descriptions of instruments and procedures that open *L'Abbé Jules*) demonstrate Mirbeau's familiarity with the medical theories and attitudes of his day, many of which, particularly those related to diet and hygiene, still owed a great deal to texts by Hippocrates and Galen. For more about Mirbeau's life see Pierre Michel and Jean-François Nivet, *Octave Mirbeau, l'imprécateur au cœur fidèle* (Paris: Séguier, 1990). Arnaud Vareille's 'Médecins', an entry in the online *Dictionnaire Octave Mirbeau*, describes Mirbeau's familiarity with medicine, his relationship to doctors, and links to a number of newspaper articles and essays evaluating the medical profession. [http://mirbeau.asso.fr/dicomirbeau/index.php?option=com_glossary&letter=M&id=385].

and 'contradictions' that refuse classification; he is not a 'type', but an individual with complex desires and needs that find no outlet in society. Jules's valiant yet futile attempts to make his behaviour conform to bourgeois expectations can be reread productively today in the light of arguments made by a twenty-first century 'neurodiversity' movement, which advocates for greater social recognition of behavioural difference and which disputes the notion of a 'normative' neural state.[9]

A Poetics of Physiological Difference

The term 'neurodiversity' is of recent coinage (1990s), particularly used to dispute the label 'autism-spectrum disorder' and to celebrate autism as but one example of the many natural variations of human neurological wiring.[10] It questions whether such a thing as 'neuronormativity' exists outside of psychological diagnostic manuals.[11] While it is, of course, anachronistic to apply such terms to the work of an author from 100 years ago, today's concept of 'neurodiversity', with its underlying belief that 'normality' itself is a convenient fiction perpetuated by the medical establishment, is already expressed within *L'Abbé Jules*. In emphasizing the pathological characteristics of both 'normal' and 'deviant' members of society, Mirbeau calls readers' attention to the arbitrary and often debilitating nature of 'normalizing' medical discourse. While he could not have advocated for a 'neurodiversity' movement that did not yet exist, his insistence on the importance of recognizing and embracing physiological difference reveals Mirbeau as a writer well ahead of his time.

In his explicit descriptions of Jules's 'volcanic' mood swings, Mirbeau clearly echoes Galen's theories of the humours, still influential in late

9 Georges Canguilhem provides a historical overview of the 'polemical' nature of the concept of 'normality' in *Le Normal et le pathologique* (Paris: PUF, 1975), p. 176.

10 'Neurodiversity' is a term originating in the 1990s and attributed to sociologist Judy Singer. 'In its broadest sense the concept of neurodiversity defines all atypical neurological development as a normal human difference that should be tolerated and respected in the same way as other human differences', write Pier Jaarsma and Stellan Welin in 'Autism as a Natural Human Variation: Reflections on the Claims of the Neurodiversity Movement', *Health Care Analysis*, 20 (2012), 20–30 (p. 23).

11 By equating Mirbeau with contemporary critics of 'neuronormativity' I am not setting him out as a proponent of 'neurodiversity' nor am I retrospectively 'diagnosing' Abbé Jules as an autist, though this could prove a fruitful reading. The priest's difficulties relating emotionally to others, his frank speech, sensorial troubles, and engagement in repetitive activities are commonly associated with autism-spectrum behaviours.

nineteenth-century medical treatises and hygiene manuals such as Father Pierre Corneille Debreyne's *Précis de physiologie humaine, suivi d'un Code abrégé d'hygiène*. This book, published in 1844, went through many editions through the end of the century, and was used widely in educational institutions (into the 1880s) because of Debreyne's impeccable credentials as priest, doctor, scholar, and member of the *Faculté de Médecine*.[12] Where Galen focused on bodily processes (an 1859 French translation describes the textures and the conditions of excess bile and attributes them to physiological or dietary factors, identifying 'epileptic' attacks like those of Jules as due to a blockage 'dans les canaux de sortie des ventricules de l'encéphale'),[13] Debreyne reads physiology largely in terms of morality: 'Étudiez l'homme physique, et vous connaîtrez l'homme moral'.[14] He thus classifes people by type ('sanguin', 'bilieux', 'lymphatique' 'mélancolique', 'nerveux', 'érotique').

In its emphasis on morality, Debreyne's manual shifts focus from Galen's descriptions of physiological processes (nouns and verbs) to moral judgements conveyed by a profusion of adjectives, as in his description of the melancholic temperament:

> Les mélancoliques ont l'imagination extrêmement *vive*, mais *très-lugubre* et *fort exaltée* [...] Le caractère du mélancolique est presque toujours *soupçonneux, méfiant, difficile, inquiet, rêveur, taciturne, fantasque, morose, misanthrope* [...] Le mélancolique est *très-vindicatif*, et souvent il nourrit dans son cœur *ulcéré* des haines *profondes, implacables, éternelles*. Aussi on le déteste et on le fuit. Ses passions sont en général *véhémentes, explosives* et souvent *dangereuses*.[15]

---

12 Debreyne's text was specifically adapted for the clergy under the title, *Physiologie catholique et philosophique, pour servir d'introduction aux études de la philosophie et de la théologie morale; suivie d'un Traité d'hygiène physique et morale: ouvrage spécialement destiné au clergé et aux séminaires* (Paris: Librairie Poussielgue frères, 1872). The opening words of the fifth edition are 'S'il est vrai, comme il n'est pas permis d'en douter, que le physique de l'homme exerce sur son moral une haute et puissante influence, n'est-il pas incontestable par là même que la physiologie catholique, qui est essentiellement la science de l'homme physique, intellectuel et moral, est une des bases les plus solides de la philosophie, de la morale et de l'éducation?' (v). The only words changed from the 1844 edition were the addition of the words 'catholique' and 'de l'éducation'.

13 Claude Galien, *Œuvres anatomiques, physiologiques et médicales de Galien*, vol. II, trans. by Dr Ch. Daremberg (Paris: J. B. Baillière, 1856), p. 563.

14 Debreyne, *Physiologie catholique et philosophique*, vi.

15 Ibid., pp. 344–45, my emphasis.

Jules Dervelle's character seems copied directly from this manual; not only do most of these italicized adjectives appear in the novel to describe his character, but Mirbeau even models Jules's physical characteristics on Debreyne's evocation of a melancholic personality: 'On y remarque une stature élevée, un corps maigre, grêle et sec, une figure pâle ou jaunâtre, allongée, amaigrie, anguleuse et osseuse' (344). Albert describes Jules as 'une chose noire, longue, anguleuse' (151).

In *L'Abbé Jules* the word *melancholy* is associated with Jules Dervelle six times, notably at moments when he contemplates suicide, a characteristic identified by Debreyne as a classic symptom of a particularly dangerous 'pathological' subset of the 'melancholic' temperament ('mélancolique-bilieux') characterized by 'une piété ou d'une dévotion peu éclairée, fausse et mal entendue' (347) that would explain Jules's remarkable swings from piety and repentance to irascibility and homicidal impulses. A calm mind set induced by a long walk in the countryside quickly gives way, for example, to a sexually induced hallucinatory fit in which he attacks a peasant woman and nearly rapes and kills her. In a comic reversal, his buxom conquest punches him and walks away: 'Quoi qu'y vous prend donc?... Ah ben!... En v'là un salaud d'curé!' (80). The epithet fits: 'soiled' by his uncontrolled physiological impulses, he becomes morally repugnant to those around him.

Although there are many ways to read *L'Abbé Jules*, the priest's struggles with social conventions are always front and centre. Looking closely at the language Mirbeau uses to evoke Jules's episodes, one remarks that they are couched in the physiological terms common to Galen's theory of a closed mind-body system in which one force or element vies with the others, thus leading to 'blockages' and 'attacks' that seek outlets.[16] Jules seems to try to follow the 'treatments' prescribed by the doctors of his time. Debreyne, for example, recommends 'les principes religieux et une bonne éducation' in order to 'réfrén[er ...] les passions de ce tempérament extraordinaire [...]'. If not, 'melancholics' risk becoming 'des hommes dangereux et insupportables à la société, ou des êtres bizarres, fantasques et visionnaires'.[17] Joining the priesthood, known for its disciplinary rigors, conforms perfectly to such recommendations. Yet, instead of submitting passively as Debreyne suggests, Jules cannot help but flex his 'muscular' willpower, thus further reinforcing the antisocial behaviour:

---

16 For an annotated translation of several of Galen's works and a discussion of their influence see *Galien: introduction générale; Sur l'ordre de ses propres livres; Sur ses propres livres; Que l'excellent médecin est aussi philosophe*, ed. and trans. by Véronique Boudon-Millot (Paris: Les Belles Lettres, 2007).

17 Debreyne, *Physiologie catholique et philosophique*, p. 345.

> [Jules] s'acharna à dompter sa nature révoltée, tenta de l'assouplir aux écœurements de la discipline, aux effacements de l'humilité, non point par la prière, et la passive observance des pratiques pieuses, comme font les faibles, mais par *un raidissement en quelque sorte musculaire de sa volonté*, par une tension pour ainsi dire physique de toutes ses facultés intellectuelles.[18] (57, my emphasis)

The reference here to 'volonté' echoes widespread scientific and philosophical debates about human behaviour that took place in the 1880s through such works as Théodule Ribot's 1883 *Les Maladies de la volonté*, which I will discuss below, and through dialogue about Arthur Schopenhauer's writings about the unconscious will, a notion that would influence Freud;[19] the passage that directly follows Jules's attempt to repress his 'nature révoltée' anticipates Freud's writings about the fraught tensions between 'super-ego' and 'id':

> Hélas! en dépit de son courage, il avait de violents retours au mal, une poussée de ses instincts mauvais, si soudaine et si formidable, qu'elle culbutait, en une minute, tous les travaux de défense, lentement, durement édifiés par lui contre lui. Et c'était à recommencer. Ce combat persistant de l'esprit et du corps, cette contraction nerveuse et morale qu'il s'imposait, empêchèrent Jules de se façonner aux manières ambiantes, d'acquérir ce qu'on appelle l'air de la maison. (57)

18 Jules is quickly disabused of his misconception; the third part of the novel provides a vicious satire of clerical education, administrative practices, and religious devotions. Indeed, in their eagerness to accept the 'miracle' of his conversion ('a new Saint Augustin'), they are willing to overlook even the most egregious and anti-clerical of Jules's behaviours.

19 Given the timing of *L'Abbé Jules*' publication, it is tempting to suggest that Mirbeau may have read Auguste Burdeau's 1885 translation of *Le Monde comme volonté et comme représentation*. It is more likely, however, that he, like many of his acquaintances, knew Schopenhauer's ideas only through excerpts of his writings translated by Jean Bourdeau in 1880: *Arthur Schopenhauer: pensées, maximes et fragments de Schopenhauer* (Paris: Germer-Baillière, 1880). Sébastien Roldan evokes the avid discussions of these extracts among Naturalist writers in *La pyramide des souffrances dans* La joie de vivre *de Zola* (Québec: Presses de l'Université du Québec, 2012). Another of Roldan's articles, '*Le Petit Chose* au pays des philosophes', provides an excellent overview of other popular concepts of 'volonté' during the 1880s, *Travaux de littérature*, 27 (2014), 65–84. I extend thanks to Dr Roldan for his insightful comments on a draft of this essay. In 'Mirbeau et Schopenhauer', *Cahiers Octave Mirbeau*, 8 (April 2001), 219–27, Annie Briaud draws parallels between ideas expressed by the two writers <http://mirbeau.asso.fr/darticlesfrancais/Briaud-OMetschopenhauer.pdf> [accessed January 2016].

In passages such as this one, Mirbeau does not simply present Jules's melancholy temperament as innate, as did Debreyne. In adopting a military vocabulary to refer to Jules's internal struggles — 'révolte', 'dompter', 'discipline', 'raidissement', 'défense', 'combat' — Mirbeau represents the priest not as predetermined by his temperament, but as a sympathetic individual struggling valiantly to repel a 'formidable' invading force. In passages describing Jules's struggles for self-control, Mirbeau calls into question the prescriptive behavioural suggestions proposed by 'hygienists' such as Debreyne who posited a direct link between lack of willpower and moral degeneration.[20]

Furthermore, terms such as 'raidissement', 'contraction', 'facultés intellectuelles' echo recent publications on what would become the field of psychology, led by Ribot, one of the major fin-de-siècle commentators of Schopenhauer.[21] The influence of Ribot's *Les Maladies de la volonté* can be detected in the military vocabulary used to describe the 'defeat' of Jules's willpower. Ribot's major conclusion is that 'la volonté' is not innate, but learned, and that those who have succeeded in 'balancing' the complex forces exerted upon them by heredity, biology, and environment have done so only after much training and effort:

> Ce n'est pas là un produit naturel. C'est le résultat de l'art, de l'éducation, de l'expérience. C'est un édifice construit lentement, pièce à pièce. L'observation objective et subjective montre que chaque forme de l'activité volontaire est le fruit d'une conquête. La nature ne fournit que les matériaux: quelques mouvements simples dans l'ordre physiologique, quelques associations simples dans l'ordre psychologique. Il faut que, à l'aide de ces adaptations simples et presque invariables, se forment des adaptations de plus en plus complexes et variables.[22]

---

20 See Robert A. Nye, *Crime, Madness, and Politics in Modern France. The Medical Concept of National Decline* (Princeton, NJ: Princeton University Press, 1984). The field of experimental psychology would develop markedly after 1890, just a few years after the publication of *L'Abbé Jules*, as the field divorced itself from philosophy and paved the way for brain-centred studies. On the development of psychology and neurophysiology see, for example, Brooks and Jeannerod.

21 Ribot's *La Philosophie de Schopenhauer* (1874) was one of the first examples of serious French engagement with the German philosopher's ideas (Paris: Librairie G.-Baillière, 1874). For a discussion of his importance for *fin-de-siècle* French debates about metaphysics, psychology, and medicine see Brooks, *The Eclectic Legacy*, who devotes a chapter to Ribot's work.

22 Ribot, *Les Maladies de la volonté* (Paris: Félix Alcan, 1888), p. 82.

Influenced by Schopenhauer's emphasis on the individual, Ribot stresses the multiplicity of factors ('complexes et variables') at play in each individual's struggle ('conquête') to find what he calls 'coordination' and 'equilibrium'.[23] Mirbeau's reference to a 'raidissement [...] musculaire de la volonté' suggests his familiarity with this work where Ribot cites a passage of William James's 'The Feeling of Effort' evoking an 'effort *musculaire*'.[24] Mirbeau thus deploys scientific vocabulary related to fluids, pressure control, and balance in his descriptions of Jules's attempts to conform to the 'manières ambiantes' of his family. They return over and over in the novel in reference to Jules's quest to master his 'nature révoltée'.

Ultimately, Jules's inability to control the competing 'mauvais instincts' inside him prevent him from achieving the expected 'air de la maison'.[25] This polite learned behaviour inculcated in children by family and school, and based on hygiene manuals such as those of Debreyne, is central to *L'Abbé Jules*, a novel which exposes the hypocrisy of this 'normal' behaviour. The hypocrisy of bourgeois social expectations is prominently displayed in the very first paragraph of the novel as the narrator, Jules's nephew (Albert Dervelle), describes his home life, dominated by the principle that: 'un enfant bien élevé ne doit ouvrir la bouche que pour manger, réciter ses leçons, faire sa prière' (28). Albert is told that children are brought by the stork ('naissaient sous des chous') despite the fact that his father, a country doctor, spends every meal describing the reproductive organs of various village women, 'des énumérations d'utérus, de placentas, de cordons ombilicaux.' He also polishes his 'redoutables instruments d'acier brillant, souffler dans les sondes, essuyer les bistouris [...] les minces lames des lancettes', giving particular care to cleaning his rusty forceps and practicing delicate manoeuvres on imaginary patients (29). Albert patiently suffers his parents' animated discussions about bloody bandages, pus, amputated limbs, and medical fees, perched 'obediently' (and ironically) on two volumes of *La Vie des Saints* (30). When his parents begin talking about the imminent arrival of Jules it is in terms diametrically opposed to Albert's identity as 'un enfant bien élevé'. Jules is resolutely 'méchant' and does not fit into society: 'un original [qui] n'a jamais pu rester en place [...] Il ne se trouve à

23 Ibid., pp. 169–72.

24 Ibid., p. 64.

25 The Dervelle family's alternating descriptions of Jules (both 'delinquent' and 'saint') provide a perfect illustration of the 'docility' demanded by legal systems in Foucault's *Surveiller et punir* and refused by Jules's body and mind.

son aise nulle part!' (31–32). Unlike Albert's saintly little body (martyred by its immobility at the dinner table atop *La Vie des Saints*), Jules's cannot stay still.

Given the novel's emphasis on biological and social pressures, willpower and balance, it is no coincidence that the novel opens with doctors and concludes with them in the Grand Guignol scene of pathological sexual madness that characterizes Jules's death. Further, in bequeathing his belongings to the first priest who will defrock himself in order to expose his colleagues' hypocrisy (231–32), Jules flummoxes Doctor Dervelle ('ce testament dépassait sa raison de bourgeois peureux [...] ce testament perpétuait jusque dans la mort cette vie d'impiété, d'ingratitude, de désordre et de mystification qui avait été celle de son frère', 232). Nonetheless, the doctor, like the other villagers and priests, cranes his neck to see the pornographic images that Jules asked to have burned (235). They, unlike Albert, do not understand that Jules's seeming madness is a product of the repressive societal system they enforce.

The entire novel, in fact, serves as a scathing critique of the 'honnêtes hommes' — the hypocritical bourgeois doctors, lawyers, and priests — who impose unnatural and unhealthy behavioural 'norms' whose rigidity creates what Freud would later term 'repression', precisely the kinds of 'blockages' and 'eruptions' that characterize Jules's behaviour:[26]

> Et je me suis demandé, quelquefois, quel homme aurait été mon oncle, si ce bouillonnement de laves, laves de pensées, laves de passion, dont tout son être était dévoré, avait pu trouver une issue à son expansion! Peut-être un grand saint, peut-être un grand artiste, peut-être un grand criminel! (143)

Albert's image of volcanic lava is apt for Jules since it is precisely what would later come to be known as 'repression' that is responsible for Jules's 'attacks': the build-up of pressures as he attempts to bring his physiological impulses in line with social constraints rather than to direct them to an external purpose. This passage closely maps the concluding chapter of Ribot's *Les Maladies de la volonté* where the most perfect 'coordination' between internal and external forces is exemplified by those like Caesar or Michelangelo who were able to marshal their passions toward a consistent outlet: 'Leur fond est une passion puissante, inextinguible, qui met les idées à son service'.[27] Others struggle to

---

26 See, for example, Cabanès, 'Le Discours sur les normes dans les premiers romans de Mirbeau', pp. 153–56.

27 Ribot, *Maladies*, p. 169.

strike a balance, from those with lives characterized by 'intermittence, dont le centre de gravité, ordinairement stable, oscille pourtant de temps en temps' or those like Jules where 'deux tendances contraires ou simplement différentes l'emportent tour à tour' or where 'il n'y a plus que des coordinations intermittentes; c'est la volonté qui devient l'exception'.[28]

The Attractions of a Volcanic Temperament

Jules Dervelle's volcanic temperament, evoked through the vague memories of his pre-adolescent nephew, is first construed as malevolent, diabolic, satanical, and detrimental to society; his *accès de colère* destroy everything in their path, inspiring fear and paralysis from those 'honnêtes hommes' affected. Yet as the nephew reconstructs his uncle's story and comes to know him, readers learn that Jules's excessive 'humours' derive not just from biology (his 'nature révoltée'), but from fissures in the seemingly stable society in which he lives. Mirbeau uses scenes where Jules erupts and then cools down to create comical situations revealing that the seemingly 'normal' bourgeois villagers — priests, judges, doctors, and parents — present much greater threats to the social fabric than the forthright Jules.

We see this specifically in the barbaric treatment of children, even those who have perfectly mastered 'les manières ambientes', like the physically 'difformé' Georges Robin, a child two years younger than Albert, whose mother keeps him locked away as her personal servant (171–72). The last image of the novel is of this saintly 'avorton' sewing patiently in his garret window (236). His father, a judge reputed for his 'incorruptibilité presque farouche', is, in reality, 'stupide, irréparablement'. He seconds his wife in sequestering their son, while accepting bribes in exchange for legal decisions (41–42). Priests are even worse: the novel provides innumerable examples of the ways in which they stifle their students' curiosity, abuse their young charges, and generally flaunt the vows they have taken (63–146).[29] Through the depiction of such 'degenerate' pillars of society Mirbeau creates sympathy for naturally occurring differences in human behaviour, often marked by uncontrollable passions or impulses that transgress strict social boundaries.

---

28 Ibid., pp. 170–71.

29 Mirbeau would provide an even more violent critique of priests' pedophilia in his next novel, *Sébastien Roch* (1890).

Such sympathy does not, however, emanate directly from Jules Dervelle and his often reprehensible speech and actions. Rather, Mirbeau builds understanding for his tremendously unpleasant character through vocabulary and imagery that stress his failed quest for balance, and through a seemingly disordered yet clever narrative technique: telling the story through the first-person voice of a narrator who evokes his childhood experiences with Jules before attempting to learn more about his uncle's life story (53). This is a clever conceit because Albert Dervelle, like many children, is a clear-eyed and brutally honest observer. He notes the practices and values of his parents without criticizing them explicitly, though his own innate dissatisfaction with their rules provides an unspoken condemnation. He regrets, for example, the strict silence, 'claustral interior', and frigid emotions of his home and longs for the intellectual and material warmth he witnesses at neighbours' houses (33–34). He passes judgment neither on his parents nor on his uncle, recording what he sees with the eyes of a child who does not yet understand what he witnesses. It is through this narration that readers understand the unnatural rigidity of the 'manières ambiantes' Jules cannot master. Mirbeau's narrative technique is doubly effective since the Jules described by the strict parents as 'monstrous' is fascinating for the obedient Albert. His uncle is presented as a bogeyman ('le diable noir', 34), held up at the beginning of the book as a terrifying 'ogre' or 'monstre', an example of what Albert will become should he diverge from the strict rules his parents have set for him: 'Laid […] sale […] gourmand […] violent […] menteur […] L'abbé Jules! c'est-à-dire tous les défauts, tous les vices, tous les crimes, toutes les hideurs' (34–35).

Yet Jules also represents 'tout le mystère', the attraction such resistance to the accepted order represents for an only child stifled by the unrelenting monotony of a nineteenth-century bourgeois upbringing. Albert knows no one who has bucked convention as has Jules, which makes him particularly fascinating. Indeed, the first time the narrator's parents talk of Jules's return to the small town of Viantais they make it clear that Albert's uncle is resolutely atypical, using labels that carry particular weight given his father's stature as medical professional: 'un original' (31), 'un mauvais parent, un mauvais prêtre, un être indécrottable' (32), 'un diable' (32), 'un fou exalté' (33). For Albert, this makes Jules the subject of fantastical reveries:

> je voyais se dresser devant moi une figure de fantôme, hérissée, sabrée de grimaces, grotesque et terrible […] À la veille de retrouver cet oncle inquiétant, je ressentais la même peur attractive qui me prenait les jours de foire, sur le seuil des ménageries et des boutiques de saltimbanques. (37–38)

It is important to note that the circus acts evoked here carried medical associations: much studied, displayed, and dissected in nineteenth-century Europe and America, the physical differences of sideshow 'freaks' excluded them from 'normal' bourgeois society. They were considered at home only in institutions such as circuses, zoos, and hospitals.[30] Albert's 'peur attractive', the repulsion and attraction characteristic of bourgeois circus audiences, thus models for readers the empathy they might derive from reading *L'Abbé Jules*. They, too, are complicit in his story and the guilty pleasure they feel in watching him struggle is not so far from the pity they might feel for a sideshow performer. Pity, for Mirbeau, is akin to solidarity; he considered it the most powerful force for initiating social justice.[31]

Throughout the novel, Albert characterizes Jules as a clown, tightrope walker, or sideshow freak, attempting to perform a balancing act between his brilliant ideas, his socially inacceptable impulses, and his inability to adhere to bourgeois norms:

> Entre ses conceptions, souvent fortes et justes, et leur réalisation, il y avait un trou, qu'il franchissait d'une grotesque culbute, comme un clown [...] être à rebours de lui-même, parodiste de sa propre personnalité, il vivait en un perpétuel déséquilibrement de l'esprit et du cœur. (73–74)

Once again, the figurative language used by Mirbeau echoes Ribot's 'coordination' and 'équilibre', synonyms of 'imbalance' that persist today in medical debates about the regulation of 'chemical imbalances'. The result is that while 'Abbé Jules' has become a code word for a rotten priest, the language of

30 There is an enormous body of critical literature related to the Western medical study and display of circus and sideshow performers and the physically and mentally 'other'. See, for example, Shoshana Feldman, *La Folie et la chose littéraire* (Paris: Seuil, 1978); Rosemarie Garland Thomson, *Extraordinary Bodies: Figuring Physical Disability in American Culture and Literature* (New York: Columbia University Press, 1997); *Human Zoos: Science and Spectacle in the Age of Colonial Empires*, ed. by Pascal Blanchard, Nicolas Bancel, Gilles Boëtsch, Eric Deroo, Sandrine Lemaire, and Charles Forsdick, and trans. by Teresa Bridgeman (Liverpool: Liverpool University Press, 2008); and, Fiona Yvette Pettit, *Freaks in Late Nineteenth-Century British Media and Medicine*, unpublished doctoral thesis (University of Exeter, 2012). Such practices have much in common with the experimentation, performance, and recording of mental illnesses at the Salpêtrière Hospital in Paris. See, for example, the spectacularity described by Asti Hustvedt, *Medical Muses: Hysteria in Nineteenth-Century Paris* (New York: W.W. Norton, 2011).

31 Pierre Michel, 'Pitié', in the *Dictionnaire Octave Mirbeau*, <http://mirbeau.asso.fr/dicomirbeau/index.php?option=com_glossary&letter=P&id=490>.

Mirbeau's novel shows an extraordinary degree of sympathy for Jules Dervelle, a 'Jules' (i.e. French for a 'normal' or 'average' guy), referred to by his nephew in the last pages of the novel as 'ce pauvre être' (228). He emerges as a troubled character negotiating the chasm between individual biological impulse and socially expected behaviour.

The seeming digression of Chapter Three does create a 'chronologie boiteuse', as Michel has called it, but it is also, as we have seen, absolutely necessary for revealing Jules as an intelligent and deeply flawed character whose attempts to fit in have only exacerbated his inner imbalance. Indeed, contrary to medical advice offered by doctors like Debreyne, it is when Jules attempts to fit into 'normal' bourgeois activities that his differences become the most pronounced. When he reunites with his family after a six-year hiatus (in Part One, Chapter Four — more than halfway through the book), the narrative returns to the time line of the initial two chapters. Importantly, readers are by now armed with a more nuanced appreciation of the hypocritical morals of Jules's bourgeois doctor brother and his family and friends. Upon his arrival in Viantais, the near-homophone of *fientais*, Jules leaves a dinner party in disgust because he thinks the family wants to display him to their neighbours as a circus freak (he is correct):

> Canaille!… Crétin!… T'z'imbécile!… […] Tu me prends donc pour une bête curieuse?… Je te sers de spectacle à toi et à tes amis… Tu leur as dit: 'L'abbé Jules… un fou, un original, un prêtre sacrilège!… vous verrez ça!… Et vous pourrez le tâter… vous rendre compte que ce n'est point une farce, mais bien une réalité vivante'… Tu espérais te payer le petit plaisir de me montrer comme un ours de ménagerie, une monstruosité de la foire, un mouton à cinq pattes!… (156)

Reacting violently to a seemingly hospitable gesture, Jules's outburst once again links him to socially marginalized sideshow acts and scientific experiments, not just through his explicit mention of caged bear, freak shows, and five-legged sheep, but also through references to 'tâter', the verb used by doctors to examine patients. Further, the 'elliptical' bursts of speech he lets out when quoted directly (always punctuated with multiple ellipses and exclamation points) mirror graphically the seemingly strange and 'epileptical' nature of his temperament, prone to violent outbursts of cursing or invective, most frequently the 'T'z'imbécile!' seen above.[32]

---

32 Pierre Michel has identified a number of Mirbeau's sources for *L'Abbé Jules*, notably the story of Mirbeau's own uncle, in 'Aux sources de *L'Abbé Jules*', *Littératures*, 30 (1994), 83–87.

After this disruptive domestic scene the novel skips forward two years and then continues chronologically thereafter, through a perfectly conventional 'Part Two', still recounted by Albert. The effect of Mirbeau's narrative experimentation is remarkable. His narrator leaps through time in Part One, providing fragments of information about the psychic condition of the protagonist as he grapples to stay balanced when confronted with a variety of different situations. These disruptive temporal shifts reflect the unstable identity of the mysterious abbé Jules and force the reader to play doctor, to try to diagnose the 'indéchiffrable énigme' (56) represented by Jules and his seemingly unpredictable behaviour.

Readers learn, in fact, that Jules, after becoming a priest, adroitly negotiated clerical politics while denouncing social corruption wherever he found it (first and foremost exposing the cupidity, moral laxity, and sexual abuse in the priesthood). But he did not do this out of a sense of duty: 'ce qui le poussait à agir, ce n'était point l'ardeur d'une foi intolérante, la grandeur d'un but entrevu, le calcul d'un intérêt particulier, c'était un besoin grossier et pervers de se divertir en terrorisant les autres' (73). Eventually, he goes too far, creating a major scandal at a banquet in honour of the bishop's feast day. As the vicar-general begins a 'sentimental and pretentious' (125) speech in honour of the bishop, Jules tells him to shut up ('Taisez-vous!'), fulminating for pages against the hypocrisy, the materialism, and the cowardliness of the priesthood, invoking his colleagues to 'retourne[r] au purin… au crottin' until the bishop breaks in and dismisses him publicly (127). He speaks the truth, even when it is inconvenient, leading the narrator to compare Jules to Robespierre and his reign of Terror (68). Incapable of using 'la diplomatie ecclésiastique', Jules causes tremendous upheaval: 'Choses, bêtes et gens, il bouleversa tout, bouscula tout' and goes so far as to chasten and terrorize the bishop himself

---

In addition to literary sources such as Zola's *La Faute de l'abbé Mouret* and *La Conquête de Plassans*, and Mirbeau's own experiences with clerical education chronicled in *Le Calvaire* and *Sébastien Roch* (already begun as he was finishing *L'Abbé Jules*), I suspect we can add medical texts of the 1880s such as Ribot's *Les Maladies de la volonté* (1883) and Gilles de la Tourette's 1885 account of nine patients at the Salpêtrière Hospital with the verbal and physical tics now known as characteristic 'Tourette's Syndrome', 'Étude sur une affection nerveuse caractérisée par de l'incoordination motrice accompagnée d'écholalie et de coprolalie (Jumping, Latah, Myriachit)', *Archives de Neurologie*, 9 (1885), 19–42, 158–200. Mirbeau himself attended dinners with Edmond de Goncourt during which recent medical developments were routinely discussed and Goncourt recalls a time just after the publication of *L'Abbé Jules* when Mirbeau attributed his own remarkable capacity for 'vomiting bile' to a hole in the canalization of his liver in a 15 June 1889 entry in his *Journal* (Paris: Robert Laffont, 1956), III, 990.

(72). Once again, his 'nature révoltée' refuses equilibrium, obliging him to 'push' and 'shake up' the established order.

This anti-social explosion is the beginning of the end of Jules's career as a priest. Though he tells the truth, it is not a truth anyone is willing to hear and he leaves his post as the bishop's secretary for a modest position in a nearby parish. But unlike most bourgeois, who would be calmed by such routine and structure ('la narcotique de l'habitude', as Albert puts it):

> sa nature s'exaspéra de jour en jour. La colère prit chez lui une forme de véritable folie furieuse. C'était un navrant spectacle que de voir cet homme éloquent en arriver à ne pouvoir plus achever une phrase, et à ne se servir que de mots grossiers, vite noyés dans une broue d'épileptique. Son opinion sur les hommes, il la résumait, dans ce bruit, pareil à un éternûment: — T'z'imbéé… ciles! des… des… des… t'z'imbéé… ciles!… (144)

Jules wanders the countryside, ranting and raving, the filth of his personal hygiene leading him to contract a typhoid fever that almost kills him. Once again such episodes are described in terms of the physiological patterns of oscillation of blockages, explosions (graphically represented in his elliptical speech), and resultant fevers (the symptoms of acute melancholia evoked by physiologists such as Debreyne). But the sympathetic language used by Albert to describe his uncle's medical condition — 'une folie furieuse', 'un navrant spectacle', 'une broue d'épileptique' — builds empathy for an otherwise reprehensible character. Albert's adjectives are not deployed to judge Jules's moral character (as they are in Debreyne's hygiene manual), but to describe his symptoms. Jules himself is 'un homme éloquent'. It is his internal 'volcanic' struggle that erupts in the 'navrant spectacle' of his 'folie furieuse'.

Jules's return to Viantais and his clashes with bourgeois society are inevitable given what readers have learned about his volatile temperament, sadism, and uncompromising frankness. His actions in the novel's second part — his decision to live in the country far from others, the sexual and anarchist education he provides the young Albert, and Jules's own repressed sexuality and erotic acts — are now understandable.[33] Interestingly, at the end of the novel,

33 In another illustration of Jules's imbalance of fluids, he is rendered orgasmically unconscious from reading George Sand's *Indiana* after introducing his nephew to the text (which also excites the younger man). The priest subsequently explains that his violent troubles with sexual fantasies are not natural, but were caused by his religious education, which, by forbidding pornographic literature and images made them more attractive

Jules's formerly uncontrollable temperament is held largely in check by his solitary life surrounded by his garden and books; it is aggravated by contact with adults: 'ces imbéciles'. Like Mirbeau's holy fool of the novel, the père Pamphile, who lives on the outskirts of society, following his dream of rebuilding the ruins of the thirteenth-century abbey of Réno, Jules chooses to become an eccentric gardener instead of a thorn in the side of *fin-de-siècle* society.

Jules's encounter with the pious père Pamphile seems, initially, to be a tangent, but is, in fact, crucial to understanding the importance 'exalted' temperaments play in *L'Abbé Jules*.[34] Unlike the sacrilegious Jules, Pamphile dreams of bringing his religious order back to its medieval glory by rebuilding a ruined chapel (95). He is 'une âme [...] si naïve, si complètement ignorante des malpropretés de la vie' (98). As a result, he is exploited by workers and by donors who promise money in exchange for the performance of humiliating acts. Another sideshow act, Pamphile earns 1200 florins in Hungary for singing the *Marseillaise* 12 times for 100 florins a performance (107). Even fellow priests exploit him (Jules plans to rob Pamphile). Likely inspired by Prince Myshkin from Dostoyevky's *The Idiot*, Pamphile's eyes are 'illuminated' by a faith (104) that is betrayed over and over again by a society that exploits, ridicules, and rejects him.[35]

Against Medical Labels: The Fiction of Normality

At first, Jules considers Pamphile a 'vieille canaille' because of the humiliations the old priest endures for money, but comes to appreciate the purity of his 'inconcevable folie', his single-minded ideal (110). 'Ce n'est pas un bandit, se dit-il... C'est quelqu'un de pire... un poète!' (111). Jules, unlike others who consider Pamphile socially deviant, recognizes and appreciates the monk's exaltation:

> Ce misérable moine, il a eu le rêve, il a eu l'amour!... Une charogne puante, dans un tas de boue!... Sur quelle déformation de la nature reposent donc

(203). His testament instructs family members to burn a trunk full of such materials upon his death.

34 Robert Ziegler has devoted a number of articles to the importance of père Pamphile, notably 'Octave Mirbeau's Cinerarium-novel: *L'Abbé Jules*', *Actes du colloque Octave Mirbeau de Cerisy* (2005) <http://mirbeau.asso.fr/darticlesetrangers/Ziegler-cinerarium.pdf> [accessed January 2016].

35 See Pierre Michel, 'Aux sources de *L'Abbé Jules*'.

> les religions et les sociétés, ces mensonges?… De quelle fiction sont donc sortis le juge et le prêtre, ces deux monstruosités morales, le juge qui veut imposer à la nature, on ne sait quelle irréelle justice, démentie par la fatalité des instincts, le prêtre, on ne sait quelle pitié baroque, devant la loi éternelle du Meurtre (132)

Pamphile, like Georges Robin, the frail and effeminate little boy locked up by his mother (172), are kindred non-conforming spirits. They are dismissed with adjectives such as 'original', 'monstrueux', and 'fou' by judges and priests who squelch creativity by imposing arbitrary labels ('mensonges', 'fiction') on behaviours and physiques that Mirbeau shows come from nature.

Curiously, Jules does not mention doctors here, though the medical profession is the third major social authority of the novel, with Doctor Dervelle forming a triumvirate alongside Judge Robin and *le curé*, the habitual dinner guests in his home. When Jules rails against the 'fictions' and 'mensonges', the 'déformation de la nature' fabricated by these social authorities, he seems to recognize and criticize what Michel Foucault would later identify as an epistemological shift that took place as doctors built a new discipline reliant on practices, definitions, and boundaries that they themselves had created.[36] Mirbeau's use of a poetics of physiological difference — a language representing the fluctuations in individual behaviour as natural phenomena — undermines medical treatises such as Debreyne's classification of all people into six 'tempéraments'. Mirbeau would be much more explicitly critical of doctors later in his career, both through monstrous fictional characters like the Doctor Triceps in *L'Epidémie* (1898) and *Les 21 jours d'un neurasthénique* (1901), who abused their power to become what Arnaud Vareille has called 'prescripteurs de la morale', labelling people healthy or sick, normal or deviant in the name of unfounded scientism.[37]

In *L'Abbé Jules* such criticisms are more implicit, with the notable exception of Jules's invective against bourgeois 'deformations of nature', one of the most-cited and well-known elements of the novel:

> 1. L'homme est une bête méchante et stupide; 2. La justice est une infâmie; 3. L'amour est une cochonnerie; 4. Dieu est une chimère (186)

36 Michel Foucault, *La Naissance de la clinique* (Paris: PUF, 1963).

37 Vareille, 'Médecins'. Mirbeau also took doctors to task in the newspapers, creating a scandal with 'Médecins du jour', a series he published in *Le Matin* from 29 May to 31 July 1907.

Should one choose to reduce the novel's conclusion to such pseudo-anarchist maxims (Albert himself called his uncle's outburst an 'anarchisme vague et sentimental', 188), one risks missing the point of all that has preceded this moment and all that follows.[38] Jules constantly changes his mind as his humour shifts, idealizing the père Pamphile before realizing the tragedy of the monk's exalted dreams, and embracing his own independence from the Church before lamenting on his deathbed his failure to fit into society (217).

In fact, as much as characters such as Jules blame social inequities, they also acknowledge the essentially personal nature of their struggles:

> — J'ai manqué ma vie, mon petit Albert… Je l'ai manquée, parce que jamais je n'ai pu dompter complètement les sales passions qui étaient en moi, passions comprimées de prêtre, passions héréditaires, nées du mysticisme de ma mère, de l'alcoolisme de mon père. J'ai lutté pourtant, va!… Elles m'ont vaincu… Je meurs de cette lutte et de cette défaite. Lorsque j'ai pensé à revenir ici dans ce calme, dans cette solitude, je m'étais promis d'oublier le passé, de vivre heureux, de travailler, car j'avais de vastes projets. Je n'ai pas pu… Ici comme partout, je me suis retrouvé face à face avec le monstre… J'ai subi d'affreuses tortures… Il est donc bon que je meure… (217)

For Jules, the struggle between body and mind is first and foremost internal, a result of hereditary instincts inflamed by an unsupportive society, which, influenced by scientific books like Debreyne's *Physiologie*, morally condemns him for not having learned to master his temperament. And yet, the figurative language used by his narrator diminishes Jules's self-criticism. Readers have seen that Jules has been 'valiant' in his long and torturous fight against the 'monster' represented by his natural passions; it is a tragedy that he has never found the 'calme' he seeks, the psychic balance he would need to achieve his 'vastes projets'.

At the end of *Les Maladies de la volonté* Ribot specifically states that strong willpower is rare and claims that he is not passing moral judgement on those unable to reconcile their instincts with the demands of the external world. Yet by calling his book *Les Maladies de la volonté* rather than *Le Mécanisme de la*

---

38 The political dimensions of his denunciation of bourgeois society were not lost on readers. Reg Carr has traced the impact of *L'Abbé Jules* on anarchist readers such as Jean Grave, and credits the novel with introducing Mirbeau to anarchist circles in *Anarchism in France: The Case of Octave Mirbeau* (Montreal: McGill-Queen's University Press, 1977), pp. 22–30.

volonté or *La Lutte de la volonté* Ribot sets out strong self-governance as normative. As a result, those like Jules who cannot achieve a balance are 'malades', defined not by the force of their resistance to internal compulsions, but by their ability to replicate 'les manières ambiantes'. Pamphile, Jules, and Georges are very different, but instead of dismissing their differences with derogative epithets ('violent', 'menteur', 'fou', 'difformé', 'avorton'), Mirbeau emphasizes process: their struggles to conform to a 'normality' that is itself a fiction.

Letters Mirbeau sent to correspondents after the publication of *L'Abbé Jules* and included by Pierre Michel in his edition, exemplify the novelist's scorn for contemporaries who labelled characters 'non-normative' without attempting to understand why they acted the way they did. He describes Jules as 'un homme très malheureux dans son débraillement moral, un de ces êtres d'exception — bien que fréquents — dont la rencontre nous étonne et dont on dit "c'est un fou!" sans chercher à découvrir le mécanisme de ces êtres déréglés'.[39] As Michel also notes, Mirbeau thought a good deal about such 'mécanismes', proposing, in his *Impressions littéraires*, that one of the worst social conventions was 'vouloir ramener l'humanité à un mécanisme régulier, tranquille et prévu, sans les cassures et sans les explosions inévitables'.[40]

Michel has identified the closeness of Mirbeau's thought here to that of Tolstoy and Dostoyevsky, who uses the poor treatment of an 'idiot', the naive and pious Prince Myshkin, to condemn the Russian society of his time (1869). Michel notes that, in an article on Tolstoy published in *Le Gaulois* of 2 July 1886 (entitled 'Un fou'), Mirbeau wrote that ordinary people call others 'madmen' because they follow different rules, without realizing that the entire concept of 'normal' is itself a construct.[41] But Mirbeau goes beyond literary models in *L'Abbé Jules* as he adopts and questions contemporary scientific discourse related to behaviour. He criticizes not just seemingly arbitrary social conventions, but especially the tendency to define without looking more closely at the biological and social forces that make people act the way they do.

Conclusion

Mirbeau's refusal of the normative discourse of his time and his intense study of a single character's behaviour is closely linked to what would become a lifelong affiliation with the anarchist movement. He did not seek to overthrow

39 Cited in *L'Abbé Jules*, p. 239. [Original letter in the Catalogue Charavay, no. 52.245].
40 Cited in *L'Abbé Jules*, p. 240, note 7.
41 *L'Abbé Jules*, p. 240, note 6.

political institutions through violence, but through strong advocacy for individual liberties.[42] He would describe his next novel, *Sébastien Roch*, to Catulle Mendès in these terms in December 1889: 'Il y a dans mon livre un souffle de révolte contre la société; une horreur presque anarchiste contre tout ce qui est régulier et bourgeois; une négation de tous les grands sentiments dont on nous berne, tout cela mêlé à des tendresses et à des élans de la nature'.[43]

It is in his refusal of systems and doctrines and in his valorization of individual differences that Mirbeau's novel has remarkable contemporary resonance. In *L'Abbé Jules* he made many of the arguments now at the heart of the twenty-first-century neurodiversity movement; he created characters who criticize society's tendency to reject anything that does not fit definitions of 'normal', revealing that the concept of 'normal' is by its nature changeable because historically and socially constructed. It is easier to apply labels such as 'fou' than to adopt a more inclusive range of behaviours based on natural observation.[44] Mirbeau, however, also refuses to provide an omniscient narrator who might draw clear scientific conclusions about Jules, his actions, and his diatribes. By delegating Albert Dervelle as narrator, Mirbeau himself does not moralize, does not fustigate, does not erupt in 'paroxysmes' of emotion and anger as many critics claim.[45] Instead, he invites readers to draw their own conclusions about the 'mechanisms' responsible for Jules's behaviour.

The remarkable modernity of Mirbeau's novel lies in this shift from a tendency to judge actions on purely moral grounds (as did Debreyne) or on largely genetic grounds (as did Zola) to advocacy for the complex processes responsible for human behaviour. Dismissing 'des êtres supérieurs' as 'dérangés' or 'méchants' and ostracizing them rather than attempting to understand and

---

42 See, for example, Michel's succinct analysis of Mirbeau's contradictory and utopian conception of anarchism in *Le Dictionnaire Octave Mirbeau*, 'Anarchie'. Reg Carr's *Anarchism in France* situates Mirbeau in the political context of his time.

43 Cited by Pierre Michel in his 'Préface' to *Sébastien Roch* (Paris: Éditions du Boucher, 2003), p. 24.

44 Mirbeau's characters use the same vocabulary with regard to naturally occurring biological differences and the artificiality of socially determined labels that have cropped up recently in debates over psychiatric definitions. See, for example, Jamie Doward, 'Medicine's Big New Battleground: Does Mental Illness Really Exist?', an article published in *The Guardian* (11 May 2013), and dedicated to battles over the diagnoses included in the fifth edition of the American Psychiatric Association's *Diagnostic and Statistical Manual* <http://www.theguardian.com/society/2013/may/12/medicine-dsm5-row-does-mental-illness-exist>.

45 See, for example, Dominque Rincé and Bernard Lecherbonnier in their 1986 Nathan anthology of nineteenth-century literature: 'Ce passionné porté naturellement au paroxysme' (551).

support their struggles deprives society of creativity.[46] When queried about presumed links between genius and madness in nineteenth-century France, Émile Zola famously responded, 'Si le génie est une névrose pourquoi vouloir le guérir?'[47] This is precisely the argument of those who argue today for the importance of recognizing 'neurodiversity'. 'Neuronormativity', far from being a desired state, may, in fact, suppress important social contributions by those restrained by adjectival labels such as 'melancholic', 'autistic' or 'mentally ill'. Unlike Caesar or Michelangelo, described by Ribot as having directed their passions into their work, Jules's obsession with fighting ('lutter') and taming ('dompter') his instincts in order to fit into society distracted him from the 'vastes projets' he might have accomplished had he found a productive outlet for his volcanic temperament. It is to Mirbeau's credit that his complex portrait of a troubled 'exalté' feels so relevant today; the questions about definitions and diagnoses raised in a fictional work from 1888 continue to haunt twenty-first-century medicine.

Bibliography

Blanchard, Pascal, Nicolas Bancel, Gilles Boëtsch, Eric Deroo, Sandrine Lemaire, and Charles Forsdick (eds), *Human Zoos: Science and Spectacle in the Age of Colonial Empires*, trans. by Teresa Bridgeman (Liverpool: Liverpool University Press, 2008)

Boudon-Millot, Véronique (ed. and trans.), *Galien: Introduction générale; Sur l'ordre de ses propres livres; Sur ses propres livres; Que l'excellent médecin est aussi philosophe*, vol. I (Paris: Les Belles Lettres, 2007)

Bowen, Ray P., 'An Analysis of the Priest Genre in the Modern French Novel', *PMLA*, 37, 4 (1922), 722–34

Briaud, Annie, 'Mirbeau et Schopenhauer', *Cahiers Octave Mirbeau*, 8 (April 2001), 219–27 <http://mirbeau.asso.fr/darticlesfrancais/Briaud-OMetschopenhauer.pdf> [accessed January 2016]

Brooks, John I., *The Eclectic Legacy: Academic Philosophy and the Human Sciences in Nineteenth-Century France* (Newark, DE: University of Delaware Press, 1998)

46 In notes to his edition of *L'Abbé Jules*, Michel has shown that contemporaries, such as Edmond de Goncourt and Stéphane Mallarmé, called Jules a 'douloureux camarade', and Mallarmé complimented Mirbeau on his character in a letter from 16 April 1888. Cited in *L'Abbé Jules*, p. 243, note 2.

47 Émile Zola, *Correspondance* VI, 1887–1890, ed. by B. H. Bakker, Colette Becker and Owen Morgan (Montreal: Les Presses de l'Université de Montréal/Paris: Éditions du CNRS, 1978–1995), p. 355, letter 341 (dated 9 December 1888).

Cabanès, Jean-Louis, 'Le Discours sur les normes dans les premiers romans de Mirbeau', in *Octave Mirbeau: Actes du colloque international d'Angers du 19 au 22 septembre 1991*, ed. by Pierre Michel and Georges Cesbron (Angers: Presses universitaires d'Angers, 1992), pp. 153–63

Carr, Reg, *Anarchism in France: The Case of Octave Mirbeau* (Manchester: Manchester University Press, 1977)

Doward, Jamie, 'Medicine's Big New Battleground: Does Mental Ilness Really Exist?', *The Guardian* (11 May 2013) <http://www.theguardian.com/society/2013/may/12/medicine-dsm5-row-does-mental-illness-exist> [accessed January 2016]

Feldman, Shoshana, *La Folie et la chose littéraire* (Paris: Seuil, 1978)

Foucault, Michel, *La Naissance de la clinique* (Paris: PUF, 1963)

——, *Surveiller et punir: naissance de la prison* (Paris: Seuil, 1975)

Galien, Claude, *Œuvres anatomiques, physiologiques et médicales de Galien*, vol. II, trans. by Dr Ch. Daremberg (Paris: J. B. Baillière, 1856)

Goodstein, Elizabeth, *Experience Without Qualities: Boredom and Modernity* (Stanford: Stanford University Press, 2005)

Hustvedt, Asti, *Medical Muses: Hysteria in Nineteenth-Century Paris* (New York: W. W. Norton, 2011)

Jaarsma, Pierr, and Stellan Welin, 'Autism as a Natural Human Variation: Reflections on the Claims of the Neurodiversity Movement', *Health Care Analysis*, 20 (2012), 20–30

Jeannerod, Marc, *The Brain Machine* (Cambridge, MA: Harvard University Press, 1985)

Jefferson, Ann, *Genius in France: An Idea and Its Uses* (Princeton: Princeton University Press, 2014)

Kagan, Jerome, *Galen's Prophecy: Temperament in Human Nature* (New York: Basic Books, 1994)

Lemarié, Yannick, 'Ovide Faujas et Jules Dervelle: deux curés en enfer', *Les Cahiers Octave Mirbeau*, 6 (1999), 100–21

——, 'Zola, Émile', *Dictionnaire Octave Mirbeau*, <http://mirbeau.asso.fr/dicomirbeau/index.php?option=com_glossary&id=550>

Michel, Pierre, 'Aux sources de *L'Abbé Jules*', *Littératures*, 30 (1994), 83–87

——, 'Pitié', *Dictionnaire Octave Mirbeau*, http://mirbeau.asso.fr/dicomirbeau/index.php?option=com_glossary&letter=P&id=490

——, 'Préface', *L'Abbé Jules* (Paris: Éditions du Boucher, 2003), pp. 3–18

——, 'Préface', *Sébastien Roch* (Paris: Éditions du Boucher, 2003), pp. 3–24

——, *Octave Mirbeau et le roman* (Angers: Société Octave Mirbeau, 2005)

Michel, Pierre, and Jean-François Nivet, *Octave Mirbeau, l'imprécateur au coeur fidèle* (Paris: Séguier, 1990)

Mirbeau, Octave, *L'Abbé Jules* (Paris: Éditions du Boucher, 2003)

Nye, Robert, *Crime, Madness, and Politics in Modern France. The Medical Concept of National Decline* (Princeton, NJ: Princeton University Press, 1984)

Pettit, Fiona Yvette, 'Freaks in Late Nineteenth-Century British Media and Medicine', unpublished doctoral thesis (University of Exeter, 2012)

Ribot, Théodule, *Les Maladies de la volonté* (Paris: G. Balliere, 1883)

Rincé, Dominique and Bernard Lecherbonnier (eds), *La Littérature du XIX*^{e} *siècle* (Paris: Nathan, 1986)

Roldan, Sébastien, *La Pyramide des souffrances dans* La Joie de vivre *de Zola* (Québec: Presses de l'Université du Québec, 2012)

——, 'Le Petit chose au pays des philosophes', *Travaux de littérature*, 27 (2014), 65–84

Thomson, Rosemarie Garland, *Extraordinary Bodies: Figuring Physical Disability in American Culture and Literature* (New York: Columbia University Press, 1997)

Tourette, Gilles de la, 'Étude sur une affection nerveuse caractérisée par de l'incoordination motrice accompagnée d'écholalie et de coprolalie (Jumping, Latah, Myriachit)', *Archives de Neurologie*, 9 (1885), 19–42, 158–200

Vareille, Arnaud, 'Médecins', *Dictionnaire Octave Mirbeau* (online edition) <http://mirbeau.asso.fr/dicomirbeau/index.php?option=com_glossary&letter=M&id=385>

Ziegler, Robert, 'Octave Mirbeau's Cinerarium-novel: *L'Abbé Jules*', *Actes du colloque Octave Mirbeau de Cerisy* (2005). <http://mirbeau.asso.fr/darticlesetrangers/Ziegler-cinerarium.pdf> [accessed January 2016]

Zola, Émile, *Correspondance*, ed. by B. H. Bakker, Colette Becker and Owen Morgan (Montreal: Les Presses de l'Université de Montréal/Paris: Éditions du CNRS, 1978–1995)

CHAPTER 10

Genius and Degeneracy: Auguste Rodin and the *Monument to Balzac*

Natasha Ruiz-Gómez

How future generations will laugh over all this buffoonery of 'nerve art'!

MAX NORDAU, *On Art and Artists* (1907)

•••

Je suis un nerveux.

AUGUSTE RODIN, quoted in *L'Éclair* (1896)

When Auguste Rodin received the commission from the *Société des gens de lettres* to create a monument to Honoré de Balzac, he was living on the *rue des Grands Augustins*, the same Parisian street where the novelist had set his celebrated *Le Chef-d'œuvre inconnu.*[1] In that fictional story, a seventeenth-century artist named Frenhofer spends ten years labouring lovingly over a painting of a nude woman. He eventually shows it to the Flemish painter Frans Po[u]rbus and a young Nicolas Poussin, who see only an indecipherable mass of colours and lines on an overworked canvas, except at one corner where a foot of the utmost beauty and perfection emerges. Having received their uncomprehending criticism, Frenhofer sets fire to his masterpiece, succumbs to madness, and dies. Surely, the coincidence of Rodin and Frenhofer's address was not lost on the well-read sculptor — and in the aftermath of the scandal that greeted his

* Quotations from the following texts are taken from their first English translation unless otherwise noted: Cesare Lombroso, *The Man of Genius* (London: Walter Scott, 1891) and Max Nordau, *Degeneration* (London: William Heinemann, 1895).

1 *Le Chef-d'œuvre inconnu* was originally published as *Maître Frenhofer* in *L'Artiste* in 1831. It was later revised and augmented by Balzac in his *Études philosophiques* (Paris, 1837). The story was integrated into *La Comédie humaine* in 1845.

 | DOI:10.1163/9789004368019_012

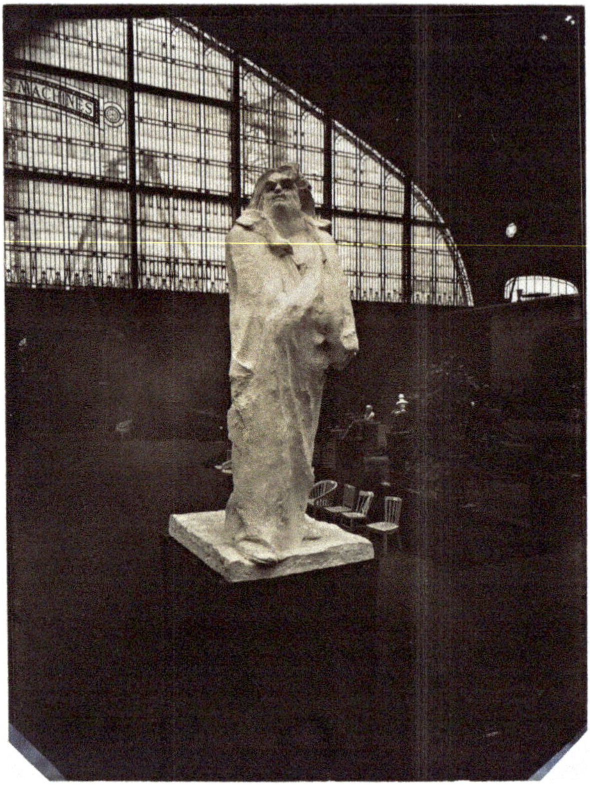

FIGURE 10.1 *Eugène Druet,* Balzac, *1898, gelatin silver print, 40 × 29.8 cm. Accession no. 1983.194.11, Iris & B. Gerald Cantor Center for Visual Arts at Stanford University; Gift of Albert E. and Patricia Elsen.*
COURTESY OF THE CANTOR ARTS CENTER AT STANFORD UNIVERSITY.

own 'misunderstood' masterpiece, the *Monument to Balzac* (1898), Rodin may well have recalled the novel's ill-fated protagonist (Fig. 10.1).

This monument was particularly important to the *Société*, as Balzac had been a founding member and its second president. Émile Zola, who was president at the time of the commission, was instrumental in awarding it to Rodin.[2] The details of the sculpture's tortuous birth and first public exhibition at the Salon of 1898 are well worn in Rodin scholarship. However, there has been insufficient recognition, let alone scrutiny, of the source of the public outrage

2 Ruth Butler, *Rodin: The Shape of Genius* (New Haven: Yale University Press, 1993), p. 253.

and the often scathing criticisms of both the work and its maker.[3] Critics savaged the sculpture, saying that it was 'grotesque' and had the appearance of an 'être informe, sorte d'ébauche couronnée d'un visage lugubre'.[4] A year later, when Rodin's planned pavilion outside the 1900 Universal Exposition began to receive attention from the press, one journalist invoked the *Monument to Balzac* and mused archly that perhaps the public was going to witness the installation of a museum of horrors.[5] By attending more closely to the language used by the critics, this chapter argues that the sculpture's provocation can be attributed to its evocation of theories of degeneration. Ignored until now in the voluminous scholarship on the *Monument to Balzac,* Rodin's exploitation of these contemporary theories also sheds light on both his working method and the concerns of the Parisian *grand public,* who, upon the unveiling of the sculpture, ridiculed its distorted visage and enshrouded body.

As an artist who articulated repeatedly over his long career that 'nature' motivated his work, Rodin struggled for seven years to produce a monument to a deceased man he had never met.[6] He searched for novel ways to model Balzac, a man who Alphonse de Lamartine famously described as having a face that 'vous charmait et vous fascinait tout entier. […] [L]es yeux noirs perçaient comme des dards émoussés par la bienveillance; […] le nez bien modelé, quoique un peu long; les lèvres découpées avec grâce, mais amples, relevées par les coins.'[7] Rodin began his research by meticulously documenting the writer from Touraine, his self-professed fidelity to 'nature' predisposing him to embrace the theories of physiognomy and regional type. In this he was following Balzac himself, in whose books Rodin would have repeatedly encountered

---

3 The most important and complete source on this sculpture is Musée Rodin, *1898: le* Balzac *de Rodin*, ex. cat. (Paris: Éditions du musée Rodin, 1998). See also Albert E. Elsen, et al., *Rodin & Balzac. Rodin's Sculptural Studies for the Monument to Balzac from the Cantor, Fitzgerald Collection*, ex. cat. (Beverly Hills: Cantor, Fitzgerald and Co., 1973).

4 Adolphe Brisson, 'Plumes et ciseaux', *La République française*, 12 May 1898, [n. pag.]; and 'Lettre de Paris, Le musée Rodin', *Le Nord maritime* [Dunkerque], 8 July 1899, [n. pag.]. Articles located in the press files for '*Balzac*', Archives du Musée Rodin, Paris (referred to hereafter as AMR).

5 *La Presse*, 14 July 1899, [n. pag.]. Article located in the press files for '*Balzac*', AMR.

6 For more on Rodin as nature's 'copyist', see the author's 'Auguste Rodin and the "Scientific Image": The Sublime Copy Versus the Photograph', in *Visions of the Industrial Age, 1830–1914: Modernity and the Anxiety of Representation in Europe*, ed. by Minsoo Kang and Amy Woodson-Boulton (Aldershot: Ashgate, 2008), pp. 109–36.

7 Alphonse de Lamartine, *Balzac et ses œuvres* (Paris: Michel Lèvy Frères, 1866), p. 17.

the cultural currency of physiognomic theories.[8] In fact, late in his career, Rodin equated the physiognomist and the artist: 'A physiognomist can easily distinguish between a cajoling air and one of real kindness, and it is precisely the rôle of the artist to show the truth, even beneath dissimulation'.[9] Yet signifiers of physiognomy and regional type proved both limiting and unconvincing, and, as this chapter demonstrates, Rodin's research over the course of the 1890s led him to abandon a naturalistic approach to his portrait of Balzac.

As his studies of the novelist developed, Rodin focused on the 'categories of difference, otherness, excess' that were part and parcel of contemporary debates around genius, madness, and degeneration.[10] Balzac was no ordinary writer, of course — he had attempted to rival Dante's *Divine Comedy* by capturing the earthly travails of contemporary society; as the Belgian poet Georges Rodenbach would write of Balzac's seemingly superhuman achievement upon seeing the finished monument: 'Pensez donc: avoir vu la comédie humaine!'[11] The monument unveiled in 1898 revealed traces of the 'stigmata' of degeneration that, for Rodin, made explicit the author's 'genius'; this caused the public and the critics discomfort, even though genius and madness were closely linked in scientific and popular discourses on degeneration at the time.[12] The sculpture focused attention on Balzac's visage, where these markers were most pronounced. In relation to his planned monument to Charles Baudelaire, another author whom Rodin deeply admired, the sculptor made a statement in the early 1890s that is equally applicable to his *Monument to Balzac*: 'What is a statue after all? A body, arms, legs, covered with banal clothing. What do these have to do with Baudelaire, who lived only by his brain? With him the head is everything.'[13] Yet Rodin did not simply replicate the 'stigmata' of

8 Graeme Tytler, *Physiognomy in the European Novel: Faces and Fortunes* (Princeton: Princeton University Press, 1982), p. 261.

9 Auguste Rodin, *Rodin on Art and Artists. Conversations with Paul Gsell* [1911], trans. by Mrs Romilly Fedden (New York: Dover Publications, 1983), p. 54.

10 Griselda Pollock, 'Artists' Mythologies and Media Genius, Madness and Art History', in *Picture This: Media Representations of Visual Art and Artists*, ed. by Philip Hayward (Luton: The University of Luton Press, 1998), pp. 101–39 (p. 109).

11 Georges Rodenbach, 'Une statue', *Le Figaro*, 17 May 1898, p. 1.

12 For an important discussion of the ways in which Rodin linked genius to sexual potency through the pose of Balzac's body, see Anne Wagner, 'Rodin's Reputation', in *Eroticism and the Body Politic*, ed. by Lynn Hunt (Baltimore: The Johns Hopkins University Press, 1991), pp. 191–242.

13 'Le Monument de Baudelaire', *La République* (22 September 1892); quoted in Albert E. Elsen with Rosalyn Frankel Jamison, *Rodin's Art: The Rodin Collection of the Iris & B. Gerald Cantor Center for Visual Arts at Stanford University*, ed. by Bernard Barryte (Oxford: Oxford

degeneration — he magnified and ultimately distorted them for expressive purposes. Rodin manipulated contemporary scientific theories in crafting the visage of a towering figure of nineteenth-century literature to show the limits of a naturalistic approach to portraiture, creating a sculpture that was utterly modern.

The Physiognomy of a *Tourangeau*

Rodin would certainly have been aware from his close reading of Balzac's extensive œuvre that the Realist writer relied on the popular tenets of physiognomy to communicate information about his characters.[14] The principles of physiognomy — defined as the study of the correspondence between an individual's physical features and his or her moral character and intelligence — had enjoyed broad popular acceptance since at least the Middle Ages.[15] By the middle of the nineteenth century, it was a multivalent term that generally referred to tenets delineated by Swiss pastor Johann Caspar Lavater (1741–1801), whose *Essays on Physiognomy, Designed to Promote the Knowledge and the Love of Mankind* was first published in French in 1781.[16] Although every element

---

University Press, 2003), p. 347. For more on the scandal, see Antoinette Le Normand-Romain, 'Pour une statue de Balzac: 1850–1891', in Musée Rodin, *1898: le* Balzac *de Rodin*, pp. 15–74 (pp. 48–57).

14 Rodin was an avid reader of Hugo, Shakespeare, and Dante in the years before this commission, but it is unclear how familiar he was with Balzac's œuvre before he began work on the monument. There are, however, a number of volumes by Balzac in Rodin's library, including *Le Député d'Arcis* (Paris, 1892–97); *Études philosophiques sur Catherine de Médicis, suivi de Louis Lambert, Les Proscrits, Séraphita* (Paris, 1864); *Histoire des Treize* (Paris, 1840); *Œuvres complètes de H. de Balzac*, XXIV: *Correspondance 1819–1850* (Paris, 1876); and *Scènes de la vie de province, deuxième série: La Vieille fille, La Grenadière* (Paris, 1839). For Balzac's indebtedness to Lavater, see Fernand Baldensperger, 'Les Théories de Lavater dans la littérature française', *Études d'histoire littéraire* (Paris: Hachette et Cie, 1910), pp. 51–91 (pp. 70–84).

15 One of the earliest works to discuss physiognomy is a medieval text entitled 'Physiognomics', which in the nineteenth century was wrongly believed to have been written by Aristotle. Aristotle, 'Physiognomics', *Minor Works*, trans. by W. S. Hett (Cambridge, MA: Harvard University Press, 1936), pp. 84–137.

16 John [Johann] Caspar Lavater, *Essays on Physiognomy, Designed to Promote the Knowledge and the Love of Mankind*, trans. by Henry Hunter, 5 vols (London: John Murray, 1789–1798). I will not be discussing here the related science of phrenology, the study of the shape of the skull as it relates to the shape of the brain and its corresponding characteristics in an individual's personality, as its tenets do not seem to have influenced the work of Rodin.

of the body was potentially a physiognomic signifier, Lavater is most famous today for his 'science' as it applied to facial features, which he discussed in the first two volumes of his treatise. '[T]o ascribe every thing to arbitrary causes, to blind chance, without rule and without law, is the philosophy of madmen', he claimed, and his system was an attempt to clarify and codify the rules of physiognomy.[17]

Balzac bought a copy of Lavater's treatise in 1822, and a careful reading of *La Comédie humaine* yields myriad clues to his reliance on physiognomic theories.[18] In his early novel *Eugénie Grandet* (1833), for instance, Balzac gives a revealing description of Monsieur Grandet, the protagonist's father:

> He had a round sun-burnt face, marked by smallpox, a firm chin, uncurving lips, white teeth. [...] His forehead, which was deeply furrowed, bulged in a fashion not without significance for the physiognomist. [...] His nose, which was thick at the end, had a veined knob on it which was popularly said, with some reason, to be full of malice. In this face [was] written a dangerous craftiness.[19]

Facial features here expose Grandet's moral character. Fernand Baldensperger asserts that, of the writers of the so-called 'generation of 1830', Balzac applied Lavater's rules the most diligently.[20] In fact, the novelist stated categorically: 'Les lois de la physiognomie sont exactes, non seulement dans leur application aux caractères, mais encore relativement à la fatalité de l'existence'.[21] It is especially fitting, then, that Rodin would bring those laws to bear on his representation of Balzac's own features.

Physiognomic theories appealed not only to nineteenth-century novelists, such as Balzac, George Sand, and Stendhal, but also to visual artists who were reacting to the codified expressions of the *École des beaux-arts*

Balzac wrote in the *avant-propos* of *La Comédie humaine* that Franz Gall, the founder of phrenology, was the '*continuateur*' of Lavater; cited in Jacques Lethève, 'Balzac et la Phrénologie', *Aesculape* (March 1951), 55–62 (p. 60).

17 Lavater, *Essays on Physiognomy*, I (1789), 30.

18 Baldensperger, 'Les Théories de Lavater dans la littérature française', p. 71.

19 Honoré de Balzac, *Eugénie Grandet* [1833], trans. by Marion Ayton Crawford (London: Penguin Books, 1955), p. 44.

20 Baldensperger, 'Les Théories de Lavater dans la littérature française', p. 84.

21 Balzac, *Une Ténébreuse affaire*, p. 3; quoted in Baldensperger, 'Les Théories de Lavater dans la littérature française', p. 77.

and Charles Le Brun's enormously influential *têtes d'expression*.[22] Moreover, painters, sculptors, and caricaturists could incorporate their widely known and accepted principles to create a visual language understood by the average consumer of culture.[23] Art critic and Realist advocate Théophile Thoré, who sought a 'beauté vivante', edited the *Dictionnaire de phrénologie et de physionomonie à l'usage des artistes* in 1836.[24] Physiognomic principles influenced the portraits painted by Jacques-Louis David and Eugène Delacroix and sculpted by Jean-Pierre Dantan, among others; these were works with which Rodin would have been intimately familiar.[25] David d'Angers, whose investment in physiognomic theories was well known, sculpted a portrait of Balzac in 1844 and apparently found a kindred spirit in the writer: Balzac said to him, 'Surtout étudiez mon nez! Mon nez est tout un monde!'[26] David, like most artists of his day, believed that the role of public sculpture was moral edification. His nude bust of Balzac, presumably through physiognomic (and phrenologic) signifiers, would demonstrate the traits of a *grand homme*.[27] Rodin, however, did not find the sculpture a useful precedent, commenting that David 'was an *idealist*; all his busts are alike, whether it is Balzac, Victor Hugo, Goethe'.[28] For Rodin, then, David's artistic agenda was more important to the final result than the sitter's individual characteristics; half a century later, the same would be true for Rodin's own *Monument to Balzac*.

When Rodin secured the commission for the monument, he wrote to Zola to say that he had 'often studied [Balzac], not only in his works but in his

---

22 See Tytler, *Physiognomy in the European Novel*, and Anthea Callen, *The Spectacular Body: Science, Method and Meaning in the Work of Degas* (New Haven: Yale University Press, 1995), p. 3.

23 See Judith Wechsler, *A Human Comedy: Physiognomy and Caricature in 19th-Century Paris* (Chicago: The University of Chicago Press, 1982).

24 Quoted in Phillipe Sorel, 'La Phrénologie et l'art', in *L'Âme au corps: arts et science, 1793–1993*, by Jean Clair, et al., ex. cat. (Paris: Éditions de la Réunion des musées nationaux, 1993), pp. 266–79 (p. 266).

25 Jean-Pierre Changeux, 'De la science vers l'art', in *L'Âme au corps*, pp. 13–39 (p. 22).

26 'Notes d'art. L'image de Balzac', *La Petite Gironde*, 6 May 1898; quoted in Musée Rodin, *1898: le* Balzac *de Rodin*, p. 346.

27 David was a founding member of the *Société phrénologique*; Jacques de Caso, *David d'Angers: Sculptural Communication in the Age of Romanticism*, trans. by Dorothy Johnson and Jacques de Caso (Princeton: Princeton University Press, 1992), p. 258, note 19.

28 Emphasis in the original. Gabriel Ferry, 'La Statue de Balzac', *Le Monde moderne* x (1899); quoted in Albert E. Elsen, et al., *Rodin & Balzac*, p. 7.

native province'.[29] He then began to collect documentary material. Rodin told a reporter from *La France* that he intended to conduct research in the Tours library and that Balzac's great-nephew was going to send him a plaster cast of the author's hand.[30] He asked the photographer Nadar for help in securing a print of the only known daguerreotype of Balzac, taken in 1842 by Louis-Auguste Bisson (see Fig. 10.2).[31] Rodin even had *père* Pion, Balzac's tailor, create a suit using the author's measurements.[32] He said that he was attempting to '*comprendre* le grand romancier'.[33] By gathering traces of the individual — including indexes like the cast and the photograph — Rodin was clearly trying to motivate his study of an individual who had died more than forty years earlier.

The sculptor's working method, however, led him to search for a live model. He therefore visited Tours, Balzac's birthplace, to find an individual with *Tourangeau* features in order to capture as accurate a likeness as possible.[34] In nineteenth-century France, physiognomic theories served as the foundation of the politically-motivated discourse of regional type, which purported to identify and assign meanings to physical attributes particular to the inhabitants of any given area of France.[35] It claimed that there was a constancy of regional features and personality — in other words, that an individual from Touraine would resemble his ancestors. Writers of the day, such as the geographer Elisée Reclus, judged the individuals from Touraine to have 'l'intelligence lucide, [...] [le] tempérament bien pondéré'.[36] Reclus also commented that the people of

29 Letter from Rodin to Zola dated 3 July 1891. Aurélien Scholl, 'La Question Rodin', *L'Écho de Paris*, 18 August 1896; quoted in Frederic V. Grunfeld, *Rodin: A Biography* (New York: Henry Holt and Co., 1987), p. 310.

30 A. B. de Farges's article appeared on 15 July 1891 in *La France*; cited in Butler, *Rodin: The Shape of Genius*, p. 254. For an illustration, see Musée Rodin, *1898: le* Balzac *de Rodin*, p. 262, cat. 11.

31 Joy Newton, 'Rodin and Nadar', *Laurels*, 52, 3 (1981–1982), 163–70 (pp. 167–68).

32 Véronique Mattiussi, '"Que de voyages j'ai faits en Touraine ..."', in Musée Rodin, *1898: le* Balzac *de Rodin*, pp. 125–32 (p. 130).

33 Emphasis in the original; Rodin quoted in Gustave Coquiot, *Rodin à Hôtel Biron et à Meudon* (Paris: Librairie Ollendorff, 1917), p. 107.

34 Letter to Zola from Toudouze dated 10 July 1891; quoted in Grunfeld, *Rodin: A Biography*, p. 310.

35 Ségolène Le Men, Luce Abélès, and Nathalie Preiss-Basset (eds), *Les Français peints par eux-mêmes*, ex. cat. (Paris: Éditions de la Réunion des musées nationaux, 1993), p. 21.

36 Elisée Reclus, *Nouvelle Géographie universelle: la terre et les hommes*, 19 vols (Paris: Librairie Hachette, 1876–1894), II: *La France* (1885), pp. 58–59.

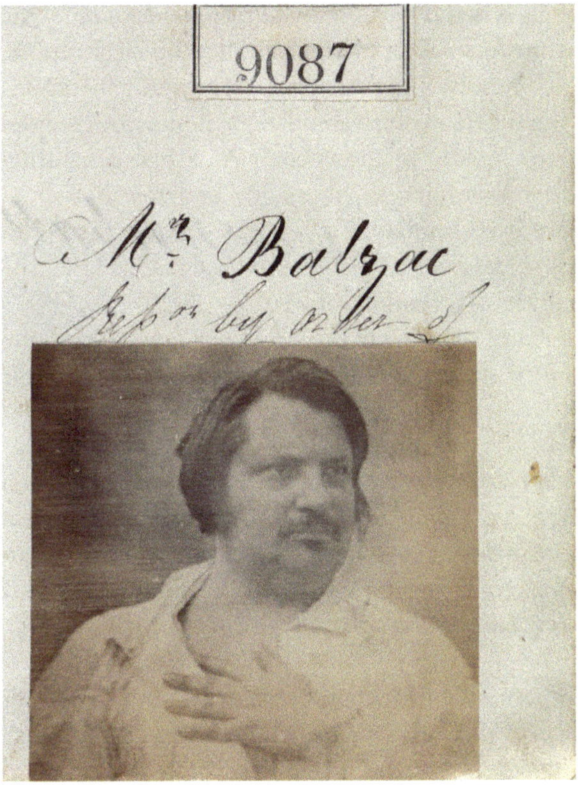

FIGURE 10.2 *Camille Silvy, after a daguerreotype by Louis Auguste Bisson,* Reproduction by order of Mr Balzac (Honoré de Balzac), *c. 1862, albumen print, 92 × 92 mm. Inventory number* NPG *Ax58909.*

the Loire valley 'se trouvent fondus dans un harmonieux ensemble de bon sens et de gaieté, d'esprit et de sérieux'.[37]

Rodin was keenly aware of physiognomic principles and theories of regional type — they would play a role not only in his studies for monuments in the 1880s and 1890s, but also in the way his sculptures were read by critics.[38] He must have understood that although the discourse of regional type was fundamentally flawed, it remained a useful entrée into his studies of Balzac. In

37 Reclus, *Nouvelle Géographie universelle*, II, p. 554.

38 See the author's 'Essence and Evanescence in the *Hands* of Rodin', *Thresholds* 31 (May 2006), 102–09.

pre-nineteenth-century France, when people rarely left their *ville natale*, the notion of regional type was more tenable; by the time Rodin was sculpting in the late nineteenth century, however, the seasonal workers of generations past who had shuttled between urban centres and their homes in agrarian communities had settled permanently in the cities.[39] As a first-generation Parisian himself — his father was born in Normandy and his mother in Lorraine — Rodin would have been intimately aware of the issues surrounding migrations within France.[40] However, he would also have realized that the public would 'recognize' the traits of a *Tourangeau.*

In fact, in an important early article on the *Monument to Balzac*, the sculptor's friend Gustave Geffroy speaks of Rodin's research in Tours in terms of regional type:

> Tout d'abord, et naturellement [...], Rodin est parti pour la Touraine, où Balzac est né, où il a reçu sa première éducation, le pays de sa formation physique et intellectuelle. Il devait se trouver, dans cette coulée de la vallée de la Loire, des mêmes traits généraux et particuliers qui se trouvent marqués et résumés sur la face de l'écrivain.

Geffroy delineates some of these qualities when he describes the search for 'quelque chose de la même corpulence, des mêmes plans de visage, du même rire des yeux, de la même lippe de la bouche'.[41] In other words, Rodin had to look for the regional features visible on the face of Balzac and of his fellow citizens of Touraine and the individual physiognomic signifiers appropriate to the great writer. Rodin's search, Geffroy asserts, was for:

> un type tourangeau qui est le type de Balzac. Il choisit quelques-uns de ceux qui portaient le plus profondément cette empreinte, et il modela leurs masques en des séances attentives, avec le soin minutieux, l'étude respectueuse qu'il apporte à la reproduction de la nature.

He then summarizes the results of the artist's two-year search for the right model: 'J'ai vu ces masques dans l'atelier du sculpteur lorsqu'il les rapporta de Touraine, je les ai revus l'autre jour, et ma stupéfaction de la première heure n'a fait que s'accroître. Avec moins de hauteur de front, moins de largeur de joues,

39 David H. Pinkney, *Napoleon III and the Rebuilding of Paris* (Princeton: Princeton University Press, 1958), pp. 154–59.

40 For more details on Rodin's family, see Butler, *Rodin: The Shape of Genius*, pp. 3–20.

41 Gustave Geffroy, 'L'imaginaire', *Le Figaro*, 29 August 1893, p. 1.

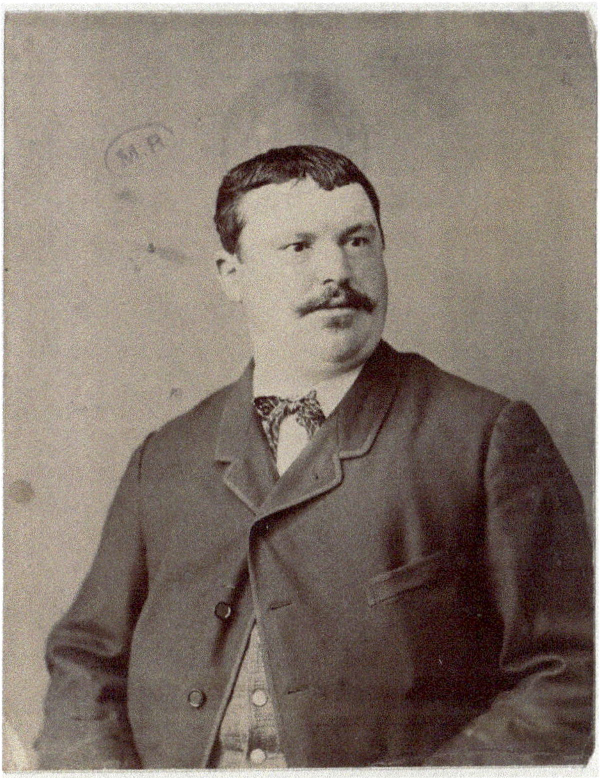

FIGURE 10.3 *Anonymous,* Portrait de M. Estager dit le Conducteur de Tours, modèle du Balzac, *épreuve sur papier albuminé, 14.4 × 11 cm. Inventory number Ph.1216, Musée Rodin, Paris.*

c'est matériellement Balzac.'[42] Rodin had found a driver by the name of Estager who ran the public coach between Azay-le-Rideau and the rail station and who bore a remarkable resemblance to his subject (Fig. 10.3 and Fig. 10.4).[43]

However, it quickly became clear in letters from Rodin's supporters that physiognomic indicators of regional type were inherently unreliable. During his stay in Tours, Rodin received surprising news from his friend Albert Pontremoli who had visited the Balzac specialist Vicomte Charles Spoelberch de Lovenjoul in Brussels: 'Selon M. de Lovenjoul, un voyage en pays tourangeau est de peu d'utilité, car si Balzac est né à Tours, c'est de parents étrangers au

42 Geffroy, 'L'imaginaire', p. 1.

43 Mattiussi, '"Que de voyages j'ai faits en Touraine ..."', p. 130.

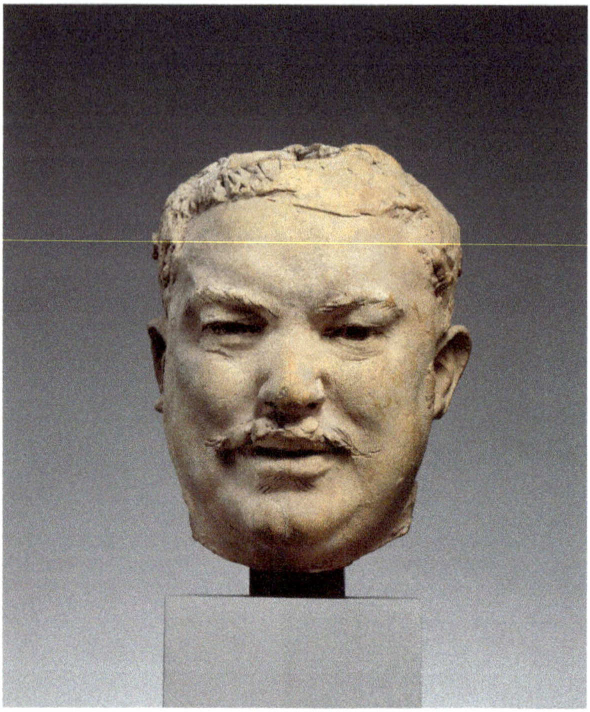

FIGURE 10.4 *Auguste Rodin,* Honoré de Balzac, *c. 1891, terracotta, height 23.5 cm. Accession number 12.11.1, Rogers Fund, 1912, Metropolitan Museum of Art, New York.*

pays tous deux, et s'il a eu le type tourangeau comme vous me le disiez ce n'est certes pas qu'il soit d'un sang des bords de la Loire.' He continued, 'je [...] me rappelle [...] avoir vu à Amboise des naturels ayant bien le même type que votre grand modèle.' Pontremoli then enumerated various photographic and drawn portraits of the author, which he believed would give Rodin a better sense of Balzac's physiognomy.[44] A few months later, in October of 1891, Geffroy also discouraged Rodin from focusing on the inhabitants of Tours: 'Je ne voudrais pas déranger vos études de têtes de tourangeaux, mais ne perdez pas de vue tout de même, cher Rodin, que Balzac est d'origine méridionale.' He asked, 'Avez-vous le volume de la *Correspondance* [?]', continuing, 'là [...] vous

44 Letter dated 29 July 1891 in the 'Albert Pontremoli' correspondence file, AMR.

connaîtrez le mieux l'admirable grand homme'.[45] Pontremoli's and Geffroy's pleas that Rodin shift his focus went unheeded. And, in another surprising turn of events, Rodin did not seek a new model after learning that Estager was himself not a native of Tours either, but of Combressol in the Limousin region.[46] Apparently, one could be a *Tourangeau* type but not from Touraine. The artist, however, could have assumed that the public would have understood the physiognomic shorthand evident in the sculpture, regardless of Balzac's true ancestral origins of which most people were not aware.

In fact, a few years later the work in progress bespoke the *Tourangeau* type to the critics who saw it. In *L'Écho de Paris* in 1894, Gaston Steigler wrote that Rodin created 'un Balzac vivant, vrai, marqué des caractères généraux de cette robuste et saine race tourangelle dont le romancier aimait à s'enorgueillir, avec une tête large et puissante où l'on devinât le grouillement de la Comédie humaine'.[47] A writer for *Le Journal de Bruxelles* recounted Rodin's search for 'des signes de race, des conformations physiques, des éléments du type qui tiennent au sol'.[48] Georges Clemenceau, writing for *La Justice*, commanded Rodin to continue with his project: 'Va en Touraine te pénétrer de la race, interroge ces têtes rustiques, modèle ces crânes solides, assemble ces traits volontaires'. Moreover, he equated the sculptor and the novelist: 'tu presses ton génie et le forces de se mesurer avec le génie de ton modèle' — an apt statement, given that the finished monument would reveal as much about the artist as it would about the model.[49]

Rodin used physiognomy and regional type to motivate his sculpture, as a way of incorporating 'nature' into his work, and to fight against staid Salon conventions.[50] After the well-known scandal of 1894, when the *Société* gave Rodin an ultimatum because they had begun to doubt that they would ever

---

45 Letter dated 4 October, probably from 1891, in the 'Gustave Geffroy' correspondence file, AMR. In fact, Balzac's father was born in the Languedoc and his mother was from Paris; Laure Surville, *Balzac, sa vie et ses œuvres d'après sa correspondance* (Paris: Librairie Nouvelle and Jaccottet, Bourdilliat et Cie., 1858), pp. 6–7.

46 Mattiussi, '"Que de voyages j'ai faits en Touraine ..."', p. 130.

47 Gaston Stiegler, 'Rodin et Balzac', *L'Écho de Paris*, 12 November 1894, [n. pag.]. Article located in the press files for '*Balzac*', AMR.

48 'Lettres parisiennes', *Le Journal de Bruxelles*, 13 November 1894, [n. pag.]. Article located in the press files for '*Balzac*', AMR.

49 G[eorges] Clemenceau, 'Balzac & Rodin', *La Justice*, 12 November 1894, [n. pag.]. Article located in the press files for '*Balzac*', AMR.

50 For a discussion of these 'well-worn poses', see Gustave Geffroy, 'The Sculptor Rodin', in *Rodin in Perspective*, ed. by Ruth Butler (Englewood Cliffs, NJ: Prentice-Hall, Inc., 1980), pp. 62–73 (p. 69). Originally published in *Arts and Letters* (London, 1889), pp. 289–304.

see the completed monument, the sculptor set aside his '[concern] with an exact resemblance' and created an almost supernatural effigy of Balzac, which transcended considerations of regional type and instead focused on the author's 'genius'.[51] Here too he was following Balzac's own musings; Gretchen Besser argues that, not only was the novelist preoccupied with the 'question of genius' throughout his life, but he even anticipated the later studies of Cesare Lombroso by '[suggesting] the possibility of making a scientific study of the heredity of great men, including their background and environment'.[52]

Genius and Neurosis

Just at the time he began manipulating Balzac's visage to make the markers of genius more evident than the 'readable' signifiers of physiognomy that had been his focus for several years, Rodin himself became the object of a study on genius. In the first days of 1896, he received a curious letter from Doctor Édouard Toulouse, a senior doctor for mental illness at the *Faculté de médecine* and a physician at the Saint-Anne Asylum. Toulouse briefly outlined a proposal: he wanted Rodin to be the subject of an 'enquête médico-psychologique' on the relationship between genius and neurosis.[53] According to the young doctor, the question of whether genius was a neurosis was the subject of a millennia-old debate to which he hoped to bring 'quelques faits précis' and 'quelques observations vérifiées et authentiques'.[54] Rodin met with him and quickly agreed to participate in the ambitious project.[55] Within a few weeks, Toulouse's team of doctors and specialists were meeting with Rodin to, among other things, measure his ears and examine his myopic eyes.[56]

By July of that year, Toulouse was preparing to publish his study of Zola, the first volume of a planned series, and he asked for permission to include Rodin's

51 Charles Chincholle, 'Balzac et Rodin', *Le Figaro*, 25 November 1894; quoted in Elsen, et al., *Rodin & Balzac*, p. 8.

52 Gretchen R. Besser, *Balzac's Concept of Genius. The theme of superiority in the 'Comédie Humaine'* (Geneva: Librairie Droz, 1969), pp. 15 and 72.

53 Letter dated 6 January 1896 in the 'Édouard Toulouse' correspondence file, AMR.

54 Ibid.

55 It is of course possible that he had already heard of this project from friends and colleagues who had agreed to participate, including Zola, Alphonse Daudet, and Jules Dalou, among others.

56 Letters dated 1 February 1896 and 9 February 1896 in the 'Édouard Toulouse' correspondence file, AMR.

name in the introduction.[57] Three months later — just one month before the book's publication — the sculptor had still not given Toulouse a final answer. The physician pointedly asked in a letter whether Rodin thought it unseemly to have his name listed alongside those of writers Zola, Alphonse Daudet, and Edmond de Goncourt, the painter Pierre Puvis de Chavannes, and the sculptor Jules Dalou, all of whom had agreed to participate in the project.[58]

The first book of the series, *Enquête médico-psychologique sur les rapports de la supériorité intellectuelle avec la névropathie*, was released with an introduction by Zola authorizing its publication.[59] Zola characterizes himself in terms familiar to both science and art, claiming, 'Mon cerveau est comme dans un crâne de verre, je l'ai donné à tous et je ne crains pas que tous viennent y lire'; he then describes himself as a 'pauvre écorché' at the hands of his critics.[60] Toulouse, in turn, considers the work and the series of which it was to be a part as 'uniquement scientifiques'.[61] He asserts that 'on pouvait s'occuper des hautes personnalités intellectuelles comme de simples matières à observation, comme de faits rares qu'on devait étudier minutieusement, sans prévention d'aucune sorte'.[62] In order to make the profile as complete as possible, the doctor includes the contributions of such notable figures as the statistician and eugenicist Francis Galton, 'qui a bien voulu noter les empreintes

57 Letter dated 3 July 1896 in the 'Édouard Toulouse' correspondence file, AMR. The second — and last — volume of this series appeared almost fifteen years later: Édouard Toulouse, *Enquête médico-psychologique sur la supériorité intellectuelle. II. Henri Poincaré* (Paris: Ernest Flammarion, 1910). Toulouse also published a short article on Berthelot; É[douard] Toulouse, 'Notes biologiques sur M. Berthelot', *Revue de psychiatrie* (*médecine mentale, neurologie, psychologie*), 4, 1 (1901), 368–71.

58 Letter dated 10 October 1896 in the 'Édouard Toulouse' correspondence file, AMR.

59 Édouard Toulouse, *Enquête médico-psychologique sur les rapports de la supériorité intellectuelle avec la névropathie. I. Introduction générale. Émile Zola* (Paris: Société d'Éditions Scientifiques, 1896). For more on Toulouse's study, see Jacqueline Carroy, '"Mon cerveau est comme dans un crâne de verre": Émile Zola sujet d'Édouard Toulouse', *Revue d'histoire du XIXe siècle*, 20/21 (2000), <http://elseminario.com.ar/biblioteca/carroy_mon_cerveau_zola.htm> [accessed 5 September 2015]; Ann Jefferson, *Genius in France: An Idea and Its Uses* (Princeton: Princeton University Press, 2015), pp. 89–122; and Agnès Sandras-Fraysse, 'La folie de l'enquête: Zola disséqué', *Fabula/Les colloques* (15 January 2008), <http://www.fabula.org/colloques/document874.php> [accessed 17 August 2015].

60 Émile Zola, 'Lettre de M. Émile Zola,' in *Enquête médico-psychologique sur les rapports de la supériorité intellectuelle avec la névropathie, I. Introduction générale. Émile Zola*, by Édouard Toulouse (Paris: Société d'Éditions Scientifiques, 1896), v–vii.

61 Toulouse, *Enquête médico-psychologique*, I, ix.

62 Ibid.

des doigts', and Alphonse Bertillon, the Paris police chief famous for inventing the mugshot and creating a photographic archive of criminals, 'qui a dressé la fiche signalétique anatomique'.[63] Other specialists checked Zola's hearing and his sense of smell, analyzed his handwriting, and measured the strength of his hand, among many other measurements. Toulouse's methods — and his and Zola's comments — reveal their inherent positivism, attributing the acquisition of knowledge to direct observation.

In the end, Rodin was acknowledged in Toulouse's book — which concluded that Zola's genius was not a result of the fact that he suffered from nervous disorders — and the book caused a scandal.[64] Articles generally ridiculing the three-hundred-page study and its subject were published in all the major newspapers; most took exception to the text's complete and often indecorous revelation of its subject: from the dimensions of Zola's skull to the composition of his urine.[65] One author speculated that Puvis de Chavannes withdrew his participation in Toulouse's study because he was not terribly interested in 'renseigner l'univers sur l'abondance de son système pileux et la régularité de ses fonctions intestinales', as Zola had done.[66] It seems that Rodin felt the same way and communication between the sculptor and the physician ceased for several years.

63 Ibid., xi–xii. For more on the methods of Galton and Bertillon, see Allan Sekula, 'The Body and the Archive', *October* 39 (Winter 1986), 3–64.

64 Toulouse, *Enquête médico-psychologique*, I, pp. 279–80. Zola's involvement in Dreyfus' defense helped the book capture the public's attention. See Michel Huteau, *Psychologie, psychiatrie et société sous la Troisième République. La Biocratie d'Édouard Toulouse (1865–1947)* (Paris: L'Harmattan, 2002), pp. 75–76. The articles that appeared around the publication of the book also attest to this. See, for example, Homodei [Arthur Huc], 'Chronique. Zola viviséqué', *La Dépêche*, 8 February 1898, [n. pag.]; L., 'Au jour le jour. Anthropologie et critique', *Le Journal des débats*, 9 June 1898, [n. pag.], and *Sunday Times* (London), 26 June 1898, [n. pag.]. Articles located in the 'personne' file for Édouard Toulouse, AMR. Later, the Dreyfus case influenced the protest that emerged when the *Société des gens de lettres* rejected the *Monument to Balzac* in 1898; see, for example, Le Normand-Romain, 'Balzac', I, 187.

65 Toulouse's methods were questioned insofar as they compared to those of other theorists, such as Lombroso. See Charles Bardin, 'Médecine & Psychologie. Génie ou folie', *Gil Blas*, 3 November 1896, [n. pag.] and Maurice de Fleury, 'Au Jour le jour. Le Livre sur Zola', *Le Figaro*, 6 November 1896, [n. pag.]. Articles located in the 'personne' file for Édouard Toulouse, AMR.

66 The anonymous author then criticizes Puvis for refusing to continue with Toulouse's study; *Le Journal des débats*, 10 November 1896, [n. pag.]. Article located in the 'personne' file for Édouard Toulouse, AMR.

In 1895, when Zola and Toulouse had begun their shared project, the novelist may have discussed it with Rodin.[67] It is intriguing to consider that it could have been Zola who proposed Rodin as a possible subject to the physician. Toulouse probably embarked on the 'vivisection'[68] of French notables as a reaction to Lombroso's theories about the connection between genius and madness, updating the Italian's nomenclature — he referred to genius as 'superior intelligence' and 'madness' as a kind of neuropathy — to fashion a more 'scientific' project.[69] The year 1889 saw the first French translation of Lombroso's *L'Uomo di genio in rapporto alla psichiatria, alla storia ed all'estetica*, a foray into the longstanding dispute on the relationship between genius and madness.[70] In France in the earlier part of nineteenth century, Louis-Francisque Lélut, Jacques-Joseph Moreau de Tours, and others had investigated the connection, but by the end of the century, there was a renewed interest in the topic with theories of hereditary degeneration circulating widely in medical and popular circles. Like the notion of regional type, theories of degeneration, too, were fed by concerns related to migrations within France from rural communities to cities.[71] As Robert Nye has noted, by the 1890s degeneracy was seen as a social pathology that explained a variety of France's ills, including, among others, depopulation, alcoholism, prostitution, and crime. The causes and symptoms of each — and of degeneration itself — became so confounded that 'they were in practice virtually interchangeable'.[72] Modernity itself could even be cast as the cause of degeneration.[73] Lombroso had already made his name with

67 Zola and Toulouse's discussions started in the summer of 1895; Henri Mitterand, *Zola*, 3 vols (Paris: Fayard, 1999–2002), III: *L'Honneur (1893–1902)* (2002), p. 229.

68 Homodei, 'Chronique', [n. pag.].

69 De Fleury, 'Au Jour le jour', [n. pag.]. Lombroso later responded critically to Toulouse's book on Zola; C[esare] Lombroso, 'Émile Zola, d'après l'étude du Docteur Toulouse et les nouvelles théories sur le génie', *La Semaine médicale* 17 (1897), 1–5. Of course, Zola was already familiar with Lombroso's work, which he read in preparation for writing *La Bête humaine*. See Mitterand, *Zola*, p. 229.

70 *L'Uomo di genio* was a revised and expanded version of Lombroso's *Genio e follia* from 1864. It was published in France as *L'Homme de génie*, trans. by Colonna D'Istria (Paris: Félix Alcan, 1889). Aristotle seemed to have begun this line of questioning, famously asking in Book XXX, 'Why is it that all men who are outstanding in philosophy, poetry or the arts are melancholic?', in his *Problems*, trans. by W. S. Hett, 2 vols (London: William Heinemann, 1936–37), II (1937), 155.

71 Daniel Pick, *Faces of Degeneration: A European Disorder, c. 1848–c. 1918* (Cambridge: Cambridge University Press, 1989), p. 53.

72 Robert A. Nye, *Crime, Madness, and Politics in Modern France: The Medical Concept of National Decline* (Princeton: Princeton University Press, 1984), p. 144.

73 Pick, *Faces of Degeneration*, p. 73.

studies on criminals — a book that examined the 'stigmata' of degeneracy in the genius seemed a natural sequel.[74] In the preface to the first English edition of *The Man of Genius*, Lombroso writes:

> Just as giants pay a heavy ransom for their stature in sterility and relative muscular and mental weakness, so the giants of thought expiate their intellectual force in degeneration and psychosis. It is thus that the signs of degeneration are found more frequently in men of genius than even in the insane.[75]

Having made this analogy, Lombroso states later in the preface that there are those who contend 'the man of genius is a monster'. He then counters: 'Very well, but even monsters follow well-defined teratologic laws'.[76]

Lombroso follows these contentious remarks with an extensive, detailed list of moral and physical 'stigmata'. The latter include: 'prominent ears, deficiency of beard, irregularity of teeth, excessive asymmetry of face and head, which may be very large or very small, sexual precocity, smallness or disproportion of the body, lefthandedness [*sic*], stammering, rickets', and so on.[77] He then delineates each symptom with the names of notable sufferers. Significantly, Balzac makes an appearance from the start, under the first sign of degeneration: 'height'. Along with Erasmus, Mozart, Hogarth, and many others, Balzac was 'famous for short stature as well as for genius', according to Lombroso.[78] Balzac reappears in the next chapter on 'Latent Forms of Neurosis and Insanity in Genius' with a long quotation from George Sand that testified to his 'megalomania'.[79] And, most importantly, Balzac is mentioned in the chapter on 'The Epileptoid Nature of Genius', where Lombroso presents his theory that 'the creative power of genius may be a form of degenerative psychosis belonging to the family of epileptic affections'.[80] He then cites a passage from Zola's *Les Romanciers Naturalistes* (1881) about Balzac's working method to prove that 'it is not only isolated paroxysms which recall the psychic phenomenology

---

74 For example, see Cesare Lombroso, *L'Uomo delinquente* (Milan, 1876).

75 Cesare Lombroso, *The Man of Genius* (London: Walter Scott, 1891), vi.

76 Ibid., viii.

77 Ibid., p. 6.

78 Ibid. See also Georges Raviart, 'Le Génie de Balzac du point de vue psychiatrique. Génie et folie', *Annales médico-psychologiques*, 2, 4 (November 1954), 481–503 (p. 493).

79 Lombroso, *The Man of Genius*, p. 47.

80 Ibid., p. 336. Toulouse's first point under his concluding comments is that Zola was not an epileptic, clearly in response to Lombroso's theory; Toulouse, *Enquête médico-psychologique*, I, p. 279.

of the epileptic, but the whole life'.[81] Interestingly, the continuation of Zola's passage — which was not included in Lombroso's text — hypothesizes about the cause of Balzac's 'temperament': 'Il y avait sans doute une lésion dans ce vaste cerveau, la fêlure du génie.'[82] Zola probably knew, as did Rodin, that at the age of fourteen Balzac had suffered a serious and unexplained nervous attack: 'une espèce de coma', according to his biographer Edmond Werdet.[83]

In the preface to the 1889 French edition of Lombroso's text, physiologist Charles Richet emphasizes that geniuses are not insane but, rather, exceptional.[84] This caveat reveals the anxiety surrounding any talk of hereditary degeneration: while it could lead to a diagnosis of genius, it could also lead to one of moral depravity. Daniel Pick has observed that the term degeneration 'served to anchor meaning, but paradoxically its own could never be fully stabilised [...]; it explained everything and nothing as it moved back and forth between the clinic, the novel, the newspaper and the government investigation'.[85] Its wide cultural currency and protean meaning facilitated its appropriation by a wide variety of interests, which could extol its connection to superior intelligence or tout its links to social and physical decay. The symptoms of cultural degeneracy, for instance, were enumerated in Max Nordau's popular diatribe, *Degeneration* (1892).[86] Also written in response to Lombroso's work, it begins with a dedication to the Italian physician in which Nordau makes clear his intent:

> Degenerates are not always criminals, prostitutes, anarchists, and pronounced lunatics; they are often authors and artists. These, however, manifest the same mental characteristics, and for the most part the same

---

81 Lombroso, *The Man of Genius*, p. 343.

82 Émile Zola, *Les Romanciers naturalistes* (Paris: G. Charpentier, 1881), p. 55.

83 Emphasis removed; Edmond Werdet, *Portrait intime de Balzac, sa vie, son humeur et son caractère* (Paris: E. Dentu, 1859; reprinted Paris: L'Arche du livre, 1970), p. 48. An annotated copy of the 1859 edition is in Rodin's library, Inv. #3548; <http://musee-rodin.bibli.fr/opac/index.php?lvl=notice_display&id=5728> [accessed 25 September 2015]. Rodin received Lemer's biography of Balzac from the author himself; Auguste Rodin, *Correspondance de Rodin*, 4 vols (Paris: Éditions du musée Rodin, 1985–1992), I: 1860–1899 (1985), p. 134. In *Louis Lambert*, the narrator, a partly autobiographical character, suffers a similar attack; Honoré de Balzac, *Louis Lambert, suivi de Séraphita* (Paris: Charpentier, 1842), p. 66.

84 Charles Richet, 'Préface', Cesare Lombroso, *L'Homme de génie*, trans. by Colonna d'Istria (Paris: Félix Alcan, 1889), vii.

85 Pick, *Faces of Degeneration*, p. 8.

86 Max Nordau, *Entartung* (Berlin: Duncker, 1892). The first French translation, *Dégénérescence*, was published in 1894.

> somatic features, as the members of the above-mentioned anthropological family, who satisfy their unhealthy impulses with the knife of the assassin or the bomb of the dynamiter, instead of with pen and pencil.[87]

And Nordau devotes a long chapter on the pernicious and corrupting influence of Zola and 'His School'.[88] Criticizing as false the precept that one can describe reality, he goes on to diagnose Zola as a 'high-class degenerate' through a reading of his works.[89] Nordau concludes: 'Zola's novels do not prove that things are badly managed in this world, but merely that Zola's nervous system is out of order'.[90] His discussion also touches on Balzac; Nordau writes that the theory of 'milieu' used by the writer of *La Comédie humaine* 'in fact, explains nothing'.[91]

In sum, over the course of the decade when Rodin was fashioning his *Monument to Balzac*, the terms 'genius', 'madness', 'neurosis', and 'degeneracy' were linked both positively and negatively to one another and also to Balzac, Zola, and even Rodin. In casting himself as a 'nerveux', as the second epigraph to this chapter illustrates, Rodin makes clear that he understood his own character through the discourses on nervous diseases in these same years.[92] Talk of genius and neurosis reached a fever pitch in his social circle around 1895 and 1896, when he, Zola, and others were involved in Toulouse's studies. It was exactly around this time that Rodin began transforming Balzac's facial features — from 'readable' physiognomic signifiers to markers of genius.

Degenerate Balzac

By 1896 the long-awaited monument to Balzac had still not materialized, and critics were growing restless; one in Bordeaux commented ominously that the public could expect from the 'mains nerveuses' of Rodin 'un Balzac de

87 Max Nordau, *Degeneration* (London: William Heinemann, 1895), vii.

88 This chapter is an about-face for Nordau; he had previously published a laudatory book on Zola, *Zola und Naturalismus Ausgewählte Pariser Briefe* (Leipzig, 1887). For more on this, see Hans-Peter Söder, *That Way Madness Lies: Max Nordau on fin-de-siècle Genius* (High Wycombe: Rivendale Press, 2009), esp. p. 142.

89 For his full diagnosis, see Nordau, *Degeneration*, pp. 499–500.

90 Nordau, *Degeneration*, p. 499.

91 Ibid., p. 488.

92 Rodin quoted in 'Balzac et Rodin. Où en est le monument du père de la "Comédie humaine"', *L'Éclair*, 28 January 1896, [n. pag.]. Article located in the press files for '*Balzac*', AMR.

cauchemar'.[93] More positively, Alexandre Hepp wrote in *Le Soir* that Rodin engaged in the 'minutieuses et passionnées enquêtes d'historien, de psychologue, d'artiste'.[94] Writing in *Le Figaro*, Rodenbach complimented Rodin's *Balzac*: 'Elle est de ce siècle, parce qu'elle offre le nu moderne, tiraillé, raviné par la névrose moderne'.[95] Roger Marx claimed that 'Rodin s'est préoccupé de chercher ce qui, sur ce visage franc, large et ouvert annonçait la puissance, la volonté, le génie, et il a visé [...] à la ressemblance statuaire [...] en accentuant les traits caractéristiques, signalétiques: l'élévation du front, l'enchassement profond de l'orbite, l'éclat aigu des yeux, la carrure du nez, la sensualité des lèvres épaisses'.[96] Like a contemporary Frankenstein, Rodin himself used the metaphor of birth in discussing the creative process: 'J'ai enfanté un Balzac dont je suis satisfait'.[97]

Also in 1896 — the year of Rodin's participation in Toulouse's study — the head of Rodin's *Balzac* began to transform dramatically. He had found a new sitter whose resemblance to Balzac he found inspiring: a man by the name of Féroux or Ferrou, who was either a bookseller or a Parisian businessman.[98] According to Antoinette Le Normand-Romain, this portrait was the 'starting point for the final head [of the *Monument to Balzac*]'.[99] *Head H*, as it is known, already shows a marked difference with earlier studies by Rodin (Fig. 10.5). The treatment of the surface is much more expressive, with pronounced dips and bumps on the forehead and the cheeks. The eyes are deeply set and the protruding eyebrows and brow give the visage a look of deep concentration and even consternation. The surviving terracotta attests to Rodin's wrestling

93 'Lettres parisiennes', *La Gironde* [Bordeaux], 29 January 1896, [n. pag.]. Article located in the press files for '*Balzac*', AMR.

94 Alexandre Hepp, 'Notes quotidiennes. L'impossible statue', *Le Soir* (Paris), 30 January 1896, [n. pag.]. Article located in the press files for '*Balzac*', AMR.

95 Georges Rodenbach, 'Encore la statue de Balzac', *Le Figaro*, 25 August 1896, [n. pag.]. Article located in the press files for '*Balzac*', AMR.

96 Emphasis removed; Roger Marx, 'Balzac et Rodin', *Le Voltaire*, 5 February 1896, [n. pag.]. Article located in the press files for '*Balzac*', AMR.

97 Rodin quoted in 'L'actualité. La Statue de Balzac et l'impatience des souscripteurs', *L'Éclair*, 20 August 1896, [n. pag.]. Article located in the press files for '*Balzac*', AMR.

98 Antoinette Le Normand-Romain, 'Balzac, head with bare forehead and cleft chin, known as Head H', *c.* 1894, in *The Bronzes of Rodin. Catalogue of Works in the Musée Rodin*, 2 vols (Paris: Éditions de la Réunion des Musées Nationaux, 2007), I, p. 174.

99 Antoinette Le Normand-Romain, 'Balzac, head with bare forehead and cleft chin, known as Head H', p. 174.

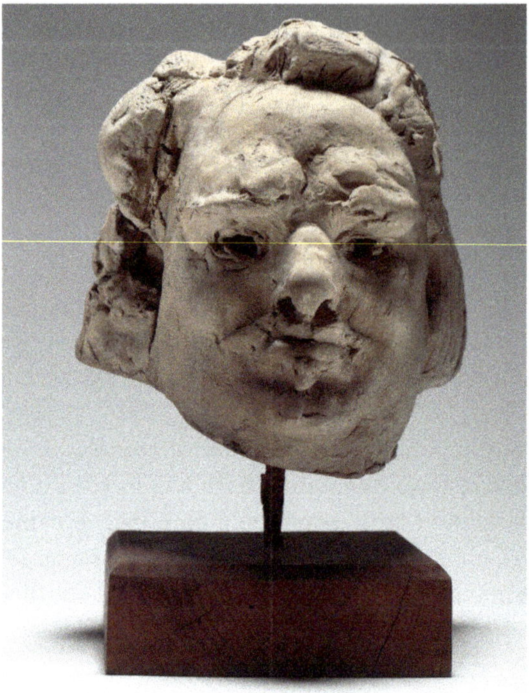

FIGURE 10.5 *Auguste Rodin,* Balzac, tête au front dégagé et au menton fendu, dite tête H, *c. 1894, terracotta, 21 × 19.9 × 22.5 cm. Inventory number S.1653, Musée Rodin, Paris.*
PHOTOGRAPHER: CHRISTIAN BARAJA.

with the material; balls of clay, the marks of the sculptor's tools, and the trace of his nails are all revealed on the surface.[100]

The penultimate study of Balzac's head reveals a further deformation of the visage (Fig. 10.6). The face has grown wider and fuller. The expression is softer and the eyes further entrenched. The features of the face — the lips, the eyes, the nose — are less symmetrical. A small cylindrical pellet of clay seems to be crawling up the bridge of the nose. Each eyebrow is modelled differently: the right has deep, slanted grooves while the flattened left evinces a central furrow created by a tool or the sculptor's finger. The lobe of the sunken left ear emerges unnaturally from the head. Balzac's moustache is more integrated into the swelling and sinking surfaces of the skin and rests, almost indistinguishable,

100 Catalogue entry for 'Balzac, tête au front dégagé et au menton fendu, dite tête H', in Musée Rodin, *1898: le* Balzac *de Rodin*, pp. 316–317 (p. 316), cat. 67.

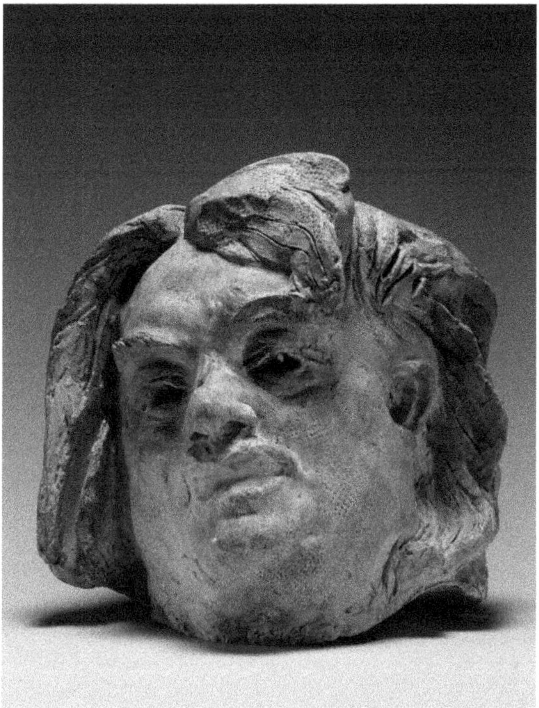

FIGURE 10.6 *Auguste Rodin,* Avant-dernière étude pour la tête de Balzac, *c. 1895–1896, plaster, 19.1 × 18.2 × 18.2 cm. Inventory number S.1652, Musée Rodin, Paris.* PHOTOGRAPHER: CHRISTIAN BARAJA.

on the thick ridge created by the uppermost contour of his upper lip. His hair swells and collapses, billowing around his head, perhaps attesting implicitly to phrenological changes in the shape of his skull.

Returning to Lombroso's list of stigmata, one finds several elements visibly heightened in Balzac's evolving visage: 'prominent ears, deficiency of beard, [...] excessive asymmetry of face and head, which may be very large or very small'. Similarly, a later variant with the same title, dated *c.* 1896–1897, cast from the penultimate head above, has a wider face and more dramatically cresting and lobed hair (Fig. 10.7). The nose appears more bulbous and the nostrils are deeply incised over a wider and fuller moustache. Two parallel scratches are visible on the forehead, calling attention to Rodin's authorship.[101] It is a cast

101 See David J. Getsy, *Rodin: Sex and the Making of Modern Sculpture* (New Haven: Yale University Press, 2010), pp. 73–100.

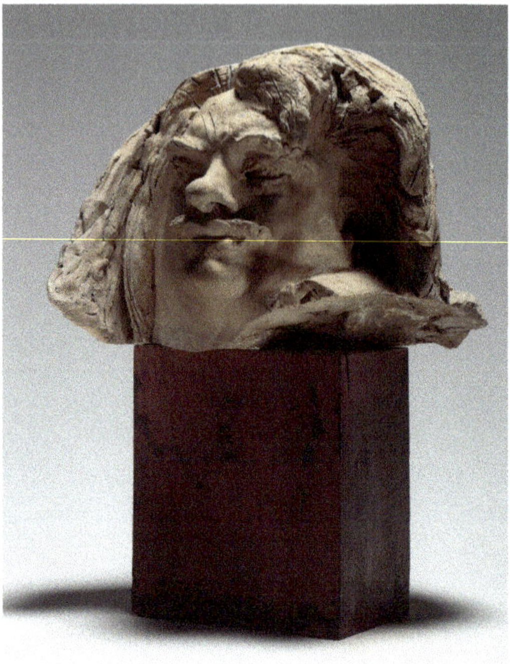

FIGURE 10.7
Auguste Rodin, Balzac, avant-dernière étude pour la tête, variante, *c. 1895–1896, terracotta, 17.7 × 24 × 20.5 cm. Inventory number S.1576, Musée Rodin, Paris.*
PHOTOGRAPHER: CHRISTIAN BARAJA.

of this version that was included in a photograph taken with two portraits of Estager (Fig. 10.8). This trio of heads, likely assembled by Rodin himself, highlights the transformation of Balzac's face in the progression of studies. Against a creased backdrop, the three sculptures stand in a pyramidal composition. The speaking portraits of Estager appear above, on a higher support, and on the right, while the cast from the penultimate head of Balzac sits on the left. The latter work appears shrivelled by comparison to the sturdy and earnest faces of the studies based on the coach driver.[102] Its unruly hair, vestige of a shoulder and bloated features make for a monstrous vision. This photograph is a personal testament to the evolution of Rodin's studies for the *Monument to Balzac*.

With the author's stout body concealed, the head of the final *Monument to Balzac* is, in fact, its only legible aspect, and it demonstrates that Rodin moved away from the physiognomic signifiers that he seemed intent on gathering

102 It is smaller because of the process of *estampage* from which it was created; for more, see Agnès Cascio, 'Approche technique de Rodin pour *Balzac*', in Musée Rodin, *1898: le* Balzac *de Rodin*, pp. 229–42 (pp. 236–37).

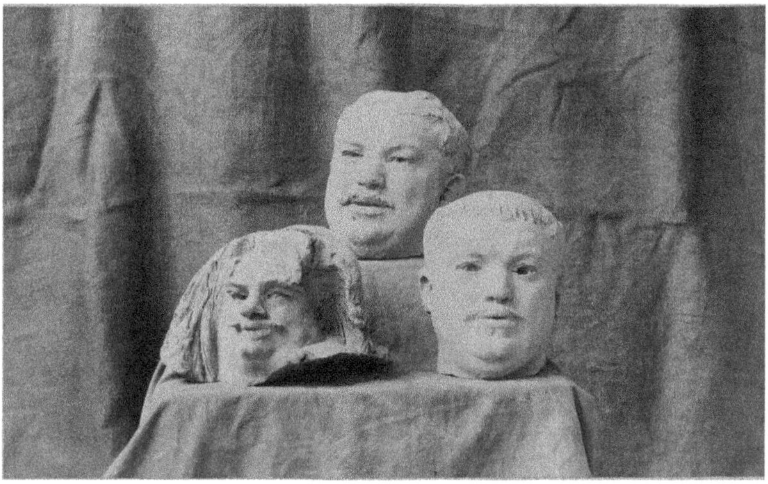

FIGURE 10.8 *Anonymous,* Trois études de têtes pour Balzac (terre). *Épreuve sur papier albuminé, 24 × 34 cm. Inventory number Ph.1213, Musée Rodin, Paris.*

in visits to the Touraine region towards those of genius (Fig. 10.9).[103] Yet even these 'stigmata' of degeneration are exaggerated, enhancing the fantastic appearance of the statue and its forceful address. Rodin has intensified the mien of the author by distorting the features of the visage: he affirmed in referring to his *Monument to Balzac,* 'Il faut amplifier la nature'.[104] And, in another interview, 'selon moi, la sculpture moderne doit exagérer […] les formes'.[105] By manipulating and exploiting scientific theories here and elsewhere, Rodin proferred a 'nerve art' that was not to Nordau's liking, as evidenced by this chapter's first epigraph, and revitalized the moribund field of sculpture.[106] He confused and angered many of the visitors to the Salon of 1898, such as the one who saw in his figure a madman: 'It's Balzac at Charenton, in his hospital

103 Wagner instead argues that in the *Monument to Balzac* '[t]he eventual decision was to equate genius with the phallus, and to subsume the particularities of history under a symbol meant to contain them'. Wagner, 'Rodin's Reputation', p. 223.

104 Rodin quoted in Ph. Dubois, 'Chez Rodin', *L'Aurore*, 12 May 1898, [n. pag.]. Article located in the press files for '*Balzac*', AMR.

105 Rodin quoted in Charles Chincholle, 'La Statue de Balzac', *Le Figaro*, 12 May 1898, [n. pag.]. Article located in the press files for '*Balzac*', AMR.

106 Max Nordau, *On Art and Artists*, trans. by W. F. Harvey (London: T. Fisher Unwin, 1907), p. 292. See also the author's 'A Hysterical Reading of Rodin's *Gates of Hell*', *Art History*, 36, 5 (November 2013), 994–1017.

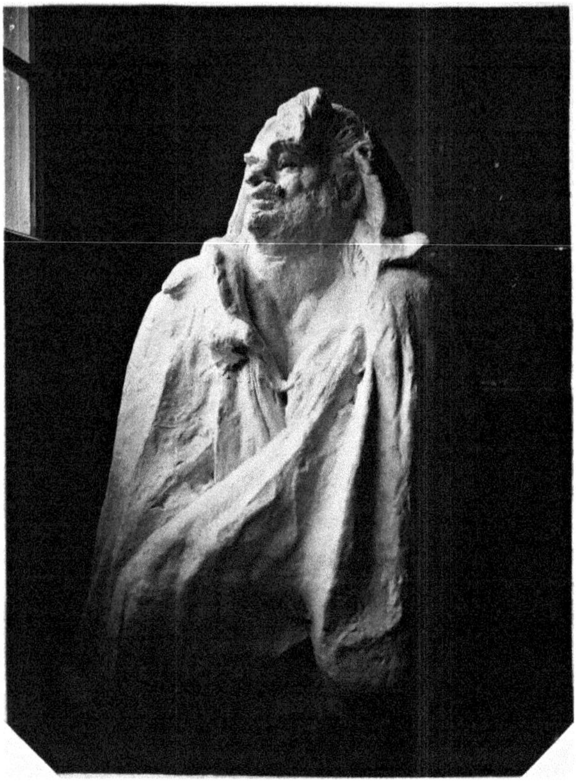

FIGURE 10.9 *Eugène Druet,* Balzac, *1898, gelatin silver print, 38.1 × 27.7 cm. Accession no. 1983.194.12, Iris & B. Gerald Cantor Center for Visual Arts at Stanford University; Gift of Albert E. and Patricia Elsen.*
COURTESY OF THE CANTOR ARTS CENTER AT STANFORD UNIVERSITY.

gown.'[107] Jean Rameau, himself a member of the *Société*, sarcastically advocated casting it in bronze and setting it on a high pedestal so that 'les siècles futurs sachent à quel degré d'aberration mentale nous étions arrivés à la fin de ce siècle-ci'.[108]

107 Jean Villemer, 'Le Vernissage' [1 May 1898], in *Rodin in Perspective*, ed. by Ruth Butler (Englewood Cliffs, NJ: Prentice-Hall, Inc., 1980), pp. 91–92 (p. 92). Originally published in *Le Figaro*.

108 Jean Rameau quoted in Arsène Alexandre, *Le Balzac de Rodin* (Paris: H. Floury, 1898), p. 10.

But for Rodin's supporters, his interpretation of theories of degeneration in the *Monument to Balzac* coalesced in a testament to genius. Clement Vautel wrote in *L'Événement* that the sculpture represented 'la matérialisation du génie énorme',[109] while Frank Harris, writing in the *The Saturday Review*, saw 'an extraordinary grotesque, a something monstrous and superhuman'. He continued, 'There is [...] something uncanny in the head. Yes, uncanny; the great jaws and immense throat that seems to rise out of the chest and form a part of it; the cavernous hollows of the eyes without eyeballs or sight, and above, the forehead, made narrow by the locks of hair — a grotesque of extraordinary power.'[110] In a long defence of the sculpture that appeared on the front page of *Le Figaro*, Rodenbach, one of the sculptor's most astute critics, writes that Rodin captured the 'visage du génie sorti de la matière et qui va rentrer dans la matière'. Echoing Balzac's own sentiment that one's destiny is written on the body, Rodenbach argues: 'La mort prématurée était là... Elle était déjà sur son visage'.[111] In a later text, he plainly articulates Rodin's vision of Balzac: 'Les génies sont moins des hommes que des monstres. Voilà ce que M. Rodin a compris et rendu si magnifiquement'.[112] It is clear, then, that the sculptor was ultimately most influenced by Balzac's conception of himself as 'an exceptional being', a notion in line, as we have seen, with Richet's formulation of genius.[113]

The implicit link between Balzac's genius and Rodin's own was difficult for some critics to ignore. Clemenceau, of course, alluded to it several years before the final monument was revealed. Gustave Schneider argued that 'l'immortel écrivain et le sculpteur m'apparaissent comme deux expressions d'un même idéal, deux génies de même puissance'.[114] Yet, for others, the implications that Rodin, too, was degenerate were disturbing. In 1917, the year of Rodin's death, his biographer Judith Cladel saw fit to dismiss the theories that linked genius with neurosis. In *Rodin, the Man and His Art*, she takes offense at the possibility that Rodin could have been considered degenerate:

109 Clément Vautel, 'Notes parisiennes, la Rodinière', *L'Événement*, 7 July 1899, [n. pag.]. Article located in the press files for '*Balzac*', AMR.

110 Frank Harris, 'A Masterpiece of Modern Art' [1898], trans. by John Anzalone, in *Rodin in Perspective*, ed. by Ruth Butler (Englewood Cliffs, NJ: Prentice-Hall, Inc., 1980), pp. 97–99 (p. 98). Originally published in *The Saturday Review* (2 July 1898).

111 Rodenbach, 'Une statue', p. 1.

112 Georges Rodenbach, *L'Élite: écrivains, orateurs sacrés, peintres, sculpteurs* (Paris: Bibliothèque Charpentier, 1899), pp. 289–90.

113 Uncited quotation, presumably by Balzac, in Elsen, et al., *Rodin & Balzac*, p. 42.

114 Gustave Schneider, 'L'Exposition privée de Rodin', *Le Petit bleu de Paris*, 19 July 1899, [n. pag.]. Article located in the press files for '*Balzac*,' AMR.

> Discredited to-day are the theories of Lombroso and his school, once so warmly welcomed by mediocre minds athirst for equality, in which great men were considered as degenerates of a superior variety, and the most sensitive spirits qualified as candidates for the madhouse! [...] Far from being half mad, this unique being [the genius], this prodigious mirror of a million facets, achieves his aim only because he possesses far more intelligence than the most brilliant of his contemporaries, because he is in touch with a more profound order of things and a more comprehensive method, because he combines the qualities of continuity in sensation and of discernment which constitute that supreme sensibility of all the senses acting together — taste. But it does not please ordinary mortals to believe things of this kind, and one can easily understand how the crowd, repudiating any such humiliating notion, are all too willing to follow the lead of exotic pseudo-scientists and look upon great men as lunatics, considering themselves far more rational.[115]

In this diatribe, Cladel tries to lay to rest a distressing possibility and claim Rodin's status as a genius for posterity. And yet his *Monument to Balzac* was a testament to the power of this link and its visual provocation.

To return to the story of *Le Chef-d'œuvre inconnu*, the similarity between Frenhofer's artistic project and Rodin's was picked up in the years when the *Monument to Balzac* was being conceived and crafted. In 1896, Paul Dolfus, wondering if the sculpture would ever be finished, stated: 'If at least, one day, Mr Rodin could give us Balzac's foot'.[116] Rodin's difficulty in bringing commissioned sculpture to completion — an issue that dogged him throughout his career — recalled Frenhofer's quixotic quest for perfection. And when the monument was being ridiculed at the Salon, his supporter Georges Duval advised the *Société* to remember the words of Balzac's protagonist: 'La mission de l'art n'est pas de copier la nature, mais de l'exprimer!'[117] Rodin echoed Frenhofer's words in those same days, asserting that his working method 'n'est pas d'imiter seulement la forme, mais d'imiter la vie. [...] Cette vie, je

115 Judith Cladel, *Rodin, the Man and His Art. With Leaves from his Note-Book*, trans. by S. K. Star (New York: The Century Co., 1917), pp. 6–7.

116 Paul Dolfus, *L'Événement*, 20 August 1896; quoted in Antoinette Le Normand-Romain, 'Balzac', in *The Bronzes of Rodin*, I, 184.

117 Georges Duval, 'Rodin et le Comité des Gens de Lettres', *L'Événement*, 13 May 1898, [n. pag.]. Article located in the press files for '*Balzac*', AMR.

la cherche dans la nature, mais en l'amplifiant.'[118] For the sculptor, 'nature' included popular notions of physiognomy and regional type and the most up-to-date scientific theories on genius, but, in the end, he interpreted and deformed it to create a modern paean to genius. Rodin's sculpture avoided the accepted conventions of the monument: easily legible features, heroic pose, and appropriate attributes. In an interview with Paul Gsell, Rodin articulated his artistic contraventions: 'Une statue sur une place publique doit représenter un grand homme dans une attitude théâtrale et capable de le faire admirer par la postérité! Mais de telles raisons sont absurdes. Je prétends, moi, qu'il n'y avait qu'une manière d'évoquer mon personnage: je devais montrer un Balzac haletant dans son cabinet de travail, les cheveux en désordre, les yeux perdus dans le rêve, un génie qui [...] reconstruit pièce à pièce toute une société.'[119] Indeed, while Rodin used contemporary scientific theories as an entrée into creating Balzac's likeness, he ultimately privileged his own subjective interpretation of the author and the traces of his hand over a naturalistic portrait. Thus the *Monument to Balzac* marks the birth of a modern public sculpture. With it, Rodin cast his genius as equal to that of Balzac's: his inner vision, too, could conjure a world.

The scholarship on Rodin has consistently emphasized the artist's own iterations about copying 'nature': for instance, Rodin claimed, 'I obey Nature in everything, and I never pretend to command her. My only ambition is to be servilely faithful to her.'[120] In general, art historians have narrowly defined the term, emphasizing in particular Rodin's practice of drawing from the nude models who, we have repeatedly been told, roamed freely around his studio, providing 'natural' poses for him to copy.[121] He wanted to create an art in which meaning was located in the form of the body and on its surface and not in the conventional poses and traditional attributes often seen in the Salon sculpture of his day. Using contemporary scientific and pseudo-scientific theories — widely discussed and popularly accepted — that attempted to understand the manifestation of morality and intelligence on the surface of the body, Rodin

---

118 Rodin quoted in X, 'M. Rodin & la Société des Gens de Lettres', *Le Journal*, 12 May 1898, [n. pag.]. Article located in the press files for '*Balzac*', AMR.

119 Paul Gsell, 'Auguste Rodin', *L'Art et les artistes*, January 1907, 410–411. Elsen calls it a 'realistically-based visionary art'; Albert E. Elsen, *Origins of Modern Sculpture: Pioneers and Premises* (London: Phaidon Press, 1974), p. 29.

120 Rodin, *Rodin on Art and Artists*, p. 11.

121 For a discussion of the ways in which Rodin's drawings also demonstrate that he did not simply 'copy' nature, see the author's 'Against the Grain: Rodin's Experiments with Paper', in *Ecstasies: Drawings by Auguste Rodin*, ed. by Thomas Lederballe, et al., ex. cat. (Copenhagen: Statens Museum for Kunst, 2016), pp. 171–202.

conceived a new way of fashioning the body with parallel goals. Just as he did not simply replicate the poses of his models, he was not 'servilely faithful' to these discourses, either. Rather, he actively engaged with them in order to serve expressive ends. Ultimately, Rodin co-opted the contentious theories of degeneration, genius, and madness to subvert and redefine naturalistic representation. His monument was a tribute not only to Balzac, but to himself and his artistic process.

Acknowledgments

I would like to express my sincere thanks to Sophie Leroy for inviting me to contribute to this volume. I am grateful to the staff at the Musée Rodin and especially to Hélène Pinet, who has provided invaluable assistance over many years; the audiences of the AHRC-funded Likeness and Facial Recognition Workshop and the Western Society for French History annual conference, who provided feedback on this work in progress; Christine Poggi, who helped coax the earliest iterations of these ideas into a meaningful form; and especially the chapter's anonymous peer reviewers, Juliet Bellow, Louis Denizet, Tania Woloshyn, and Raffi Yegparian for their attentive readings and incisive criticism.

Bibliography

'L'actualité. La Statue de Balzac et l'impatience des souscripteurs', *L'Éclair*, 20 August 1896, [n. pag.]

Alexandre, Arsène, *Le Balzac de Rodin* (Paris: H. Floury, 1898)

Aristotle, 'Physiognomics', *Minor Works*, trans. by W. S. Hett (Cambridge, MA: Harvard University Press, 1936), pp. 84–137

——, 'Physiognomics', *Problems*, trans. by W. S. Hett, 2 vols (London: William Heinemann, 1936–37)

Baldensperger, Fernand, 'Les Théories de Lavater dans la littérature française', *Études d'histoire littéraire* (Paris: Hachette et Cie, 1910), pp. 51–91

'Balzac et Rodin. Où en est le monument du père de la "Comédie humaine"', *L'Éclair*, 28 January 1896, [n. pag.]

Balzac, Honoré de, *Eugénie Grandet* [1833], trans. by Marion Ayton Crawford (London: Penguin Books, 1955)

Balzac, Honoré de, *Louis Lambert*, trans. by Katharine Prescott Wormeley (Boston: Roberts Brothers, 1888)

Bardin, Charles, 'Médecine & Psychologie. Génie ou folie', *Gil Blas*, 3 November 1896, [n. pag.]

Besser, Gretchen R., *Balzac's Concept of Genius. The theme of superiority in the 'Comédie Humaine'* (Geneva: Librairie Droz, 1969)

Brisson, Adolphe, 'Plumes et ciseaux', *La République française*, 12 May 1898, [n. pag.]

Butler, Ruth, *Rodin: The Shape of Genius* (New Haven: Yale University Press, 1993)

Callen, Anthea, *The Spectacular Body: Science, Method and Meaning in the Work of Degas* (New Haven: Yale University Press, 1995)

Carroy, Jacqueline, '"Mon cerveau est comme dans un crâne de verre"': Émile Zola sujet d'Édouard Toulouse', *Revue d'histoire du XIXe siècle*, 20/21 (2000), <http://elseminario.com.ar/biblioteca/carroy_mon_cerveau_zola.htm>

de Caso, Jacques, *David d'Angers: Sculptural Communication in the Age of Romanticism*, trans. by Dorothy Johnson and Jacques de Caso (Princeton: Princeton University Press, 1992)

Chincholle, Charles, 'La Statue de Balzac', *Le Figaro*, 12 May 1898, [n. pag.]

Cladel, Judith, *Rodin, the Man and His Art. With Leaves from his Note-Book*, trans. by S. K. Star (New York: The Century Co., 1917)

Clair, Jean, et al., *L'Âme au corps: arts et science, 1793–1993*, ex. cat. (Paris: Éditions de la Réunion des musées nationaux, 1993)

Clemenceau, G[eorges], 'Balzac & Rodin', *La Justice*, 12 November 1894, [n. pag.]

Coquiot, Gustave, *Rodin à Hôtel Biron et à Meudon* (Paris: Librairie Ollendorff, 1917)

Dubois, Ph., 'Chez Rodin', *L'Aurore*, 12 May 1898, [n. pag.]

Duval, Georges, 'Rodin et le Comité des Gens de Lettres', *L'Événement*, 13 May 1898, [n. pag.]

Elsen, Albert E., *Origins of Modern Sculpture: Pioneers and Premises* (London: Phaidon Press, 1974)

Elsen, Albert E., et al., *Rodin & Balzac. Rodin's Sculptural Studies for the Monument to Balzac from the Cantor, Fitzgerald Collection*, ex. cat. (Beverly Hills: Cantor, Fitzgerald and Co., 1973)

Elsen, Albert E. with Rosalyn Frankel Jamison, *Rodin's Art: The Rodin Collection of the Iris & B. Gerald Cantor Center for Visual Arts at Stanford University*, ed. by Bernard Barryte (Oxford: Oxford University Press, 2003)

Fleury, Maurice de, 'Au jour le jour. Le Livre sur Zola', *Le Figaro*, 6 November 1896, [n. pag.]

Geffroy, Gustave, 'L'imaginaire', *Le Figaro*, 29 August 1893, 1

Getsy, David J., *Rodin: Sex and the Making of Modern Sculpture* (New Haven: Yale University Press, 2010)

Grunfeld, Frederic V., *Rodin: A Biography* (New York: Henry Holt and Co., 1987)

Gsell, Paul, 'Auguste Rodin', *L'Art et les artistes*, January 1907, 393–415

Hepp, Alexandre, 'Notes quotidiennes. L'impossible statue', *Le Soir* (Paris), 30 January 1896, [n. pag.]

Homodei [Arthur Huc], 'Chronique. Zola viviséqué', *La Dépêche*, 8 February 1898, [n. pag.]

Huteau, Michel, *Psychologie, psychiatrie et société sous la Troisième République. La Biocratie d'Édouard Toulouse (1865–1947)* (Paris: L'Harmattan, 2002)

Jefferson, Ann, *Genius in France: An Idea and Its Uses* (Princeton: Princeton University Press, 2015)

Le Journal des débats, 10 November 1896, [n. pag.]

L., 'Au jour le jour. Anthropologie et critique', *Le Journal des débats*, 9 June 1898, [n. pag.]

Lamartine, Alphonse de, *Balzac et ses œuvres* (Paris: Michel Lèvy Frères, 1866)

Lavater, John [Johann] Caspar, *Essays on Physiognomy, Designed to Promote the Knowledge and the Love of Mankind*, trans. by Henry Hunter, 5 vols (London: John Murray, 1789–1798)

Lethève, Jacques, 'Balzac et la Phrénologie', *Aesculape* (March 1951), 55–62

'Lettre de Paris, Le musée Rodin', *Le Nord maritime* [Dunkerque], 8 July 1899, [n. pag.]

La Presse, 14 July 1899, [n. pag.]

'Lettres parisiennes', *La Gironde* [Bordeaux], 29 January 1896, [n. pag.]

——, *Le Journal de Bruxelles*, 13 November 1894, [n. pag.]

Lombroso, C[esare], 'Émile Zola, d'après l'étude du Docteur Toulouse et les nouvelles théories sur le génie', *La Semaine médicale* 17 (1897), 1–5

——, *L'Homme de génie*, trans. by Colonna D'Istria (Paris: Félix Alcan, 1889)

——, *The Man of Genius* (London: Walter Scott, 1891)

——, *L'Uomo delinquente* (Milan, 1876)

Marx, Roger, 'Balzac et Rodin', *Le Voltaire*, 5 February 1896, [n. pag.]

Le Men, Ségolène, Luce Abélès, and Nathalie Preiss-Basset, *Les Français peints par eux-mêmes*, ex. cat. (Paris: Éditions de la Réunion des musées nationaux, 1993)

Mitterand, Henri, *Zola*, 3 vols (Paris: Fayard, 1999–2002)

Musée Rodin, *1898: le* Balzac *de Rodin*, ex. cat. (Paris: Éditions du musée Rodin, 1998)

Newton, Joy, 'Rodin and Nadar', *Laurels*, 52, 3 (1981–1982), 163–70

Pick, Daniel, *Faces of Degeneration: A European Disorder, c. 1848–c. 1918* (Cambridge: Cambridge University Press, 1989)

Nordau, Max, *On Art and Artists*, trans. by W.F. Harvey (London: T. Fisher Unwin, 1907)

——, *Degeneration* (London: William Heinemann, 1895)

——, *Zola und Naturalismus Ausgewählte Pariser Briefe* (Leipzig, 1887)

Nye, Robert A., *Crime, Madness, and Politics in Modern France: The Medical Concept of National Decline* (Princeton: Princeton University Press, 1984)

Pinkney, David H., *Napoleon III and the Rebuilding of Paris* (Princeton: Princeton University Press, 1958)

Pollock, Griselda, 'Artists' Mythologies and Media Genius, Madness and Art History', in *Picture This: Media Representations of Visual Art and Artists*, ed. by Philip Hayward (Luton: The University of Luton Press, 1998), pp. 101–39

Raviart, Georges, 'Le Génie de Balzac du point de vue psychiatrique. Génie et folie', *Annales médico-psychologiques*, 2, 4 (November 1954), 481–503

Reclus, Élisée, *Nouvelle Géographie universelle: la terre et les hommes*, 19 vols (Paris: Librairie Hachette, 1876–1894)

Rodenbach, Georges, *L'Élite: écrivains, orateurs sacrés, peintres, sculpteurs* (Paris: Bibliothèque Charpentier, 1899)

——, 'Encore la statue de Balzac', *Le Figaro*, 25 August 1896, [n. pag.]

——, 'Une Statue', *Le Figaro*, 17 May 1898, p. 1

Rodin, Auguste, *Correspondance de Rodin*, 4 vols (Paris: Éditions du musée Rodin, 1985–1992)

——, *Rodin on Art and Artists. Conversations with Paul Gsell* [1911], trans. by Mrs Romilly Fedden (New York: Dover Publications, 1983)

Ruiz-Gómez, Natasha, 'Against the Grain: Rodin's Experiments on Paper', in *Ecstasies: Drawings by Auguste Rodin*, ed. by Thomas Lederballe et al., ex. cat. (Copenhagen: Statens Museum for Kunst, 2016), pp. 171–201

——, 'Auguste Rodin and the "Scientific Image": The Sublime Copy Versus the Photograph', in *Visions of the Industrial Age, 1830–1914: Modernity and the Anxiety of Representation in Europe*, ed. by Minsoo Kang and Amy Woodson-Boulton (Aldershot: Ashgate, 2008), pp. 109–136

——, 'Essence and Evanescence in the *Hands* of Rodin', *Thresholds* 31 (May 2006), 102–109

——, 'A Hysterical Reading of Rodin's *Gates of Hell*', *Art History*, 36, 5 (November 2013), 994–1017

Sandras-Fraysse, Agnès, 'La folie de l'enquête: Zola disséqué', *Fabula/Les colloques* (15 January 2008), <http://www.fabula.org/colloques/document874.php>

Schneider, Gustave, 'L'Exposition privée de Rodin', *Le Petit bleu de Paris*, 19 July 1899, [n. pag.]

Sekula, Allan, 'The Body and the Archive', *October* 39 (Winter 1986), 3–64

Söder, Hans-Peter, *That Way Madness Lies: Max Nordau on fin-de-siècle Genius* (High Wycombe: Rivendale Press, 2009)

Sorel, Philippe, 'La Phrénologie et l'art', in *L'Âme au corps: arts et science, 1793–1993*, ed. by Jean Clair, et al., ex. cat. (Paris: Éditions de la Réunion des musées nationaux, 1993), pp. 266–79

Stiegler, Gaston, 'Rodin et Balzac', *L'Écho de Paris*, 12 November 1894, [n. pag.]

Sunday Times (London), 26 June 1898, [n. pag.]

Surville, Laure, *Balzac, sa vie et ses œuvres d'après sa correspondance* (Paris: Librairie Nouvelle and Jaccottet, Bourdilliat et Cie., 1858)

Toulouse, Édouard, *Enquête médico-psychologique sur les rapports de la supériorité intellectuelle avec la névropathie. I. Introduction générale. Émile Zola* (Paris: Société d'Éditions Scientifiques, 1896)

——, *Enquête médico-psychologique sur la supériorité intellectuelle. II. Henri Poincaré* (Paris: Ernest Flammarion, 1910)

——, 'Notes biologiques sur M. Berthelot', *Revue de psychiatrie* (*médecine mentale, neurologie, psychologie*), 4, 1 (1901), 368–71

Tytler, Graeme, *Physiognomy in the European Novel: Faces and Fortunes* (Princeton: Princeton University Press, 1982)

Vautel, Clément, 'Notes parisiennes, la Rodinière', *L'Événement*, 7 July 1899, [n. pag.]

Wagner, Anne, 'Rodin's Reputation', in *Eroticism and the Body Politic*, ed. by Lynn Hunt (Baltimore: The Johns Hopkins University Press, 1991), pp. 191–242

Wechsler, Judith, *A Human Comedy: Physiognomy and Caricature in 19th-Century Paris* (Chicago: The University of Chicago Press, 1982)

Werdet, Edmond, *Portrait intime de Balzac, sa vie, son humeur et son caractère* (Paris: E. Dentu, 1859; repr. Paris: L'Arche du livre, 1970)

X., 'M. Rodin & la Société des Gens de Lettres', *Le Journal*, 12 May 1898, [n. pag.]

Zola, Émile, *Les Romanciers naturalistes* (Paris: G. Charpentier, 1881)

CHAPTER 11

Courbes névrosées, lignes asthmatiques : usages de la métaphore médicale dans la réception de l'Art Nouveau

Cyril Barde

> Art nouveau : c'est neurasthénie,
> Névrosisme et Névropathie.[1]

∵

Le XIXe siècle positiviste et hygiéniste fut le siècle des médecins, siècle où les discours et les imaginaires médicaux ont investi de nombreuses sphères de la société. Susan Sontag et Judith Schlanger ont réfléchi dans leurs travaux respectifs sur les usages et les enjeux des métaphores médicales, en particulier dans le domaine socio-politique.[2] Schlanger écrit :

> la maladie est une expression analogique fondamentale du mal. Souillure, infection, engluement caractérisent ainsi le mal comme une détérioration radicale qui est une altération ; à quoi s'ajoute toute la charge répressive que véhicule le langage morbide, instrument particulièrement expressif d'une attitude qui n'est jamais neutre.[3]

La fin du XIXe siècle, marquée par la hantise de la décadence, est particulièrement friande d'un imaginaire médical qui s'empare de la sphère esthétique, si tant est qu'on puisse radicalement la séparer de la sphère politique. La seconde moitié du siècle voit s'affirmer un processus de pathologisation de l'art et de

---

1 Ralph de Chanlas [Charles Alphand], 'Le Modern style', *La Revue mondaine*, 5 janvier 1902, p. 354.

2 Voir Susan Sontag, *La Maladie comme métaphore : le sida et ses métaphores*, trad. par Marie-France de Paloméra, *Œuvre complètes*, 9 vols (Paris : Christian Bourgois, 2009), III (1989), p. 99 ; Judith Schlanger, *Les Métaphores de l'organisme* (Paris : L'Harmattan, 1995).

3 Schlanger, *Les Métaphores de l'organisme*, p. 177.

 | DOI:10.1163/9789004368019_013

l'artiste d'avant-garde, qui rompt avec les principes académique et la *mimesis*.[4] Rappelons-en les grandes lignes. Dès le milieu du siècle, Moreau de Tours affirme que le génie est une forme de la névrose :

> le génie, comme toute disposition quelconque du dynamisme intellectuel, a nécessairement son *substratum* matériel ; ce substratum, c'est un état semi-morbide du cerveau, véritable éréthisme nerveux dont la source nous est désormais bien connue.[5]

Lecteur de Moreau de Tours, l'italien Cesare Lombroso fait du génie une figure de la dégénérescence et compare, dans *L'Homme de génie*, l'inspiration artistique à la crise d'épilepsie.[6] Alors que Lombroso reconnaît l'importance des œuvres du génie dans la marche de l'humanité, Max Nordau radicalise et pousse le propos jusqu'au délire dans son célèbre *Dégénérescence*.[7] Il y fustige les diverses tendances de l'art 'fin-de-siècle' (du naturalisme au symbolisme en passant par l'impressionnisme et la musique de Wagner) comme autant de créations maladives et dégénérées, entraînant la régression des sociétés plutôt que leur progrès. Le contexte polémique qui accompagne la naissance des avant-gardes picturales et artistiques en cette fin de siècle est propice au réinvestissement de ces métaphores médicales. Les nouvelles esthétiques en rupture avec l'Académisme et le régime de la *mimesis* vont être analysées au prisme de la pathologie.

Nous proposons de voir comment se cristallisent et se reconfigurent ces discours autour de 1900, dans le champ des arts décoratifs qui connaissent alors un véritable renouveau et suscitent autant d'intérêt que de polémiques. L'Art Nouveau, qui essaime dans toute l'Europe, se propose de mettre fin à l'historicisme et à l'imitation des styles anciens qui ont prévalu pendant tout le XIXe siècle. De fait, il se pose d'emblée comme une esthétique de la renaissance et de l'énergie qui puise son inspiration et son vocabulaire ornemental dans une observation minutieuse de la nature. Émile Gallé, célèbre verrier et ébéniste de Nancy, exhorte les artistes-artisans modernes à transposer

---

4 Voir par exemple Jean-Pierre Guillerm, 'Psychopathologie du peintre', *Romantisme*, 66 (1989), 75–86.

5 Jacques-Joseph Moreau de Tours, *La Psychologie morbide dans ses rapports avec la philosophie de l'histoire, ou De l'influence des névropathies sur le dynamisme intellectuel* (Paris : Masson, 1859), p. 465.

6 Cesare Lombroso, *L'Homme de génie*, trad. de l'italien par Fr. Colonna d'Istria (Paris : Alcan, 1889).

7 Max Nordau, *Dégénérescence* (Paris : Alcan, 1894).

la structure des végétaux dans leurs meubles, seule garantie d'un 'art plein de naturelle santé, vivant, humain et vrai'[8] tandis que Gabriel Mourey, féru de préraphaélisme et des théories de Morris, loue le pavillon Bing de l'Exposition universelle de 1900 en félicitant les artistes de la 'la s*anté* de leurs tendances'.[9] L'isotopie de la maladie n'est donc pas seulement mobilisée par les opposants au nouveau style. Le sain et le malsain deviennent les critères qui permettent à ses partisans de distinguer le bon Art Nouveau du 'modern style', expression française souvent péjorative, utilisée pour discréditer un Art Nouveau dévoyé, extravagant, maniéré et cosmopolite.

Si l'Art Nouveau s'attire les foudres de certains critiques dès son apparition en France en décembre 1895, lorsque Siegfried Bing ouvre la Maison de l'Art Nouveau rue de Provence, son triomphe à l'Exposition universelle de 1900 est presque aussitôt suivi de vives contestations qui amorcent et accompagnent son rapide déclin dans la première décennie du siècle. Nous proposons d'étudier trois types de pathologies régulièrement évoquées dans les textes, sérieux ou ludiques, sèchement polémiques ou plus légèrement satiriques, qui prennent l'Art Nouveau — ou son double grimaçant 'modern style' — pour cible.[10] Nous tenterons de mettre au jour les stratégies rhétoriques qui les sous-tendent et de dégager les enjeux spécifiques à chaque type de maladie convoqué par les auteurs.

Asthme, anémie, parasitisme : maladies de l'épuisement

Asthme, anémie, neurasthénie

Le décor linéaire de l'Art Nouveau, surtout lorsqu'il est stylisé comme celui de Van de Velde,[11] est souvent raillé comme un art fatigué et fatigant, un art de l'anémie et de l'épuisement vital. En 1905, Serge de Chessin publie dans *L'Ermitage* une diatribe féroce contre le 'modern style' qui porte à incandescence un certain nombre des accusations qui visent fréquemment le

8 Émile Gallé, *Écrits pour l'art : floriculture, art décoratif, notices d'exposition (1844–1889)* (Marseille : Jeanne Laffitte, 1999), p. 243.

9 Gabriel Mourey, 'L'Art nouveau de M. Bing à l'Exposition universelle', *Revue des arts décoratifs*, t. XX (1900), 278–84 (p. 283).

10 Notre corpus se constitue pour l'essentiel de textes publiés entre 1900 et 1907, auxquels s'ajoutent en amont l'article d'Arsène Alexandre sur la Maison Bing en 1895 (*Le Figaro*) et en aval l'essai de Paul Morand, publié en 1931.

11 Henry Van de Velde est l'un des artistes majeurs qui exposent chez Bing en décembre 1895.

style nouveau. Il y fustige ses 'formes asthmatiques',[12] thème que Paul Morand reprendra en 1931, évoquant notamment les thèmes floraux d'Alphonse Mucha : 'C'est une léthargie, une syncope'.[13] On suffoque, on étouffe au milieu de ces végétations décoratives. Loin d'insuffler une nouvelle vigueur aux objets et aux intérieurs, les formes Art Nouveau déclinent, s'affaissent dans les discours des détracteurs. Sous la plume de Chessin et Morand, les lignes onduleuses du style nouveau n'évoquent pas le dynamisme végétal de la plante en croissance mais la détumescence et la décomposition. Pis, elles décrivent un mouvement d'involution, un retour à des formes primaires, protozoaires ou larves. Un imaginaire du gluant et du visqueux se déploie pour dénoncer le déficit d'énergie d'un art familièrement qualifié de 'style nouille'. Serge de Chessin analyse les 'molles et glissantes courbes' comme les symptômes de ce style mourant à la recherche désespérée d'une 'illusion de vitalité'.[14] Le propos associe la sensation d'étouffement causée par l'invasion végétale aux images de l'amorphe qu'Évanghelia Stead[15] a étudiées comme une véritable 'obsession fin-de-siècle' :

> Tandis que d'autres styles, pour couronner les meubles et les édifices de feuillages et de guirlandes, se sont attachés à l'imitation des plantes saines [...] le Style Moderne a choisi comme modèle le bourgeonnement scarieux, le fouillis des plantes, moitié végétaux, moitié larves [...] On connaît les théières couleur influenza, les divans marécageux et moisis, le cendrier où se dessèche un crachat de poitrinaire. [...] On comprend que les fleurs étouffent dans cette atmosphère empoisonnée.[16]

Comme le note Stead, l'organique, loin de célébrer ici les retrouvailles des arts décoratifs avec la nature, 'envahit les descriptions toujours saisies sous l'angle de la décomposition, de la maladie et de la mort'.[17] Le crachat de poitrinaire concrétise cette double image de l'asthme et du résidu visqueux. Version dégradée et décadente du poète phtisique romantique, l'artiste 'modern style' crache ses poumons. Paul Morand file la métaphore du mou

---

12 Serge de Chessin, 'Philosophie du "modern-style"', *L'Ermitage*, 32 (1905), 166–79 (p. 178).

13 Paul Morand, *1900* (Paris : Flammarion, 1931), p. 89.

14 Chessin, 'Philosophie du "modern-style"', p. 178.

15 Évanghelia Stead, 'Gélatine, poumon marin et poème amorphe. Sens et valeurs d'une obsession fin-de-siècle', *Poétique*, 159 (2009), 339–557.

16 Chessin, 'Philosophie du "modern-style"', p. 173.

17 Stead, 'Gélatine, poumon marin et poème amorphe', p. 347.

pour rejeter un style 'mauve et guimauve'[18] débilitant, émollient, un style 'élastique et fondant' qui 'infecte'[19] toutes les autres formes d'art, dont la littérature. Le critique Robert de la Sizeranne s'en prenait dès 1900 au 'grand vermicelle belge',[20] style sous-marin faisant la part belle aux mollusques : 'c'est un minimum de volonté, comme chez les mollusques'.[21] Art invertébré, aboulique, l'Art Nouveau rejoint la grande cohorte des névroses de la fin du siècle.[22] La reprise de ce *topos* décadent est d'autant plus efficace qu'elle permet d'attaquer le nouveau style sur son propre terrain en prenant l'exact contre-pied de ses promoteurs qui, à la manière de Roger Marx, veulent en faire une réponse vitaliste à 'l'imagination anémiée des peuples'.[23]

Pire encore, cet art débile rend malade ceux qui se trouvent à son contact. Estelle Thibault retrace dans un ouvrage[24] récent la généalogie d'une idée qui, au carrefour de la psychologie, de la physiologie et de l'esthétique, prête aux formes et aux lignes un pouvoir expressif qui affecte l'observateur. Cette emprise des formes sur la psyché de l'individu est très présente dans la critique d'art autour de 1900. Dès 1895, Arsène Alexandre écrit être sorti de la Maison Bing, condamnée pour son cosmopolitisme, 'fatigué, malade, exaspéré'.[25] La rotonde décorée par Besnard, la salle à manger conçue par Van de Velde le plongent dans un état de malaise et de langueur qui n'est pas sans rappeler celui de l'esthète décadent : 'la migraine commence à gagner, l'énervement me court au bout des doigts, je suis à point pour goûter l'art nouveau'[26] raille le critique, qui persiste et signe en 1900, au retour de l'Exposition universelle : 'la décoration et l'ameublement de notre époque ont un style, — et [...] ce style est malade'.[27] Sur un ton plus humoristique *Le Temps* publie en août 1901 une fiction où le narrateur, un jeune homme, raconte être atteint d'une maladie nouvelle, une 'crise d'artistisme' contractée lors d'un séjour chez une

18 Paul Morand, *1900*, p. 133.
19 Ibid., p. 157.
20 Robert de la Sizeranne, 'L'Art à l'Exposition de 1900. Avons-nous un style moderne ?', *Revue des Deux-Mondes*, 15 octobre 1900, p. 876.
21 Ibid., p. 874.
22 Voir Albert Deschamps et Jean Vinchon, *Les Maladies de l'énergie* (Paris : Alcan, 1927 [1908]).
23 Roger Marx, *La Décoration et les industries d'art à l'Exposition universelle de 1900* (Paris : Librairie Ch. Delagrave, 1902), p. 80.
24 Estelle Thibault, *La Géométrie des émotions : les esthétiques scientifiques de l'architecture en France, 1860–1950* (Wavre : Maradag, 2010).
25 Arsène Alexandre, 'L'Art nouveau', *Le Figaro*, 28 décembre 1895, p. 1.
26 Ibid., p. 1.
27 Arsène Alexandre, 'Modern style', *Le Figaro*, 1 septembre 1900, p. 1.

amie, Madame Norbert. Son hôtesse l'accueille 'voilée d'étoffes anémiées sur lesquelles pâlissaient des floraisons morbides'.[28] Esthète, elle s'entoure d'objets que le lecteur devine très proches de l'esthétique Art Nouveau. Leur profusion et leur effet déprimant oppressent le jeune homme, accablé par cette 'débauche d'art'[29]. Le même malaise étreint l'ingénieur Dietzch dans le roman *L'Emprise* de Pierre l'Ermite lorsqu'il arrive chez Alberte Harmmester. La décoration Art Nouveau de son hôtel particulier 'ne laisse[e] jamais un moment à l'esprit pour se reposer sur un objet qui ne le fasse pas travailler'.[30] L'ingénieur lance à la jeune femme :

> votre papier, votre ameublement, agissent certainement sur votre cerveau. Je reviens généralement à pied de chez vous ; le grand air et la marche me font du bien, cela me remet de votre neurasthénie ; et pourtant j'ai la tête solide ...[31]

À rebours des envolées lyriques qu'esquissent certains de ses plus ardents défenseurs, les détracteurs de l'Art Nouveau font le portrait d'une esthétique qui étouffe, accable. Son effet sur le spectateur, purement négatif, se caractérise par le manque et l'épuisement.

Parasitisme

Le parasitisme est l'autre grande figure de l'épuisement que l'on trouve dans les discours polémiques et satiriques qui ciblent l'Art Nouveau, également surnommé 'style ténia'. Le ténia, plus communément connu sous le nom de 'vers solitaire', est ce parasite qui colonise les intestins sans que son hôte ne s'en aperçoive. Sa présence peut entraîner chez le sujet parasité fatigue, troubles de l'appétit, amaigrissement rapide. Proche de l'imaginaire du mou et de l'amorphe que nous venons d'évoquer, le ténia vient sous le plume d'Émile Gallé, pour s'opposer à une ornementation linéaire abstraite qui ne procèderait pas du modèle végétal :

> Par contre, la nature, qui, elle, ne fournit pas les festons et les astragales, prête à l'artiste bien autres choses que les lombrics et les ténias, les

28 Frump, 'À Bâtons rompus : une crise "d'artistisme"', *Le Temps*, 28 août 1901, p. 2.

29 Ibid., p. 2.

30 Pierre L'Ermite, 'L'Emprise. Chapitre IX', *Le Mois littéraire et pittoresque* (janvier-juin 1903), 438–52 (p. 441).

31 L'Ermite, 'L'Emprise', p. 443.

> pseudo-varechs et les vermicelles affolés dont on a pensé faire, avec beaucoup de talent, à l'occasion de 1900, un berceau où abriter le vingtième siècle, un style helminthique et 'larveux'. Si c'est là le mobilier moderne, nous consentons à reprendre la perruque et la queue ![32]

Léonce Bénédite, directeur du Musée du Luxembourg, dénonce dans la section 'arts décoratifs' du rapport de jury de l'Exposition de 1900 une tendance dangereuse du style nouveau caractérisée par 'tous ces contournements et ces enchevêtrements de ténias surexcités et de nouilles tumultueuses'.[33] Précisons que ce style ténia est attribué par Bénédite aux Anglais et aux Belges. Dans un contexte où s'affirment les nationalismes européens, le ténia, corps étranger qui colonise le corps national et le fait dépérir, s'oppose à la recherche d'un style proprement français. Dans un climat politique dominé par l'affaire Dreyfus, l'action silencieuse, sourde et sournoise fait du parasite une métaphore privilégiée du vocabulaire antisémite : 'Le thème rebattu de l'envahissement sournois s'exprime par de nombreuses métaphores — *complot juif, reptile juif, envahisseur de Judée, marée, gangrène* — dont se détachent les groupes *péril juif* et *parasite juif*, commente Jean-Paul Honoré.[34]

Sans nécessairement s'inscrire dans une perspective antisémite, les caricatures de l'Art Nouveau mobilisent beaucoup les motifs de la perte d'appétit et de l'amaigrissement, comme si le style nouveau infectait le corps de l'amateur à la manière d'un ténia. Le jeune homme du *Temps* atteint d'une crise d'artistisme a justement remarqué sur le papier peint de son hôtesse 'une lutte éperdue de vers solitaires'[35] qui lui ont coupé l'appétit. Dans un numéro entièrement consacré à l'Art Nouveau, le journal satirique *L'Assiette au beurre* explique que les adeptes du style moderne 'ont perdu tout appétit'.[36] Le dessin qu'accompagne cette légende nous montre un amateur d'Art Nouveau attablé, la main sur l'estomac et l'air crispé. Les couverts qu'utilise le personnage parodient les formes contournées des objets Art Nouveau, et certaines fourchettes évoquent des instruments de torture. L'Art Nouveau apparaît comme un art littéralement dégoûtant (Fig. 11.1) :

---

32 Gallé, *Écrits pour l'art*, p. 251. L'helminthe appartient à la classe des vers parasites.

33 Léonce Bénédite, *Rapports du jury international* (Paris : Imprimerie nationale, 1905), p. 676.

34 Jean-Paul Honoré, 'Le Vocabulaire de l'antisémitisme en France pendant l'affaire Dreyfus', *Mots* (1981), 73–92 (p. 86).

35 Frump, 'À Bâtons rompus', p. 2.

36 *L'Assiette au beurre*, 28 septembre 1907, p. 430.

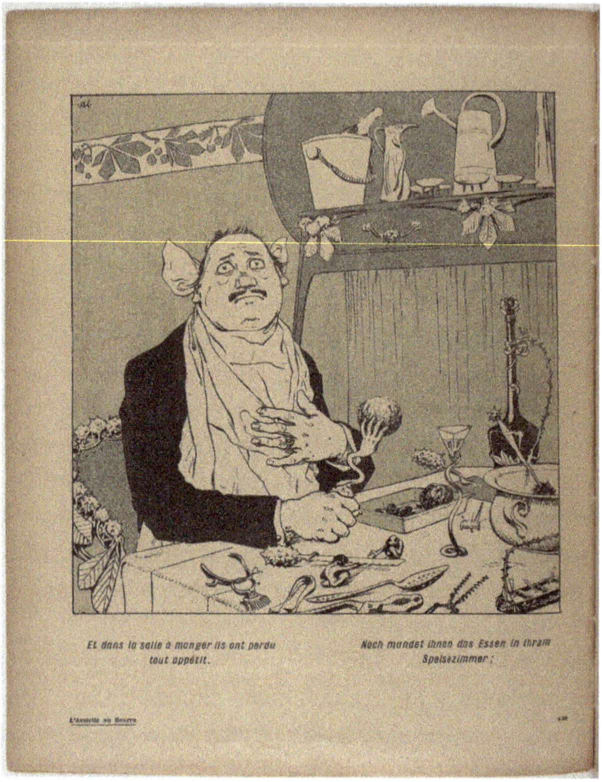
Et dans la salle à manger ils ont perdu tout appétit.
Noch mundet ihnen das Essen in ihrem Speisezimmer ;
L'Assiette au Beurre
430

FIGURE 11.1 L'Assiette au beurre, *28 septembre 1907, p. 430, Bibliothèque nationale de France (BnF)-Gallica.*

Octave Mirbeau va encore plus loin dans un article publié dans *Le Journal* en décembre 1901. Le texte se présente comme un dialogue entre le chroniqueur et un certain M.C., présenté comme un promoteur du style moderne. M.C. a conçu une pendule sur le modèle d'une plante, dont il décrit le socle au journaliste :

> Le socle de ma pendule, ce sont les racines du soleil, mais des racines tellement tordues, emmêlées, enchevêtrées, qu'on dirait les intestins d'un homme malade d'une entérite infectieuse … C'est superbe ![37]

Ici, le thème végétal de la décoration Art Nouveau est totalement détourné. On passe des racines aux viscères, du végétal à l'animal, du (pseudo)poétique

37 Octave Mirbeau, 'Art nouveau', *Le Journal*, 22 décembre 1901, p. 310.

au trivial. L'Art Nouveau est présenté comme un art indigeste, au sens propre du terme, un art à faire vomir qui érige la laideur en valeur suprême. Cette projection d'une intériorité malade et déréglée sur les formes des meubles et objets du style moderne se retrouve également sous la plume de ceux qui identifient les chantournements des courbes 1900 aux complications de cerveaux détraqués.

Cérébralités tortueuses

L'Art Nouveau ne pouvait échapper à la grande maladie de cette fin-de-siècle, la névrose dont la figure protéiforme et labile se profile derrière bien des détraquements, des dérèglements et des déséquilibres qu'on ne saurait nommer autrement. Parce qu'il surexcite le système nerveux, le style moderne devient 'l'emblème de la névrose dont la plupart des gens sont affectés'.[38] Ses courbes capricieuses rappellent les contorsions des corps et des cerveaux malades et donnent prise à un discours qui croise esthétique et psychiatrie.

Hystérie

Ne faut-il pas voir dans ces formes convulsées et contractées les contorsions du corps hystérique, ce corps dont Charcot scrute les moindres mouvements et les moindres réactions à la Salpêtrière ? C'est en tout cas ce que prétendent plusieurs observateurs du temps. On ne fera jamais assez remarquer que les années 1890 voient coexister deux écoles de Nancy : celle d'Émile Gallé et des artisans lorrains, celle du psychiatre Hippolyte Bernheim, pionnier des travaux sur la suggestion. Ces pistes de recherche ont déjà été empruntées par Rae Beth Gordon,[39] Debora Silverman,[40] ou Céline Eidenbenz.[41] Leurs études ont montré les parallèles et les analogies que l'on peut établir entre l'iconographie de l'hystérie telle qu'elle se constitue autour de 1900 (contractures, cambrures) et l'esthétique tout en courbes de l'Art Nouveau.

---

38 J.-H. Morel Lacordaire, 'Chronique de l'Exposition. L'Art nouveau III', *Le National*, 21 août 1900, p. 1.

39 Rae Beth Gordon, *Ornament, Fantasy and Desire in Nineteenth-Century French Literature* (Princeton : Princeton University Press, 1992).

40 Debora Silverman, *L'Art nouveau en France : politique, psychologie et style fin-de-siècle* (Paris : Flammarion, 1994).

41 Céline Eidenbenz, 'L'Âme renversée. L'Arc hystérique et ses corps à rebours autour de 1900', dans *Pulsion(s) : art et déraison* (Waterloo, Belgium : Renaissance du Livre, 2012), pp. 51–89 et Eidenbenz, 'Les Mots de l'hystérie : de la Salpêtrière au serpentinisme', dans *Pulsion(s)*, pp. 91–169.

Nous suggérons un autre point commun qui rapproche les formes décoratives des formes du corps féminin malade : la maigreur. Jean de Palacio a consacré un chapitre de ses *Configurations décadentes* à ce qu'il appelle une 'poétique de l'hystérie, ou de la maigreur en littérature'.[42] Le personnage de la femme maigre, héritier des danses macabres baudelairiennes, constituerait une figure de l'hystérique dans la littérature fin-de-siècle. Jean de Palacio rappelle que l'anorexie était considérée comme un symptôme de l'hystérie. Or, les lignes Art Nouveau sont parfois accusées d'être trop maigres et, implicitement, de ne pas présenter la saine rondeur de formes plus charnues. Alors que les discours sur les styles décoratifs associent de manière topique la forme des meubles et la forme des corps féminins d'une époque, la maigreur du mobilier Art Nouveau renvoie aux corps émaciés et androgynes que la fin du siècle fantasme comme le symptôme d'une décadence. Notre amateur d'Art Nouveau de *L'Assiette au beurre* est flanqué d'une compagne qui transgresse toutes les frontières de genre : sans formes, portant lunettes et cheveux courts, une cigarette entre les doigts, elle incarne une émancipation féminine considérée en cette fin-de-siècle comme un empiètement sur les territoires du masculin.

Émile Molinier dénonce la maigreur du mobilier[43] du Castel Béranger d'Hector Guimard tandis que Louis de Fourcaud reproche au 'modern style' cosmopolite son 'ameublement paradoxal, lourd et maigre'.[44] André Hallays, très sévère à l'égard du style nouveau, s'en prend à un décor qui 's'amincit et se déséquilibre selon la mode nouvelle. Du nord et du sud de l'Europe, ce sont les mêmes formes grêles et vacillantes'.[45] Avec la maigreur, c'est de nouveau l'instabilité et la silhouette torturée d'un corps tendu par la maladie qui est mise en avant. Rae Beth Gordon voit dans le motif de la torsion et dans le processus d'extériorisation d'une force intérieure le point de contact entre l'hystérie et la ligne coup de fouet :

> The eruption of hysteria in the body is an attempt to express and exorcize fears, but perhaps also to exhibit and glorify pain and 'ugliness'. In its will to express an unnameable desire, the body breaks the bounds assigned to it, and its life force contorts and extends to fill the space around it, exhibiting the inside (the psyche) on the outside. An analogy with Art

---

42 Jean de Palacio, 'Poétique de l'hystérie, ou de la maigreur en littérature', in *Configurations décadentes*, (Belgique : Peeters, 2007), pp. 215–24.

43 Émile Molinier, 'Le Castel Béranger', *Art et Décoration*, 5 (janvier-juin 1899), 76–81 (p. 80).

44 Louis de Fourcaud, 'Les Arts décoratifs au Salon de 1899 : les objets d'art (fin)', *Revue des arts décoratifs*, XIX (1899), 321–34 (p. 327).

45 André Hallays, *À travers l'Exposition de 1900* (Paris : Perrin, 1901), p. 256.

> Nouveau's architectures contortionist twisting of space readily comes to mind. The inside (nerves, organic growth, cellular expansion) is now on the outside in wood, walls, ironwork, and so on, providing a mirror for the psyche and for the drives within.[46]

L'architecte Henry Van de Velde, figure de l'Art Nouveau belge, est sans doute celui qui formule le plus clairement cette conception de la ligne-force dans ses cours et ses écrits. Selon l'architecte, les ornements linéaires doivent exprimer 'des tensions, compressions, flexions, torsions, que leur position et leur fonction suscitent dans l'architecture comme dans l'objet'.[47] Cette conception de la ligne n'est pas si éloignée de certaines interprétations critiques de l'ornementation Art Nouveau. Arsène Alexandre dénonce une décoration linéaire qui a perdu de vue la nature et ressemble aux 'coups de fouet tumultueux décochés par un charretier névropathe',[48] Serge de Chessin évoque les 'courbures névrosées'[49] et les lis aux 'gestes d'épileptique'[50] du 'modern style'. Les détracteurs de l'Art Nouveau recourent fréquemment à l'image de l'hystérie pour mettre en garde contre le délire des lignes d'un art ornemental illogique ou étranger. Gabriel Mourey vante le mobilier du pavillon Bing évitant 'les complications, les contorsions, les épileptiques gestes décoratifs'[51] tandis que Léonce Bénédite note dans son rapport sur l'Exposition de 1900 que certains motifs décoratifs étranges et excentriques du style moderne semblent 'avoir été conçus à la Salpêtrière ou à Bicêtre'.[52] Charles Saunier, dans les pages de *La Plume*, dénonce pour sa part une décoration qui consisterait dans 'un enchevêtrement de lignes bizarres, illogiques, vrai travail de pensionnaire d'asiles d'aliénés'.[53]

La redécouverte surréaliste de l'Art Nouveau contribuera à renforcer cette interprétation de la ligne convulsée, mais pour en célébrer le pouvoir subversif et anti-bourgeois. Lorsque Salvador Dalí publie 'De la beauté terrifiante et comestible de l'architecture Modern' Style' dans la revue *Minotaure*, il souligne une coïncidence entre l'avènement de ce qu'il nomme 'le décorativisme

---

46 Rae Beth Gordon, *Ornament, Fantasy and Desire*, p. 34.

47 Henry Van de Velde, *Déblaiement d'art* (Bruxelles : Éditions des Archives d'Architecture Moderne, 1979), p. 22.

48 Alexandre, 'Modern style', p. 1.

49 Chessin, 'Philosophie du "modern-style"', p. 178.

50 Ibid., p. 173.

51 Mourey, 'L'Art nouveau de M. Bing à l'Exposition universelle', p. 283.

52 Bénédite, *Rapports du jury international*, p. 676.

53 Charles Saunier, 'Les Arts du Foyer : une série d'expositions au *Salon de La Plume*', *La Plume*, 15 septembre 1901, pp. 697–99 (p. 697).

psychique'[54] de 1900 et la 'sculpture hystérique' représentant des 'contractions et attitudes sans antécédents dans l'histoire de la statuaire (il s'agit des femmes découvertes et connues après Charcot et l'école de la Salpêtrière)'.[55] Les lignes tortueuses de l'Art Nouveau semblent la transcription décorative des psychismes torturés.

Complexions et complications psychiques

Dans le sillage de la 'méthode graphique' d'Étienne-Jules Marey, dont les appareils de mesure (sphygmographe, myographe ...) transcrivent des phénomènes physiologiques internes sous la forme de courbes et de graphiques, la ligne de l'Art Nouveau est lue comme la trace abstraite d'un état d'âme, l'extériorisation graphique d'une intériorité torturée ou aberrante. Il s'agit d'établir un rapport d'analogie entre les circonvolutions tortueuses d'un cerveau malade et les lignes coups de fouet des meubles et tapisseries d'un style décoratif. 'Quelle cervelle embrouillée et enfantine devait avoir cette petite dame qui s'entourait d'un fouillis frissonnant d'algues marines'[56] s'exclame notre homme victime de la crise d'artistisme. Si Arsène Alexandre avance railleusement que les artistes du décor semblent avoir pris 'pour modèle les circonvolutions mêmes de leur cerveau',[57] Serge de Chessin esquisse dans son article une petite théorie de psychologie architecturale : 'Par son ornementation, un style dénonce son origine psychologique comme un visage porte les traces de la maladie ou de la santé'.[58] Ainsi pour lui 'les longues et fuyantes courbes semblent esquisser des mouvements psychologiques'.[59] Il faut prendre au sérieux cette image du décor Art Nouveau comme analogie ou transposition des replis d'une cervelle. Comme l'a montré Pierre Citti dans *Contre la décadence*,[60] les discours esthétiques, politiques et sociaux du tournant 1900 exaltent un principe vital anti-intellectualiste délesté des pesanteurs de l'analyse cérébrale qui ne cesse de disséquer, de ramifier, de figer. Alors que l'Art Nouveau est censé participer de ce vitalisme, il est pourtant décrit par ses opposants comme un art trop intellectuel, incapable de renouer avec la vie et le monde extérieur. Un art

---

54 Salvador Dalí, 'De la beauté terrifiante et comestible de l'architecture *modern'style*', *Minotaure*, 1 (3–4), (1933), 69–76 (p. 70).

55 Ibid., p. 73.

56 Frump, 'À Bâtons rompus', p. 2.

57 Arsène, 'Modern style', p. 1.

58 Chessin, 'Philosophie du "modern-style"', p. 179.

59 Ibid., p. 172.

60 Pierre Citti, *Contre la décadence : histoire de l'imagination française dans le roman 1890–1914* (Paris : PUF, 1987).

du pli et du repli sur soi, un art de l'autisme où l'artiste n'offre que le miroir de ses tourments psychiques. En somme, tout l'inverse de l'art social, de l'art dans la vie qu'il prétend être. Là encore, la métaphore de la maladie n'est pas seulement un *topos*, elle porte en elle un contre-discours qui attaque le style moderne sur son propre terrain.

Cauchemar, emprise, hantise

L'influence de ce décor malsain sur son occupant est là encore un motif récurrent des détracteurs de l'Art Nouveau. La maison Art Nouveau se retourne contre son habitant. Le jeune homme souffrant de crise d'artistisme évoque sa 'nuit troublée de mauvais rêves'[61] dans la demeure décorée comme à l'exposition universelle. Les nuits des adeptes de l'Art Nouveau sont perturbées 'par d'horribles cauchemars'[62] prévient *L'Assiette au beurre*.

Les meubles Art Nouveau, souvent jugés incommodes, illogiques et inconfortables ne torturent pas seulement les corps, ils affectent aussi les esprits, travaillent les cerveaux, assaillent, harcèlent l'imagination. Après avoir comparé les meubles du 'modern style' aux instruments de torture de l'Inquisition, Gabriel Mourey écrit :

> S'endormir, dormir, s'éveiller, être malade, mourir au milieu de ces formes hostiles, parmi la menace perpétuelle et affolante de ces lignes exaspérées, les sentir dans l'obscurité braquées vers soi, fleurs tordues, feuilles acérées, arabesques serpentines au dard toujours tendu… l'affreux cauchemar ![63]

Le décor Art Nouveau se lance à l'assaut de l'individu qui l'habite. Les lignes onduleuses deviennent des armes ou des dards. Qu'il coupe l'appétit ou empêche le repos, l'Art Nouveau s'en prend au fonctionnement naturel du corps et de l'esprit. À la fin d'une conférence donnée en 1899 pour *Le Figaro*, Guimard s'amuse des craintes suscitées par son tout récent Castel Béranger :

> Ainsi les gens qui vont habiter le Castel, me suis-je dit alors, vont avoir le cauchemar. Eh bien ! je vais y vivre moi-même, non pas pour y voir probablement tous les jours des gens évanouis sur les planchers, mais

61 Frump, 'À Bâtons rompus', p. 2.

62 *L'Assiette au beurre*, p. 431.

63 Mourey, 'L'Art nouveau de M. Bing à l'Exposition universelle', p. 268.

> pour suivre de près cette impression. J'ai cherché des gens évanouis, je n'en ai point trouvé [...]
>
> Un monsieur, visitant le Castel Béranger (ce n'était pas une dame, et je le regrette, car j'ai une préférence pour le goût des dames) a l'air tout à coup de blêmir ; la concierge, une très brave femme, s'empresse, lui offre d'aller chercher un verre d'eau, et lui demande avec sollicitude s'il n'est pas malade. 'Oui, répond le visiteur, je me sens un peu mal, en effet. — Qu'avez-vous donc ? reprend cette bonne concierge. — Je ne sais pas ... c'est ce papier ... je ne sais pourquoi, il me produit un drôle d'effet ... Bref, il s'est remis, sans même avoir besoin d'un verre d'eau, je vous l'assure. Voilà un fait.[64]

Guimard fait peut-être référence à l'article d'Émile Molinier paru dans les pages de la revue *Art et Décoration* :

> si cette complication apparaissait successivement sur vingt ou trente façades d'immeubles se suivant, j'imagine qu'on éprouverait un violent mal de tête et qu'on demanderait à s'aller cacher au fond d'un désert pour fuir ce cauchemar.[65]

Émile Molinier dénonce une trop grande recherche de lignes, une dissymétrie trop accusée, autant de déséquilibres que l'auteur reproche à Guimard d'être allé chercher en Belgique, en particulier chez Victor Horta. La menace d'invasion des rues par les lignes Art Nouveau répond à une autre contagion, celle de l'art français par les esthétiques étrangères. Abel Fabre, s'inquiétant des exubérances de Guimard et d'une ornementation linéaire émancipée de la référence végétale, compare un motif de ses papiers peints à 'un microbe grossi au microscope'.[66]

---

64 Hector Guimard, 'La Renaissance de l'art dans l'architecture moderne', *Le Moniteur des arts*, 7 juillet 1899, p. 470.

65 Molinier, 'Le Castel Béranger', p. 79.

66 Abel Fabre, 'Du Gothique au moderne', *Le Mois littéraire et pittoresque*, septembre 1901, 291–302 (p. 296).

Contagion, virus et suggestion

Un virus venu de l'étranger

Dans un ouvrage récent, Sophie Basch revient sur les discours qui dénoncèrent l'Art Nouveau, dès l'ouverture de la Maison Bing à Paris en 1895, comme un art cosmopolite, 'art interlope, art métèque'.[67] L'Art Nouveau est alors accusé d'être un art de l'étranger qui viendrait corrompre le bon goût français, un corps étranger qui viendrait infecter le corps national. Dans un essai de 1906 intitulé 'La Maladie contemporaine', Émile de Lacombe décrit explicitement le style moderne comme un virus :

> Et l'art décoratif? il commence à être infecté par une sorte d'influenza venue aussi de l'Asie ou tout au moins des pays Danubiens, qui s'intitule *art nouveau*, ou mieux *modern style*, sans doute pour bien marquer qu'elle n'est pas française.[68]

On reconnaît dans les différents foyers du virus mentionnés par Lacombe les différentes sources et formes de ce phénomène européen, qui doit à l'art japonais comme aux *Arts and Crafts* anglais, connaît en Belgique comme en Allemagne et en Autriche des développements flamboyants. Le numéro que *L'Assiette au beurre* consacre à L'Art Nouveau en 1907 est bilingue : la légende de chaque dessin est donnée au lecteur en français et en allemand pour s'adapter au caractère cosmopolite de l'objet. La page de couverture présente le bacille de l'Art Nouveau conservé dans du formol et désigné un son nom savant parodique, 'Bacillus Ars Nova'.[69] La représentation de ce bacille parodie le répertoire formel de l'Art Nouveau : silhouette d'un corps féminin élancé tout en courbe, traitement décoratif d'une chevelure dont les méandres se confondent avec l'élément liquide. Telle est la muse malade du style moderne (Fig. 11.2). Les premières lignes annoncent : 'Le bacille a été découvert il y a quelques années, par plusieurs artistes indépendants, et il s'est répandu rapidement à travers l'Europe'.[70] Le cosmopolitisme est donc clairement envisagé comme l'effet d'une contagion généralisée. Les cibles du journal satiriques sont certainement diverses et les niveaux de lecture multiples. En

---

67 Sophie Basch, *Rastaquarium : Marcel Proust et le 'modern style', arts décoratifs et politique dans* À la recherche du temps perdu (Turnhout : Brepols, 2014), p. 38.

68 Émile de Lacombe, *La Maladie contemporaine : examen des principaux problèmes sociaux au point de vue positiviste* (Paris : Alcan, 1906), p. 179.

69 *L'Assiette au beurre*, p. 421.

70 Ibid., p. 422.

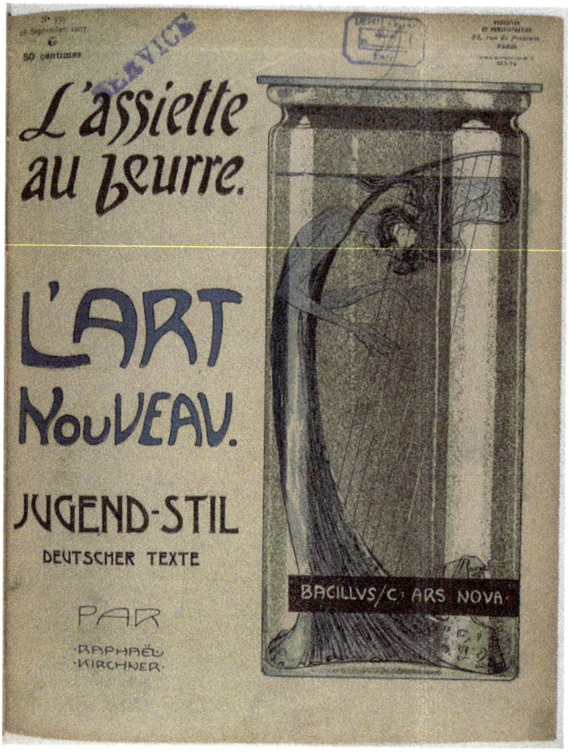

FIGURE 11.2
L'Assiette au beurre, *28 septembre 1907, page de couverture, dessin de Raphaël Kirchner, BnF-Gallica.*

effet, Raphaël Kirchner, dessinateur d'origine autrichienne très influencé par l'Art Nouveau, est l'auteur du texte allemand et de certaines illustrations (au moins celle de la couverture) du numéro. Il s'agit peut-être autant de caricaturer l'Art Nouveau que les discours nationalistes qui le prennent pour cible …

La suggestion, le snobisme et la mode

Parce qu'elle demeure toujours — au moins en partie — obscure, mystérieuse et difficilement contrôlable, la contagion est la dimension de la maladie qui suscite le plus l'imaginaire. En cette fin de XIXe siècle, les recherches en psychiatrie ont mis en avant le concept de 'suggestion' qu'Hippolyte Bernheim, médecin de Nancy, définit minimalement comme 'l'acte par lequel une idée est introduite dans le cerveau et acceptée par lui'.[71] L'état d'hypnose s'avère un puissant adjuvant de la suggestion. Bernheim, qui affirme contre Charcot que cet état n'est pas le propre des sujets hystériques, le définit comme un 'état

71 Hippolyte Bernheim, *Hypnotisme, suggestion, psychothérapie : études nouvelles* (Paris : Octave Doin, 1891), p. 24.

psychique particulier susceptible d'être provoqué, qui met en activité ou exalte à des degrés divers la suggestibilité'.[72] Reprenant les théories de l'école de Nancy au service de son travail sociologique, Gabriel Tarde construit son concept central d'imitation sur le modèle de la suggestion et conçoit le phénomène d'imitation dans la vie sociale comme :

> une suggestion de personne à personne [...] L'état social, comme l'état hypnotique, n'est qu'une forme de rêve, un rêve de commande et un rêve en action. N'avoir que des idées suggérées et les croire spontanées : telle est l'illusion propre au somnambule, et aussi bien à l'homme social.[73]

Dans le sillage de Bernheim, il ne s'agit pas de concevoir cet état hypnotique comme un fait pathologique, mais au contraire comme un fait normal. Cependant, l'imaginaire pathologique est à l'œuvre dans le texte de Tarde qui parle à plusieurs reprises de 'contagion imitative' pour penser la mode, la propagation des idées et des croyances. Dès lors, la contagion de l'Art Nouveau peut se penser sur le mode de la suggestion et de l'état hypnotique. *L'Assiette au beurre* s'en amuse : 'Une variété de cette maladie, qui fait horriblement souffrir celui qui en est atteint, est connue sous le nom de "ars nova suggestiva", et se transmet par contagion directe'.[74] La scène qu'accompagne cette légende présente des personnages hallucinés, aux yeux exorbités et aux gestes désordonnés. Les lignes verticales qui structurent l'arrière-plan de l'image évoquent les barreaux d'une prison ou d'un asile. Les personnages semblent enfermés dans une idée fixe. La caricature ramène la suggestion sur le terrain de la maladie, également suggérée par les couleurs froides et les tons verdâtres. La notion de suggestion, circulant entre esthétique, psychiatrie et science sociale, remet en cause l'idée même d'un libre choix et de goûts individuels. Si mes goûts me sont suggérés, alors ce ne sont plus mes goûts, ce sont les goûts des autres que j'imite, que je reproduis et que je suggère à d'autres d'imiter. Dans une perspective polémique ou satirique, évoquer la propagation de l'Art Nouveau comme suggestion, c'est donc se moquer de la crédulité d'esprits faibles qui croient jeter volontairement leur dévolu sur les dernières innovations de l'art décoratif alors qu'ils sont les jouets de phénomènes subconscients ou inconscients qu'ils ne maîtrisent pas. C'est désigner l'amour de l'Art Nouveau comme le symptôme d'une maladie sociale, le snobisme.

---

72 Ibid., p. 76.

73 Gabriel Tarde, *Les Lois de l'imitation : étude sociologique* (Paris : Alcan, 1890), pp. 82–83.

74 *L'Assiette au beurre*, p. 428.

Au terme de ce parcours, nous voudrions souligner que l'imaginaire de la maladie déployé contre l'Art Nouveau autour de 1900 n'est pas le simple alignement de clichés ou de figures stéréotypées visant à discréditer une nouvelle esthétique. La rhétorique qui recourt à ces métaphores (qui sont parfois plus que des métaphores) est fondamentalement ironique en ce sens qu'elle contrecarre, de manière implicite mais ciblée, les discours qui valorisent l'Art Nouveau comme un art sain du retour à la nature et de la régénérescence. En outre, la rhétorique de la maladie n'est pas seulement mise au service d'un combat esthétique, elle est aussi le moyen de porter un discours d'ordre politique ou sociopolitique. Elle peut soutenir un discours nationaliste lorsqu'il s'agit de dénoncer les influences corruptrices de l'étranger et du cosmopolitisme. Elle participe du discours anti-intellectualiste qui se constitue au tournant du siècle lorsqu'elle fustige les contorsions de cerveaux trop alambiqués. Elle s'articule à une réflexion sur les modes qui fait la part belle aux théories psychiatriques. En somme, il s'agit bien pour ses détracteurs de faire de l'Art Nouveau un art décadent, au même titre que la littérature du même nom, cible d'attaques similaires au tournant du siècle. Le parallèle est explicitement avancé par Émile Bayard, inspecteur au ministère des Beaux-Arts :

> La littérature aidant, dont la quintessence inclina souvent au maladif, à travers les subtilités de l'analyse et de l'inquisition du 'soi', l'art tout entier fut sensitif et troublé. Son charme désordonné s'affirmait néanmoins volontaire comme son orientation d'une originalité séduisante.[75]

Nous avons vu que cet art pathétique, pathologique est aussi un art pathogène, qui rend malade un spectateur passif. Or, cette emprise ne tient pas au sujet représenté : les motifs des papiers peints, les courbes des architectures, les galbes des objets sont sans sujet, et n'ont plus grand-chose de figuratif ni de narratif. Comme l'écrit l'historien d'art Éric Michaud, 'le XIXe siècle [découvre] que la puissance de l'image ne tient pas tant à '[l]'idée' qu'elle figure, par le moyen de corps représentés, qu'à la forme et à la matière qui en sont le véhicule'.[76] Dans ce monde des formes qui déforment ou réforment l'individu — à son insu voire contre son gré — le régénèrent ou le font dégénérer, l'art décoratif, plus tout à fait figuratif et pas totalement abstrait, tient une place importante, cristallise les espoirs, les angoisses et les fantasmes d'une époque auxquels l'imaginaire de la maladie donne un accès privilégié.

75 Émile Bayard, *Le Style moderne* (Paris : Garnier Frères, 1919), p. 50.
76 Éric Michaud, *Histoire de l'art. Une discipline à ses frontières* (Paris: Hazan, 2005), p. 128.

Bibliographie

Alexandre, Arsène, 'L'Art nouveau', *Le Figaro*, 28 décembre 1895, p. 1

——, 'Modern style', *Le Figaro*, 1 septembre 1900, p. 1

Basch, Sophie, *Rastaquarium : Marcel Proust et le 'modern style', arts décoratifs et politique dans* À la Recherche du temps perdu (Turnhout : Brepols, 2014)

Bayard, Émile, *Le Style moderne* (Paris : Garnier Frères, 1919)

Bénédite, Léonce, *Rapports du jury international* (Paris : Imprimerie nationale, 1905)

Bernheim, Hippolyte, *Hypnotisme, suggestion, psychothérapie : études nouvelles* (Paris : Octave Doin, 1891)

Chessin, Serge de, 'Philosophie du "modern-style"', *L'Ermitage*, 32 (1905), 166–79

Citti, Pierre, *Contre la décadence : histoire de l'imagination française dans le roman 1890–1914* (Paris : PUF, 1987)

Dalí, Salvador, 'De la beauté terrifiante et comestible de l'architecture *modern'style*', *Minotaure*, 1 (3–4) (1933), 69–76

Eidenbenz, Céline, 'L'Âme renversée : l'Arc hystérique et ses corps à rebours autour de 1900', in *Pulsion(s) : art et déraison*, Catalogue d'exposition (Waterloo, Belgium : Renaissance du Livre, 2012), 51–89

——, 'Les Mots de l'hystérie : de la Salpêtrière au serpentinisme', (as previous), pp. 91–169

Fabre, Abel, 'Du Gothique au moderne', *Le Mois littéraire et pittoresque*, 33 (septembre 1901), 291–302

Fourcaud, Louis de, 'Les Arts décoratifs au Salon de 1899 : les objets d'art (fin)', *Revue des arts décoratifs*, XIX (1899), pp. 321–34

Frump, 'À Bâtons rompus : une crise « d'artistisme »', *Le Temps*, 28 août 1901, p. 2

Gallé, Émile, *Écrits pour l'art : floriculture, art décoratif, notices d'exposition (1844–1889)* (Marseille : Jeanne Laffitte, 1999)

Gordon, Rae Beth, *Ornament, Fantasy and Desire in Nineteenth-Century French Literature* (Princeton : Princeton University Press, 1992)

Guillerm, Jean-Pierre, 'Psychopathologie du peintre', *Romantisme*, 66 (1989), 75–86

Guimard, Hector, 'La Renaissance de l'art dans l'architecture moderne', *Le Moniteur des arts*, 7 juillet 1899, pp. 1465–71

Hallays, André, *À travers l'Exposition de 1900* (Paris : Perrin, 1901)

Honoré, Jean-Paul, 'Le Vocabulaire de l'antisémitisme en France pendant l'affaire Dreyfus', *Mots* (1981), 73–92

Lacombe, Émile de, *La Maladie contemporaine : examen des principaux problèmes sociaux au point de vue positiviste* (Paris : Alcan, 1906)

La Sizeranne, Robert de, 'L'Art à l'Exposition de 1900. Avons-nous un style moderne ?', *Revue des Deux-Mondes*, 15 octobre 1900, section IV, pp. 866–97

L'Ermite, Pierre, 'L'Emprise', *Le Mois littéraire et pittoresque*, 12 vols (Paris : Maison de la Bonne Presse, 1903), IX, pp. 169–88

Lombroso, Cesare, *L'Homme de génie*, trad. par Fr. Colonna d'Istria (Paris : Alcan, 1889)

Marx, Roger, *La Décoration et les industries d'art à l'Exposition universelle de 1900* (Paris : Librairie Ch. Delagrave, 1902)

Michaud, Éric, *Histoire de l'art : une discipline à ses frontières* (Paris : Hazan, 2005)

Mirbeau, Octave, 'Art nouveau', *Le Journal*, 22 décembre 1901, p. 310

Molinier, Émile, 'Le Castel Béranger', *Art et Décoration*, 5 (janvier-juin 1899), 76–81

Morand, Paul, *1900* (Paris : Flammarion, 1931)

Moreau de Tours, Jacques-Joseph, *La Psychologie morbide dans ses rapports avec la philosophie de l'histoire, ou De l'influence des névropathies sur le dynamisme intellectuel* (Paris : V. Masson, 1859)

Morel Lacordaire, J.-H., 'Chronique de l'Exposition : l'Art nouveau III', *Le National*, 21 août 1900, p. 1

Mourey, Gabriel, 'L'Art nouveau de M. Bing à l'Exposition universelle', *Revue des arts décoratifs*, XX (septembre 1900), 278–84

Nordau, Max, *Dégénérescence* (Paris : Alcan, 1894)

Palacio, Jean de, 'Poétique de l'hystérie, ou de la maigreur en littérature', dans *Configurations décadentes* (Belgique : Peeters, 2007), pp. 215–24

Ralph de Chanlas [Charles Alphand], 'Le Modern style', *La Revue mondaine*, 5 janvier 1902, pp. 352–54

Saunier, Charles, 'Les Arts du Foyer : une série d'expositions au *Salon de La Plume*', *La Plume*, 15 septembre 1901, pp. 697–99

Schlanger, Judith, *Les Métaphores de l'organisme* (Paris : L'Harmattan, 1995)

Silverman, Debora, *L'Art nouveau en France : politique, psychologie et style fin-de-siècle* (Paris : Flammarion, 1994)

Sontag, Susan, *La Maladie comme métaphore : le sida et ses métaphores*, trad. par Marie-France de Paloméra, *Œuvre complètes*, 9 vols (Paris : Christian Bourgois, 2009), III (1989)

Stead, Évanghelia, 'Gélatine, poumon marin et poème amorphe : sens et valeurs d'une obsession fin-de-siècle', *Poétique*, 159 (2009), 339–557

Tarde, Gabriel, *Les Lois de l'imitation : étude sociologique* (Paris : Alcan, 1890)

Thibault, Estelle, *La Géométrie des émotions : les esthétiques scientifiques de l'architecture en France, 1860–1950* (Wavre : Maradag, 2010)

Van de Velde, Henry, *Déblaiement d'art* (Bruxelles : Éditions des Archives d'Architecture Moderne, 1979)

Index

www.ingramcontent.com/pod-product-compliance
Ingram Content Group UK Ltd.
Pitfield, Milton Keynes, MK11 3LW, UK
UKHW022209051026
15624UKWH00001B/73

9 789004 367999